Heart Failure in Children

Guest Editor

JEFFREY A. TOWBIN, MD, FACC, FAAP, FAHA

HEART FAILURE CLINICS

www.heartfailure.theclinics.com

Consulting Editors
RAGAVENDRA R. BALIGA, MD, MBA
JAMES B. YOUNG, MD

Founding Editor
JAGAT NARULA, MD, PhD

October 2010 • Volume 6 • Number 4

SAUNDERS an imprint of ELSEVIER, Inc.

W.B. SAUNDERS COMPANY
A Division of Elsevier Inc.

1600 John F. Kennedy Boulevard • Suite 1800 • Philadelphia, Pennsylvania 19103-2899

http://www.theclinics.com

HEART FAILURE CLINICS Volume 6, Number 4
October 2010 ISSN 1551-7136, ISBN-13: 978-1-4377-2457-8

Editor: Barbara Cohen-Kligerman
Developmental Editor: Jessica Demetriou

Heart Failure Clinics (ISSN 1551-7136) is published quarterly by Elsevier Inc., 360 Park Avenue South, New York, NY 10010-1710. Months of publication are January, April, July, and October. Business and editorial offices: 1600 John F. Kennedy Boulevard, Suite 1800, Philadelphia, PA 19103-2899. Periodicals postage paid at New York, NY, and additional mailing offices. Subscription prices are USD 207.00 per year for US individuals, USD 326.00 per year for US institutions, USD 70.00 per year for US students and residents, USD 248.00 per year for Canadian individuals, USD 374.00 per year for Canadian institutions, USD 264.00 per year for international individuals, USD 374.00 per year for international institutions, and USD 89.00 per year for Canadian and foreign students/residents. To receive student and resident rate, orders must be accompanied by name of affiliated institution, date of term, and the *signature* of program/residency coordinator on institution letterhead. Orders will be billed at individual rate until proof of status is received. Foreign air speed delivery is included in all *Clinics* subscription prices. All prices are subject to change without notice. **POSTMASTER:** Send address changes to *Heart Failure Clinics*, Elsevier Health Sciences Division, Subscription Customer Service, 3251 Riverport Lane, Maryland Heights, MO 63043. **Customer Service: 1-800-654-2452 (US and Canada). From outside of the US and Canada, call 314-447-8871. Fax: 314-447-8029. For print support, e-mail: JournalsCustomerService-usa@elsevier.com. For online support, e-mail: JournalsOnlineSupport-usa@elsevier.com.**

Reprints. For copies of 100 or more of articles in this publication, please contact the Commercial Reprints Department, Elsevier Inc., 360 Park Avenue South, New York, NY 10010-1710. Tel.: 212-633-3812; Fax: 212-462-1935; E-mail: reprints@elsevier.com.

Heart Failure Clinics is covered in *MEDLINE/PubMed (Index Medicus)*.

Cover artwork courtesy of Umberto M. Jezek.

Printed and bound in the United Kingdom

Transferred to Digital Print 2011

Contributors

CONSULTING EDITORS

RAGAVENDRA R. BALIGA, MD, MBA
Professor of Internal Medicine, Vice Chief
and Assistant Division Director, Division
of Cardiovascular Medicine, The Ohio State
University, Columbus, Ohio

JAMES B. YOUNG, MD
Professor of Medicine and Executive Dean,
Cleveland Clinic Lerner College of Medicine;
George and Linda Kaufman Chair, Chairman,
Endocrinology and Metabolism Institute,
Cleveland Clinic, Cleveland, Ohio

GUEST EDITOR

**JEFFREY A. TOWBIN, MD, FACC,
FAAP, FAHA**
Executive Co-Director, The Heart Institute;
Professor and Chief, Pediatric Cardiology;
Director, Heart Failure, Cardiomyopathy
and Heart Transplant Service, Cincinnati
Children's Hospital Medical Center,
Cincinnati, Ohio

AUTHORS

MICHAEL J. ACKERMAN, MD, PhD
Division of Cardiovascular Diseases,
Department of Medicine; Division of Pediatric
Cardiology, Department of Pediatrics;
Department of Molecular Pharmacology and
Experimental Therapeutics, Windland Smith
Rice Sudden Death Genomics Laboratory,
Mayo Clinic, Rochester, Minnesota

STUART BERGER, MD
Professor of Pediatrics, Children's Hospital
of Wisconsin, Medical College of Wisconsin,
Milwaukee, Wisconsin

MICHAEL BURCH, MD, FRCP, FRCPCH
Director of Cardiothoracic Transplantation;
Chief, Department of Cardiology, Great
Ormond Street Hospital, London,
United Kingdom

CHARLES E. CANTER, MD
Professor, Department of Pediatrics,
Washington University; Division of Pediatric
Cardiology, St Louis, Missouri

STEVEN D. COLAN, MD
Professor of Pediatrics, Harvard Medical
School; Associate Chief, Department of
Cardiology, Children's Hospital Boston,
Boston, Massachusetts

GERALD F. COX, MD, PhD
Children's Hospital Boston, Boston,
Massachusetts

SUSAN W. DENFIELD, MD
Associate Professor of Pediatrics, Lillie Frank
Abercrombie Division of Pediatric Cardiology,
Texas Children's Hospital, Baylor College
of Medicine, Houston, Texas

ANNE I. DIPCHAND, MD
Associate Professor of Pediatrics, Division of Cardiology, Labatt Family Heart Centre, Hospital for Sick Children, Toronto, Ontario, Canada

ANNE M. DUBIN, MD
Associate Professor of Pediatrics, Lucile Packard Children's Hospital, Stanford University Medical School, Palo Alto, California

DAPHNE T. HSU, MD
Professor, Department of Pediatrics, Albert Einstein College of Medicine; Division Chief and Co-Director, Department of Pediatrics, Pediatric Heart Center, Children's Hospital at Montefiore, Bronx, New York

TIMOTHY M. HOFFMAN, MD
Division of Pediatric Cardiology, Nationwide Children's Hospital, Columbus, Ohio

JOHN LYNN JEFFERIES, MD, MPH, FAAP, FACC
Director, Cardiomyopathy and Heart Failure; Co-Director, Cardiovascular Genetics Service; Assistant Professor, Pediatric Cardiology, Texas Children's Hospital; Assistant Professor, Adult Cardiovascular Diseases, Texas Heart Institute at St Luke's Episcopal Hospital, Baylor College of Medicine, Houston, Texas

PAUL F. KANTOR, MB, BCh, DCH, FRCPC
University of Toronto, Division of Cardiology, Hospital for Sick Children, Toronto, Ontario, Canada

UWE KÜHL, MD, PhD
Department of Cardiology and Pneumology, University Medicine Berlin, Campus Benjamin-Franklin, Medical Clinic II, Berlin, Germany

DAVID C. LANDY, MPH
Department of Pediatrics, Leonard M. Miller School of Medicine, University of Miami, Miami, Florida

STEVEN E. LIPSHULTZ, MD
Department of Pediatrics, Leonard M. Miller School of Medicine, University of Miami, Miami, Florida

DAVID L.S. MORALES, MD, FACS, FACP
Surgical Director, Mechanical Circulatory Support; Director, Clinical and Industrial Research, Congenital Heart Surgery; Associate Surgeon, Congenital Heart Surgery Service, Texas Children's Hospital; Associate Professor, Surgery and Pediatrics, Baylor College of Medicine, Houston, Texas

DAVID P. NELSON, MD, PhD
Division of Cardiology, The Heart Institute at Cincinnati Children's Hospital Medical Center, Cincinnati, Ohio

MATTHEW J. O'CONNOR, MD
Fellow, Division of Cardiology, The Children's Hospital of Philadelphia; University of Pennsylvania School of Medicine, Philadelphia, Pennsylvania

E. JOHN ORAV, PhD
Division of General Internal Medicine, Brigham and Women's Hospital, Boston, Massachusetts

ELFRIEDE PAHL, MD
Professor of Pediatrics, Department of Pediatrics, Children's Memorial Hospital, Northwestern Feinberg School of Medicine, Chicago, Illinois

DANIEL J. PENNY, MD, PhD
Professor and Chief, Section of Pediatric Cardiology, Departments of Pediatrics, Baylor College of Medicine, Texas Children's Hospital, Houston, Texas

JACK F. PRICE, MD
Assistant Professor of Pediatrics (Cardiology), Texas Children's Hospital, Baylor College of Medicine, Houston, Texas

ANDREW N. REDINGTON, MD, FRCP
University of Toronto, Division of Cardiology, Hospital for Sick Children, Toronto, Ontario, Canada

DAVID N. ROSENTHAL, MD
Associate Professor of Pediatrics, Stanford University Medical Director, Pediatric Cardiology, Pediatric Advanced Cardiac Therapies Program, Lucile Packard Children's Hospital, Stanford, California

HEINZ-PETER SCHULTHEISS, MD
Head, Department of Cardiology and
Pneumology, University Medicine Berlin,
Campus Benjamin-Franklin, Medical Clinic II,
Berlin, Germany

ROBERT E. SHADDY, MD
Chief, Division of Cardiology, The Children's
Hospital of Philadelphia; Professor of
Pediatrics, University of Pennsylvania
School of Medicine, Philadelphia,
Pennsylvania

LYNN A. SLEEPER, ScD
New England Research Institutes, Watertown,
Massachusetts

**JEFFREY A. TOWBIN, MD, FACC,
FAAP, FAHA**
Executive Co-Director, The Heart Institute;
Professor and Chief, Pediatric Cardiology;
Director, Heart Failure, Cardiomyopathy
and Heart Transplant Service, Cincinnati
Children's Hospital Medical Center,
Cincinnati, Ohio

MATTEO VATTA, PhD
Director of Pediatric Cardiology Research
and Assistant Professor, Department
of Pediatrics (Cardiology), Texas Children's
Hospital, Baylor College of Medicine;
Department of Molecular Physiology
and Biophysics, Texas Children's Hospital,
Baylor College of Medicine, Houston, Texas

GILES WESLEY VICK III, MD, PhD
Associate Professor, Section of Pediatric
Cardiology, Department of Pediatrics, Baylor
College of Medicine, Texas Children's
Hospital, Houston, Texas

STEVEN A. WEBBER, MBChB, MRCP
Professor of Pediatrics, University of
Pittsburgh School of Medicine; Chief, Division
of Cardiology; Co-Director, Heart Center;
Medical Director, Pediatric Heart and
Heart-Lung Transplantation, Children's
Hospital of Pittsburgh of UPMC, Pittsburgh,
Pennsylvania

JAMES D. WILKINSON, MD, MPH
Department of Pediatrics, Leonard M. Miller
School of Medicine, University of Miami,
Miami, Florida

Contents

> Cardiomyopathy is a serious disorder of the heart muscle and, although rare, is a common cause of heart failure in children and the most common cause for heart transplantation in children older than 1 year of age. Funded by the National Heart Lung and Blood Institute since 1994, the Pediatric Cardiomyopathy Registry (PCMR) has followed more than 3500 North American children with cardiomyopathy. Early analyses determined estimates for the incidence of pediatric cardiomyopathy (1.13 cases per 100,000 children per year), risk factors for cardiomyopathy (age <1 year, male sex, black race, and living in New England as opposed to the central southwestern states), the prevalence of heart failure at diagnosis (6%–84% depending on cause), and 10-year survival (29%–94% depending on cause). More recent analyses explored cause-specific functional status, survival and transplant outcomes, and risk factors in greater detail. For many topics these analyses are based on the largest and best-documented samples of children with disease such as the muscular dystrophies, mitochondrial disorders, and Noonan syndrome. Data from the PCMR continue to provide valuable information that guides clinical management and the use of life-saving therapies, such as cardiac transplantation and approaches to treating heart failure, and prepares children, their families, and their caregivers to deal with this serious condition.

> This article describes the causes and outcomes of dilated cardiomyopathy in children. Genetic, infectious, metabolic, and acquired causes of dilated cardiomyopathy are discussed. The predictors for better and worse outcomes are reviewed. Guidelines for the use of medical and surgical therapies to treat heart failure in children are summarized.

> Hypertrophic cardiomyopathy has important differences in children compared with adults, particularly with regard to the range of causes and the outcomes in infants. Survival is highly dependent on etiology, particularly in the youngest patients, and pursuit of the specific cause is therefore necessary. The clinical utility of defining the genotype in children with familial hypertrophic cardiomyopathy exceeds that at other ages and has a highly favorable cost/benefit ratio. Although most of the

available information concerning treatment and prevention of sudden death is derived in adults, management of children requires consideration of the differences in age-specific risk/benefit ratios.

Depending on the part of the world one lives in, restrictive cardiomyopathy is either one of the rarest forms of cardiomyopathy in childhood, with no cause usually identified, or it is secondary to a poorly understood disease, endomyocardial fibrosis, that is endemic in some populations. Regardless of the underlying cause, the outcome is poor once symptoms develop. This article reviews the definitions, epidemiology, etiologies, genetics, "overlap" phenotypes, clinical presentation, diagnostic evaluation, outcome, and management of pediatric patients with restrictive cardiomyopathy.

In this article the newly classified cardiomyopathy known as left ventricular noncompaction is discussed. This genetic inherited form of heart disease has substantial risk of heart failure, stroke, metabolic derangement, arrhythmias, and sudden cardiac death. The disorder seems to occur because of an arrest of the normal process of development, and the genes identified to date seem to encode for cytoskeletal or sarcomeric proteins. These features are outlined.

There are various underlying causes of tachycardia-induced cardiomyopathy (TIC), and it is critical that it be considered in any patient who presents with a newly diagnosed dilated cardiomyopathy. Unlike most other forms of cardiomyopathy, TIC should be considered a treatable form of cardiomyopathy and it is imperative that the diagnosis be fully considered. A 12-lead ECG should be obtained in all patients with a dilated cardiomyopathy. Prompt diagnosis and therapy of this relatively uncommon cause of heart failure is critical and has the potential to completely reverse the ventricular dysfunction that may be present in this abnormality.

Myocarditis is an inflammatory disease of the cardiac muscle caused by myocardial infiltration of immunocompetent cells following any kind of cardiac injury. Acute myocarditis in childhood is often a result of a viral infection that produces myocardial necrosis and triggers an immune response to eliminate the infectious agent. Chronic myocardial injury may develop by postinfectious immune or autoimmune processes or be associated with systemic autoimmune diseases, which, in the long run, are responsible for persistent or progressive ventricular dysfunction, arrhythmias, and cardiac complaints. The disease often presents as an acute form of dilated cardiomyopathy, but because of its broad spectrum of presentation the clinical diagnosis is frequently misleading. If the underlying infectious or immune-mediated causes of the disease are carefully defined by clinical and biopsy-based tools, specific immunosuppressive and antiviral treatment options in addition to basic symptomatic therapy may avoid unnecessary interventions and improve prognosis in many patients with acute and chronic disease.

published by the International Society for Heart and Lung Transplantation the American College of Cardiology, and the American Heart Association. The primary aim of heart failure therapy is to reduce symptoms, preserve long-term ventricular performance, and prolong survival primarily through antagonism of the neurohormonal compensatory mechanisms. Because some medications may be detrimental during an acute decompensation, physicians who manage these patients as inpatients must be knowledgeable about the medications and therapeutic goals of chronic heart failure treatment. Understanding the mechanisms of chronic heart failure may foster improved understanding of the treatment of decompensated heart failure.

Despite optimization of standard medical therapy, some patients with chronic heart failure will deteriorate to the point that they require hospitalization for intravenous therapies and inpatient monitoring. Once the condition is recognized, the therapeutic goals are to reverse hemodynamic derangements, correct metabolic abnormalities, and provide symptomatic relief. Achievement of these goals requires individualized care and a familiarity with the risks and benefits of particular therapies.

Heart transplantation has become standard therapy for end-stage heart failure in children with cardiomyopathy as well as complex congenital heart disease, and has a significant effect on survival and quality of life. The indications for listing and referral for transplantation are outlined. Evaluation for heart transplantation is discussed, including full pretransplant assessment. ABO incompatible listing and HLA sensitization are discussed, and listing algorithms are outlined for different countries.

Heart failure is an important cause of morbidity and mortality in individuals of all ages. The many-faceted nature of the clinical heart failure syndrome has historically frustrated attempts to develop an overarching explanative theory. However, much useful information has been gained by basic and clinical investigation, even though a comprehensive understanding of heart failure has been elusive. Heart failure is a growing problem, in both adult and pediatric populations, for which standard medical therapy, as of 2010, can have positive effects, but these are usually limited and progressively diminish with time in most patients. If we want curative or near-curative therapy that will return patients to a normal state of health at a feasible cost, much better diagnostic and therapeutic technologies need to be developed. This review addresses the vexing group of heart failure etiologies that include cardiomyopathies and other ventricular dysfunctions of various types, for which current therapy is only modestly effective. Although there are many unique aspects to heart failure in patients with pediatric and congenital heart disease, many of the innovative approaches that are being developed for the care of adults with heart failure will be applicable to heart failure in childhood.

Heart Failure Clinics

VISIT THE CLINICS ONLINE!

Access your subscription at:
www.theclinics.com

Editorial

Giant Strides and Baby Steps in Pediatric Cardiac Disease and Heart Failure in Children

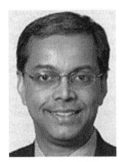
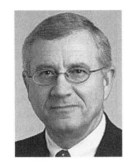

Ragavendra R. Baliga, MD, MBA   James B. Young, MD
Consulting Editors

In the past six decades giant strides have been made in the management of complex congenital cardiac defects resulting in survival to adulthood. Coarctation of the aorta and patent ductus arteriosus were the only correctable lesions in 1950 and in 1960 the likelihood that an infant who had heart disease would survive 12 months was about 60%.[1] Between 1979 and 1997 the reduction infant mortality rates due to heart disease was nearly 40%.[2] The 1-year survival for infants undergoing heart surgery now exceeds 95%.[3] These advances in pediatric cardiology have resulted in the rather dramatic growth of "adult congenital heart disease" as a cardiology subspecialty with several hundred patients being followed up in these specialized clinics.

Pediatric patients have complex cardiovascular physiology, and the natural history of heart failure in these individuals has a different trajectory than that of patients with more common causes of heart failure in the adult heart failure management programs. Even the New York Heart Association classification does not apply to most children, who instead require the use of the modified Ross Heart Failure classification that incorporates growth problems, feeding difficulties, and symptoms of exercise intolerance (**Table 1**). The management of pediatric heart failure in 1962, when rheumatic fever, endocarditis and myocarditis were predominant etiologies, included propping up the infant in an upright position (**Fig. 1**) to improve ventilation.[4] Nowadays, congenital heart disease or cardiac surgery account for 61% of all pediatric cases and for 82% of cases of heart failure in infants.[5] In contrast, in adults less than 1% of heart failure discharges are due to congenital heart disease. It is estimated that heart failure caused by congenital heart disease and cardiomyopathy affects about 12,000 to 35,000 children below age 19 in the United States every year.[6]

As the burden of heart failure in children continues to grow and with the increasing need to develop specific heart failure therapies for these patients with unique and complex cardiovascular physiology, the National Heart Lung and Blood Institute (NHLBI) set up a Pediatric Cardiomyopathy registry to better understand the natural history.[7] This registry reported that only 58% of all children with cardiomyopathy were given therapy for heart failure, with 83% of those with dilated cardiomyopathy receiving such treatment. Not all medications useful in adult heart failure, however, are efficacious in children. For example, a recent study demonstrated that angiotensin converting enzyme inhibitors, are not useful in heart failure due to single ventricle.[8] Meanwhile, the mortality rate or the need for cardiac

Heart Failure Clin 6 (2010) xiii–xv
doi:10.1016/j.hfc.2010.08.001

heartfailure.theclinics.com

Table 1
Modified Ross Heart Failure Classification for Children

Class I	Asymptomatic
Class II	Mild tachypnea or diaphoresis with feeding in infants Dyspnea on exertion in older children
Class III	Marked tachypnea or diaphoresis with feeding in infants Marked dyspnea on exertion Prolonged feeding times with growth failure
Class IV	Symptoms such as tachypnea, retractions, grunting, or diaphoresis at rest

From Hsu DT, Pearson GD. Heart failure in children: part I: history, etiology, and pathophysiology. Circ Heart Fail 2009;2(1):63–70; with permission.

transplantation in children remains high with almost 40% of children with symptomatic cardiomyopathy eventually dying due to heart failure or requiring orthotopic heart transplantation.[3,9] This arena of sub-sub-specialization has been challenged with unique complexities as well. Indeed, when one remembers that the first attempts at orthotopic cardiac transplantation in North America were largely in infants with congenital heart disease using anencephalic newborns for donors, the challenges of this approach are highlighted. Indeed, donor hearts for infants are rare and the development of adequate mechanical circulatory assist devices is challenged by requirements for miniaturization of vital machines. Nonetheless, despite the limitations of presently available devices and the fact that transplanted hearts rarely function well after 20 years (often necessitating re-transplantation in the pediatric group), this is an arena of important "baby steps."[10]

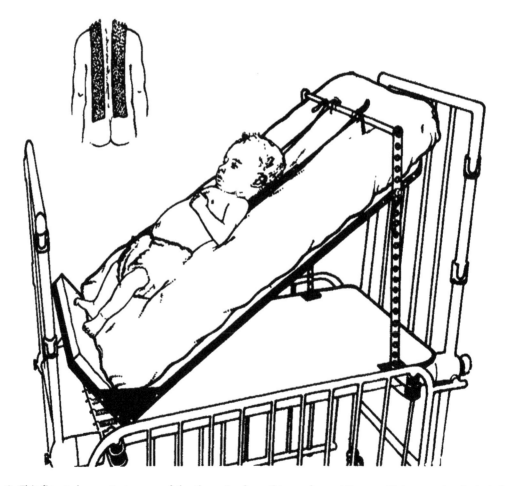

Fig. 1. This figure demonstrates one of the therapies from this era for assisting ventilatory mechanics in infants with heart failure. The figure shows a device for nursing infants in an upright position. (Inset shows the straps on the infant's back. Tincture of benzoin was used to prepare the skin). (*From* Goldblatt E. The treatment of cardiac failure in infancy: a review of 350 cases. *Lancet:* 1962;2:212–5; with permission.)

Table 2
Cardiovascular Causes of Heart Failure in Children

Congenital cardiac malformations
  Volume overload
    Left-to-right shunting
      Ventricular septal defect
      Patent ductus arteriosus
    Atrioventricular or semilunar valve
      insufficiency
      Aortic regurgitation in bicommissural
        aortic valve
      Pulmonary regurgitation after repair
        of tetralogy of Fallot
  Pressure overload
    Left sided obstruction
      Severe aortic stenosis
      Aortic coarctation
    Right-sided obstruction
      Severe pulmonary stenosis
  Complex congenital heart disease
    Single ventricle
      Hypoplastic left heart syndrome
        Unbalanced atrioventricular septal
          defect
    Systemic right ventricle
      L-transposition ("corrected
        transposition") of the great arteries
Structurally normal heart
  Primary cardiomyopathy
    Dilated
    Hypertrophic
    Restrictive
  Secondary
    Arrhythmogenic
    Ischemic
    Toxic
    Infiltrative
    Infectious

From Hsu DT, Pearson GD. Heart failure in children: part 1: history, etiology, and pathophysiology. Circ Heart Fail 2009;2(1):63–70; with permission.

Because only baby steps have been made in decreasing heart failure mortality in children, much more work must be done. The lack of success in the management of pediatric heart failure has several causes, including the disparate natural history of heart failure, a multitude of etiological factors (**Table 2**),[6] accompanying congenital defects, and physiological changes brought about by surgical correction. In this issue Dr Jeffrey A Towbin has assembled a panel of international experts who discuss important challenges that are faced in the management heart failure in children and how best to meet these challenges. We hope that these articles will stimulate research that results in making giant strides in the management of heart failure in children.

Ragavendra R. Baliga, MD, MBA
Division of Cardiovascular Medicine
The Ohio State University
Columbus, OH, USA

James B. Young, MD
Division of Medicine and
Lerner College of Medicine
Cleveland Clinic
Cleveland, OH, USA

E-mail addresses:
Ragavendra.Baliga@osumc.edu
youngj@ccf.org

REFERENCES

1. Report of the New England Regional Infant Cardiac Program. Pediatrics 1980;65(2 Pt 2):375–461.
2. Boneva RS, Botto LD, Moore CA, Yang Q, Correa A, Erickson JD. Mortality associated with congenital heart defects in the United States: trends and racial disparities, 1979–1997. Circulation 2001;103(19): 2376–81.
3. Strauss A, Lock JE. Pediatric cardiomyopathy—a long way to go. N Engl J Med 2003;348(17):1703–5.
4. Goldblatt E. The treatment of cardiac failure in infancy. A review of 350 cases. Lancet 1962;2 (7249):212–5.
5. Webster G, Zhang J, Rosenthal D. Comparison of the epidemiology and co-morbidities of heart failure in the pediatric and adult populations: a retrospective, cross-sectional study. BMC Cardiovasc Disord 2006;6:23.
6. Hsu DT, Pearson GD. Heart failure in children: part I: history, etiology, and pathophysiology. Circ Heart Fail 2009;2(1):63–70.
7. Lipshultz SE, Sleeper LA, Towbin JA, Lowe AM, Orav EJ, Cox GF, Lurie PR, McCoy KL, McDonald MA, Messere JE, Colan SD. The Incidence of Pediatric Cardiomyopathy in Two Regions of the United States. New England Journal of Medicine 2003;348(17):1647–55.
8. Hsu DT, Zak V, Mahony L, Sleeper LA, Atz AM, Levine JC, Barker PC, Ravishankar C, McCrindle BW, Williams RV, Altmann K, Ghanayem NS, Margossian R, Chung WK, Border WL, Pearson GD, Stylianou MP, Mital S. Enalapril in Infants With Single Ventricle: Results of a Multicenter Randomized Trial. Circulation 122(4):333–40.
9. Lipshultz SE. Ventricular dysfunction clinical research in infants, children and adolescents. Prog Pediatr Cardiol 2000;12(1):1–28.
10. Young J, Baumgartner WA, Reitz BA, Ohler L. Magic moments in heart transplantation. In: Kirklin JK, Mehra M, West LJ, editors. History of International Heart and Lung Transplantation, ISHLT Monograph Serries 2010;4:45–90.

Preface
Heart Failure in Children

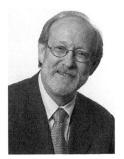

Jeffrey A. Towbin, MD, FACC, FAAP, FAHA
Guest Editor

Heart failure is a common and sometimes devastating disorder that affects an estimated 4.8 million Americans, including 2% of Americans between the ages of 40 and 59 years, 5% between 60 and 69 years, and 10% over the age of 70 years. The incidence is approximately 400,000 annually. Lacking over the years has been a focus on children and young adults, who are also affected by this problem; limited statistics have been published. The National Institutes of Health–National Heart, Lung, and Blood Institute Pediatric Cardiomyopathy Registry has published the largest series on this disorder in childhood, but the field has continued to be underrepresented and has been underfunded. Hence, our knowledge regarding the diagnostic, etiologic, and therapeutic approaches has lagged behind that for adult counterparts until the present.

There now appears to be a momentum for training specialists in pediatric cardiomyopathies and heart failure, in both the clinical and the research aspects of these disorders. Unlike adult patients with heart failure, children are rarely afflicted by ischemic heart disease, toxicities such as alcohol-related disease, or the common comorbidities seen in adults with these disorders. Instead, children have primary genetic disease (including genes causing primary cardiomyopathies, syndromes, neuromuscular disease, metabolic disorders, and chromosomal disorders), acquired diseases such as viral-induced myocarditis, or chemotherapy-induced disease as the most common known causes. Importantly, a large percentage of these children are now surviving well into adulthood, and in many cases these disorders are not well known by the adult heart failure community. Therefore, the information on childhood heart failure requires broad distribution and frequent updates as the field is now moving quickly into new areas of knowledge. This special issue of *Heart Failure Clinics* is dedicated to childhood forms of heart failure and approaches to the care and the science of these disorders.

In this issue we have assembled the world leaders in these childhood disorders and cover all of the forms of childhood cardiomyopathies, including dilated, hypertrophic, restrictive, and arrhythmogenic forms, as well as left ventricular noncompaction. This discussion is kicked off by the article that describes the data generated in the Pediatric Cardiomyopathy Registry. In addition, other causes of heart failure in children are discussed, including myocarditis in childhood as well as heart failure associated with congenital heart disease. The genetic basis of cardiomyopathies and heart failure and the metabolic causes of heart failure in children are described in detail and facilitate a current understanding of the etiologic basis of disease. This better understanding of the causes of disease can also impact therapy and outcome and therefore

Heart Failure Clin 6 (2010) xvii–xviii
doi:10.1016/j.hfc.2010.06.006

outpatient care and treatment, inpatient care and treatment in the intensive care unit, as well as mechanical support in children, heart transplantation in children, and novel therapies now and on the horizon are covered in separate articles. It is the intent of the Editor and the authors that after reading this issue, the reader will gain a better understanding of heart failure in children and that this important problem will become better known in the community by families and caregivers alike.

Jeffrey A. Towbin, MD, FACC, FAAP, FAHA
The Heart Institute
Pediatric Cardiology, Heart Failure,
Cardiomyopathy & Heart Transplant Service
Cincinnati Children's Hospital Medical Center
3333 Burnet Avenue
Cincinnati, OH 45229, USA

E-mail address:
jeffrey.towbin@cchmc.org

The Pediatric Cardiomyopathy Registry and Heart Failure: Key Results from the First 15 Years

James D. Wilkinson, MD, MPH[a], David C. Landy, MPH[a], Steven D. Colan, MD[b], Jeffrey A. Towbin, MD[c], Lynn A. Sleeper, ScD[d], E. John Orav, PhD[e], Gerald F. Cox, MD, PhD[b], Charles E. Canter, MD[f], Daphne T. Hsu, MD[g,i], Steven A. Webber, MBChB[h], Steven E. Lipshultz, MD[a,*]

KEYWORDS
- Cardiomyopathy • Pediatrics • Heart failure
- Pediatric cardiomyopathy registry

Cardiomyopathy is a serious disorder of the heart muscle and, although rare, is a common cause of heart failure in children, and it is also the most common cause of heart transplantation in children older than 1 year of age.[1–4] Although cardiomyopathy has various functional types, the vast majority of children with this diagnosis have either a dilated or a hypertrophic type, both of which are associated with abnormal cardiac structure and function and poor outcomes. The true incidence, prevalence, risk factors, causes, and natural history of the various types of pediatric cardiomyopathy were not known before the mid-1990s.

Accurately estimating the incidence of this rare and heterogeneous disease required applying a rigorous recruitment strategy over a large geographic area to collect a sufficiently large and unbiased population-based sample. The varied and often prolonged clinical course of the disease also required regular long-term follow-up of these children to better document their diagnosis, treatment, clinical course, and outcomes. Thus, in

Funding support: This work was supported by the National Heart Lung and Blood Institute (HL53392) and the Children's Cardiomyopathy Foundation.

[a] Department of Pediatrics (D820), Leonard M. Miller School of Medicine, University of Miami, PO Box 016820, Miami, FL 33101, USA

[b] Department of Cardiology, Children's Hospital Boston, 300 Longwood Avenue, Boston, MA 02115, USA

[c] The Heart Institute, Pediatric Cardiology, Heart Failure, Cardiomyopathy & Heart Transplant Service, Cincinnati Children's Medical Center, 3333 Burnet Avenue, Cincinnati, OH 45229, USA

[d] New England Research Institutes, 9 Galen Street, Watertown, MA 02472, USA

[e] Division of General Internal Medicine, Brigham and Women's Hospital, 3rd Floor, 1620 Tremont Street, Boston, MA 02115, USA

[f] Department of Cardiology and Cardiothoracic Surgery, St Louis Children's Hospital, One Children's Place 2nd Floor, Suite F, St Louis, MO 63110, USA

[g] Department of Pediatrics, Pediatric Heart Center, Children's Hospital Montefiore, 3415 Bainbridge Avenue, Rosenthal Pavilion, Room 3, Bronx, NY 10467, USA

[h] Department of Cardiothoracic Surgery and Heart Transplantation, Children's Hospital of Pittsburgh, 45th Street and Penn Avenue, Pittsburgh, PA 15201, USA

[i] Department of Pediatrics, Albert Einstein College of Medicine, 3415 Bainbrige Avenue, Bronx, NY 10467, USA

* Corresponding author.

E-mail address: slipshultz@med.miami.edu

Heart Failure Clin 6 (2010) 401–413

doi:10.1016/j.hfc.2010.05.002

1994, the National Heart, Lung and Blood Institute (NHLBI) funded the Pediatric Cardiomyopathy Registry (PCMR), a large, multicenter observational study of primary and idiopathic cardiomyopathies in children. The PCMR was designed to study the epidemiology and clinical course of selected cardiomyopathies in children and adolescents as well as to promote the development of cause-specific prevention and treatment strategies. Currently, data from more than 3500 children with cardiomyopathy have been collected in the PCMR database with annual follow-up continuing from enrollment until death, heart transplant, or loss to follow-up.

Some of the aims of the PCMR have evolved over the past 15 years in response to registry findings and changing clinical challenges. The original aims were primarily epidemiologic: to describe the incidence and presentation of cardiomyopathy in all patients by functional types and within demographic subgroups. Adding a retrospective cohort of children strengthened the ability to describe clinical outcomes and predictors of such outcomes. This clinical focus was emphasized in the second funding cycle by including prospectively collected, parent-reported functional status data to better characterize the effect of cardiomyopathy on the daily lives of affected children and their families.

In the current funding cycle, study aims were expanded by collaborating with the Pediatric Heart Transplant Study Group to examine the effect of cardiac transplantation on the clinical course of cardiomyopathy, as well as to describe long-term changes in functional status and their relationship to clinical events and outcomes, including heart transplantation. Also, for the first time since the establishment of the PCMR, blood and cardiac tissue specimens were collected to investigate the relationship of genetic and viral markers to clinical and functional outcomes.

The PCMR has helped establish reliable estimates of the incidence of cardiomyopathy in children and has provided unbiased assessments of typical clinical presentations and outcomes. It has led to refined descriptions of functional types of disease and even descriptions by cause with the identification of risk factors for cardiac transplantation and death. It has also provided the most complete accounts of how cardiomyopathy is diagnosed and treated providing an evidence-based background on which to create diagnostic and treatment algorithms.

We review here the most important PCMR findings and describe current PCMR investigations, focusing especially on findings related to pediatric heart failure.

THE DESIGN AND OPERATION OF THE PCMR

The design and implementation of the PCMR are detailed elsewhere.[5] In brief, children up to 18 years old diagnosed with cardiomyopathy at participating centers are eligible for inclusion if they meet specific quantitative echocardiographic criteria, if the pattern of cardiomyopathy conforms to a defined semi-quantitative pattern, or if the diagnosis is confirmed by tissue analysis (**Box 1**). Each case of cardiomyopathy is then classified morphologically as dilated, hypertrophic, restrictive, mixed, or other. Children are excluded if they have specific secondary causes of myocardial abnormalities, including potential causes of myocardial hypertrophy, such as congenital heart disease and exposure to drugs known to cause cardiac hypertrophy (**Box 2**).

The original PCMR design consisted of 2 cohorts. The first was a retrospective cohort of children who were diagnosed between January 1, 1990, and December 31, 1995, and identified by chart review from 39 tertiary care centers in the United States and Canada. The purpose of this cohort was to identify potential predictors of outcome as well as diagnostic approaches. The second cohort was a population-based prospective cohort of children diagnosed after January 1, 1996, by pediatric cardiologists at 98 pediatric cardiac centers in 2 geographically distinct regions of the United States (New England [Connecticut, Maine, Massachusetts, New Hampshire, and Rhode Island] and the central southwest [Arkansas, Oklahoma, and Texas]). These geographic areas were selected because of the local referral patterns, which should identify essentially all incident cases of pediatric cardiomyopathy. The purpose of this cohort was to estimate accurately the incidence of cardiomyopathy in children. Standardized data collection in both regions was performed by an outreach team that regularly traveled to the participating centers to enroll new cases and to abstract data from medical records.

Collected data included demographic characteristics, quantitative echocardiographic measurements, a brief family history, vital and transplant status, and clinical findings. More detailed data were collected from the retrospective cohort. These data included a complete family history, qualitative echocardiographic studies (eg, mitral regurgitation), electrocardiographic data, therapy, and hospitalizations. The clinical and echocardiographic characteristics and clinical outcomes were similar between cohorts (**Fig. 1**).[1] Therefore, for most PCMR analyses, with the exception of estimating incidence rate, the 2 cohorts are combined.

Box 1
Inclusionary echocardiographic criteria for the PCMR

Measurements

- Left ventricular fractional shortening or ejection fraction greater than 2 standard deviations below the normal mean for age (left ventricular fractional shortening is acceptable in children with a normal ventricular configuration and without abnormal regional wall motion; abnormal ejection fractions detected by echocardiography, radionuclide or contrast angiography, or magnetic resonance imaging (MRI) are acceptable alternatives but age-appropriate norms for the individual laboratory must be applied)
- Left ventricular posterior wall thickness at end diastole greater than 2 standard deviations above the normal mean for body-surface area
- Left ventricular posterior wall thickness at end-systole greater than 2 standard deviations below the normal mean for body-surface area
- Left ventricular end-diastolic dimension or volume greater than 2 standard deviations above the normal mean for body-surface area (dimension data are acceptable under the conditions outlined for left ventricular fractional shortening, and volume data may be derived from the imaging methods as above)

Patterns

- Localized ventricular hypertrophy: such as, septal thickness greater than 1.5 × left ventricular posterior wall thickness with at least normal left ventricular posterior wall thickness, with or without dynamic outflow obstruction
- Restrictive cardiomyopathy: 1 or both atria enlarged relative to the ventricles of normal or small size with evidence of impaired diastolic filling and in the absence of marked valvular heart disease
- Contracted form of endocardial fibroelastosis: similar to restrictive cardiomyopathy plus an echo-dense endocardium
- Ventricular dysplasia or Uhl congenital anomaly: a very thin right ventricle with a dilated right atrium (usually better assessed by MRI than by echocardiography)
- Concentric hypertrophy in the absence of a hemodynamic cause: a single measurement of left ventricular posterior wall thickness at end diastole greater than 2 standard deviations suffices
- Left ventricular myocardial noncompaction: highly trabeculated spongiform left ventricle myocardium with multiple interstices

Box 2
Exclusionary criteria for the PCMR

- Endocrine disease known to cause heart muscle disease (including infants of diabetic mothers)
- A history of rheumatic fever
- Toxic exposures known to cause heart muscle disease (eg, anthracyclines, mediastinal radiation, iron overload, or heavy metal exposure)
- Human immunodeficiency virus (HIV) infection or born to an HIV-positive mother
- Kawasaki disease
- Congenital heart defects unassociated with malformation syndromes (eg, valvar heart disease or congenital coronary artery malformations)
- Immunologic disease
- Invasive cardiothoracic procedures or major surgery during the preceding month except those specifically related to cardiomyopathy including left ventricular assist device, extracorporeal membrane oxygenation, and automated implantable cardioverter defibrillator placement
- Uremia, active or chronic
- Abnormal ventricular size or function that can be attributed to intense physical training or chronic anemia
- Chronic arrhythmia unless there are studies documenting inclusion criteria before the onset of arrhythmia (except a patient with chronic arrhythmia, subsequently ablated, whose cardiomyopathy persists after 2 months is not to be excluded)
- Malignancy
- Pulmonary parenchymal or vascular disease (eg, cystic fibrosis, cor pulmonale, or pulmonary hypertension)
- Ischemic coronary vascular disease
- Age less than 18 years
- Association with drugs known to cause hypertrophy (eg, growth hormone, corticosteroids or cocaine)
- Left ventricular assist device; extracorporeal membrane oxygenation; automatic implantable cardioverter defibrillator

In the current award period (2005 to the present), 397 additional children from the 11 pediatric cardiology centers that provided the majority of PCMR cases were prospectively enrolled and followed. Data on these children are the most detailed and include medications and echocardiographic and other cardiac studies. Blood specimens were also obtained and tested for mutations in the G4.5 (taffazin) gene, which has been assumed to be associated with boys with Barth syndrome.[6,7] Also, biopsy or heart explant

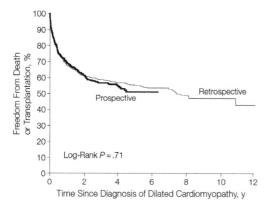

Fig. 1. Freedom from death or transplant for 491 children in the retrospective cohort and 935 children in the prospective cohort with pure dilated cardiomyopathy (*P* = .71). Data are from the Pediatric Cardiomyopathy Registry for the period between 1990 and 2002. (*From* Towbin JA, Lowe AM, Colan SD, et al. Incidence, causes, and outcomes of dilated cardiomyopathy in children. JAMA 2006;296:1869; with permission.)

tissue was obtained from a subset of these children to determine the prevalence of viral causes of cardiomyopathy with polymerase chain reaction analysis.

An adjunct study to the PCMR is the NHLBI-funded Pediatric Cardiomyopathy Specimen Repository (J. Towbin, principal investigator), which stores blood and tissue specimens from PCMR participants so that the genetic and viral causal associations with cardiomyopathy can be explored. Repository specimens (and a de-identified PCMR dataset) are made available to interested investigators on request.

THE INCIDENCE OF PEDIATRIC CARDIOMYOPATHY

Between 1996 and 1999, 467 children with a new diagnosis of cardiomyopathy meeting PCMR criteria were identified in the 2 geographic regions described above. Completeness of case capture by the 18 pediatric cardiology centers in New England and the 20 centers in the central southwest was assessed in multiple ways. We estimate that fewer than 5 cases per year were missed.[8] The estimated annual incidence of pediatric cardiomyopathy in the United States based on these 2 regions is 1.13 cases per 100,000 children aged 18 years or younger, a result similar to that reported for Finland and Australia.[8–10]

The annual incidence was significantly higher in infants less than 1 year of age (8.34 cases per 100,000, 95% confidence interval 7.21 to 9.61).

The incidence was higher in boys than in girls (1.32 vs 0.92 per 100,000 children, *P*<.001), higher in blacks than in whites (1.47 vs 1.06 per 100,000, *P* = .02), and in New England than in the central southwest (1.44 cases vs 0.98 per 100,000; *P*<.001). The annual incidence of dilated cardiomyopathy was 0.58 cases per 100,000 children and of hypertrophic cardiomyopathy, 0.47 per 100,000 children. These variations in incidence by sex, race, and geographic region were found in both the dilated and hypertrophic functional subgroups. The incidence may be underestimated because children with sudden death as a presenting symptom may not have been identified: pathologists and medical examiners were not contacted in the original protocol. Children with asymptomatic left ventricular dysfunction would also not be identified until they sought medical evaluation; however, the PCMR definition of cardiomyopathy is based on clinically present disease.

CAUSES OF PEDIATRIC CARDIOMYOPATHY

Examinations of more than 1400 children with dilated cardiomyopathy and more than 800 children with hypertrophic cardiomyopathy revealed that, for the most common types of cardiomyopathy, most cases lack a known cause.[1,11] In the more than 1400 children with a newly diagnosed pure form of dilated cardiomyopathy, only 34% had a known cause: 16% of children with myocarditis, 9% with a neuromuscular disorder, 5% with familial cardiomyopathy, 4% with inborn errors of metabolism, and 1% with malformation syndrome. In total, 71% of children with dilated cardiomyopathy presented with congestive heart failure at diagnosis, and although the causes varied greatly, all groups presented with severely reduced left ventricular fractional shortening (**Table 1**). In the more than 800 children with newly diagnosed hypertrophic cardiomyopathy, only 26% had a known cause: 9% with malformation syndrome, 9% with inborn errors of metabolism, and 8% with a neuromuscular disorder.[11] Only 13% of children hypertrophic cardiomyopathy presented with congestive heart failure at diagnosis, although again, the causes varied greatly (see **Table 1**).

In a separate study of only the retrospective cohort, among 916 children with any type of cardiomyopathy, only one-third had a known cause for their cardiomyopathy at the time of diagnosis.[12] Patient demographics and presentation, including heart failure at presentation, family history, echocardiographic findings, laboratory testing, and biopsy, were analyzed for possible associations with specific causal diagnoses for

Table 1
Prevalence of heart failure and left ventricular fractional shortening z score at diagnosis of pediatric cardiomyopathy, by type and cause of cardiomyopathy

Type of Cardiomyopathy, by Cause	Heart Failure, n	Mean Left Ventricular Fractional Shortening z Score (95% CI) [Standard Deviation]
Dilated		
Idiopathic	74	−9.62 (−11.42 to −7.16)
Myocarditis	84	−9.11 (−11.05 to −6.67)
Neuromuscular disorders	35	−5.88 (−8.02 to −3.32)
Familial	53	−7.07 (−9.63 to −3.68)
Inborn errors of metabolism	60	−8.94 (−10.30 to −5.33)
Malformation syndromes	67	−5.95 (−9.49 to −5.10)
Hypertrophic		
Inborn errors of metabolism	40.3	−1.11 [5.65]
Malformation syndromes	23.4	5.42 [4.31]
Neuromuscular disorders	6.4	3.01 [3.40]
Infantile	9.9	3.62 [5.15]

Data are from the Pediatric Cardiomyopathy Registry.

each type of cardiomyopathy. Children with a family history of cardiomyopathy were more likely to have a causal diagnosis regardless of cardiomyopathy type, and children with either dilated or hypertrophic cardiomyopathy and a family history of sudden death or a genetic syndrome were more likely to have a known causal diagnosis.

For children with dilated cardiomyopathy, older age at diagnosis, smaller left ventricular dimensions, and a higher left ventricular fractional shortening were associated with a causal diagnosis. For children with hypertrophic cardiomyopathy, female sex, decreased height and weight for age, and increased left ventricular posterior wall thickness were also associated with a causal diagnosis. After adjusting for age at diagnosis, congestive heart failure, and geographic region and excluding cases with neuromuscular disease, familial isolated cardiomyopathy, and malformation syndromes, analyses found that children with hypertrophic cardiomyopathy who had metabolic blood and urine test results were more likely to have a causal diagnosis than were children without such test results (odds ratio, 4.15). In patients with dilated cardiomyopathy, this same type of analysis identified endomyocardial biopsy and viral serology or culture as significant independent predictors of a causal diagnosis (odds ratios 4.84 and 1.81, respectively).

TREATMENT OF PEDIATRIC CARDIOMYOPATHY

Treatment at diagnosis for 350 children with idiopathic dilated cardiomyopathy diagnosed between 1990 and 1995 in the retrospective cohort was compared with that of similar children diagnosed between 2000 and 2006 in the prospective cohort.[13] Of the children from the retrospective cohort, 43% were less than 1 year old and 73% had heart failure at diagnosis. Within 1 month of diagnosis, 84% of those in the retrospective cohort were started on anti–heart-failure therapy (digoxin, a diuretic, or both), 66% were started on an angiotensin-converting enzyme inhibitor (ACE-I), and 4% were started on a β-blocker. These proportions were similar for children in the prospective cohort, except that β-blocker use increased to 18%. Predictors of both anti–heart-failure and ACE-I therapy were worsening left ventricular dilation and left ventricular fractional shortening. In addition, children with asymptomatic heart failure were frequently treated with anti–heart-failure therapy, and 47% were not started on ACE-I therapy. Such practice does not conform to current guidelines based on expert consensus, which recommend starting anti–heart-failure therapy only for symptomatic relief, whereas ACE-I therapy is recommended for nearly all children with heart failure, regardless of symptoms.[14]

OUTCOMES OF PEDIATRIC CARDIOMYOPATHY

Analyses of the PCMR database have identified cause-specific outcomes and predictors of outcome for children with cardiomyopathy. The clinical outcomes examined were death and cardiac death (either death or heart transplantation).

Of the more than 1400 cases of pure dilated cardiomyopathy, the 1- and 5-year rates of death or heart transplantation were 31% and 46%, respectively. These rates varied greatly by the cause of disease (**Fig. 2**).[1] Children aged 6 years or older were more likely to die or to undergo heart transplantation than were younger children (P<.001). After excluding children with neuromuscular disease and inborn metabolic errors, Cox regression modeling showed that for children with idiopathic dilated cardiomyopathy (as opposed to cardiomyopathy with a known diagnosis), the presence of congestive heart failure at diagnosis and decreased left ventricular fractional shortening were significant predictors of the composite end point of death or heart transplantation. Thus, outcomes for children with dilated cardiomyopathy depend on cause, age at diagnosis, and heart failure at presentation. Most children do not have an identified cause for dilated cardiomyopathy, which limits the application of disease-specific therapy.

An analysis of nutritional status in children with dilated cardiomyopathy showed that those diagnosed before 1 year of age were more likely to have growth retardation than older children with the same type of disease.[15] Cardiac dysfunction was associated with low height and body mass index, and low height was associated with increased risk of death.

Sudden death is less common in children with dilated cardiomyopathy than it is in adults with non-ischemic dilated cardiomyopathy, accounting for only 12% of deaths in these children enrolled in the PCMR. Heart failure and the use of anti-arrhythmic medications are associated with increased risk of sudden death. This knowledge should guide the use of automatic implantable cardiac defibrillators in these children.

Myocarditis accounts for 10% to 20% of the cardiomyopathies in children. An analysis of PCMR data found no difference in outcomes between children diagnosed with biopsy and those diagnosed clinically. More than two-thirds of these children are alive and have not received a heart transplant 2 years after diagnosis, and left ventricular size returns to almost normal in nearly half of these children during the same time. However, dilation and decreased left ventricular fractional shortening at diagnosis are associated with increased risk of death or transplant.

A separate PCMR study compared children with the 2 most common types of muscular dystrophy, Duchenne (DMD) and Becker (BMD).[16] All 128 children with DMD and 15 with BMD had dilated cardiomyopathy with roughly one-third of each group presenting with heart failure and both groups receiving similar treatment at diagnosis. Median follow-up time was 3.3 years during which 47 children with DMD died and 6 children with BMD underwent heart transplant. Of the 47 deaths, 30 had a known cause and 20 of these

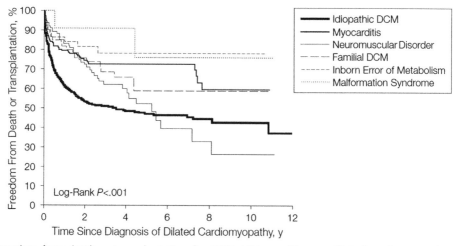

Fig. 2. Freedom from death or transplantation for 1423 children with pure dilated cardiomyopathy, by cause. Data are from the Pediatric Cardiomyopathy Registry for the period between 1990 and 2002. (*From* Towbin JA, Lowe AM, Colan SD, et al. Incidence, causes, and outcomes of dilated cardiomyopathy in children. JAMA 2006;296:1873; with permission.)

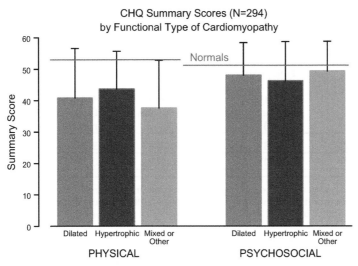

Fig. 5. Physical and psychosocial function, as measured by the Child Health Questionnaire, of 294 children with cardiomyopathy, by functional type. Data are from the Pediatric Cardiomyopathy Registry for the period between 1990 and 2002. (*From* Sleeper LA, Towbin JA, Colan SD, et al. Functional status is impaired and correlated with clinical status in pediatric cardiomyopathy. In: Proceedings of the 5th World Congress on Pediatric Cardiology and Cardiac Surgery 2009;5:134 (abstract).)

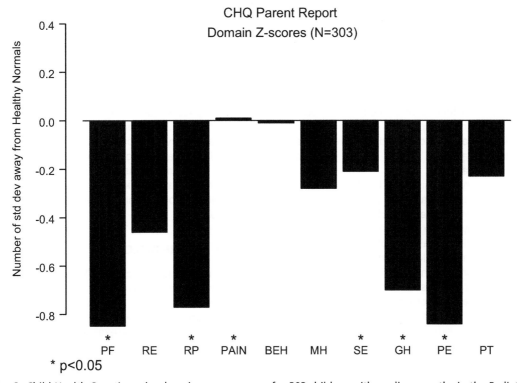

Fig. 6. Child Health Questionnaire domain mean z scores for 303 children with cardiomyopathy in the Pediatric Cardiomyopathy Registry. Scores for the physical domains, general health, self-esteem, and parental impact-emotional domains were significantly below the average for healthy children. Scores for mental health and behavior did not differ significantly from those of healthy children. BEH, behavior; GH, general health perception; MH, mental health; PAIN, bodily pain; PE, parental impact-emotional; PF, physical functioning; PT, parental impact-time; RE, role/social limits-emotional; RP, role/social limits-physical; SE, self-esteem. Data are from the Pediatric Cardiomyopathy Registry for the period between 1990 and 2002. (*From* Sleeper LA, Towbin JA, Colan SD, et al. Functional status is impaired and correlated with clinical status in pediatric sardiomyopathy. In: Proceedings of the 5th World Congress on Pediatric Cardiology and Cardiac Surgery 2009;5:134 (abstract).)

Table 2
G4.5 gene variants found in 37 of 158 children enrolled in the Pediatric Cardiomyopathy Registry[a]

Sex	n/N (%)	Hemizygous Single Nucleotide Polymorphism, n/N (%)	Intronic Substitution, Single Nucleotide Polymorphism, n/N (%)	Missense Substitution, Unclassified, n/N (%)	Hemizygous Mutation,[a] n/N (%)
Boys	27/110 (25)[b]	22/27 (81)	24/27 (89)	3/27 (11)	2/27 (7)
Girls	10/48 (22)[b]	3/10 (30)	10/10 (100)	0/10 (0)	0/10 (0)

[a] The number of children with G4.5 gene variants as a proportion of all children with the same diagnosis were: 9 of 45 (20%) children with pure hypertrophic cardiomyopathy; 19 of 79 (24%) with pure dilated cardiomyopathy; 3 of 10 (30%) with pure restrictive cardiomyopathy; 4 of 22 (18%) with other or mixed forms of cardiomyopathy; and 2 of 2 with unknown forms.

[b] Causes of cardiomyopathy in boys: idiopathic disease (n = 6); Barth syndrome or probably myocarditis (n = 2 each); Cori disease, Noonan syndrome, or familial dilated cardiomyopathy (n = 1 each). Causes in girls: idiopathic disease (n = 6); familial hypertrophic cardiomyopathy or confirmed myocarditis (n = 2 each). Children with Barth syndrome patients each had 2 variants, denoted here as hemizygous mutations (hemizygous single nucleotide polymorphisms were not counted).

From Towbin JA, Sleeper L, Jefferies JL, et al. Genetic and viral genome analysis of childhood cardiomyopathy: the PCMR/PCSR experience [abstract]. J Am Coll Cardiol 2010;55;A43.E409.

positively associated with longer time since diagnosis, suggesting that many children improve over time. Physical functioning in children with dilated cardiomyopathy or hypertrophic cardiomyopathy was associated with increased left ventricular size and the left ventricular posterior wall thickness to end-diastolic dimension ratio, respectively. Poorer functional status is a risk factor for later death or transplant in children with dilated cardiomyopathy and mixed or other types of cardiomyopathy, but not hypertrophic cardiomyopathy.

Preliminary analysis of the G 4.5 mutation in 160 children showed that more than 20% had gene variants and that, unexpectedly, these were similar for both boys and girls (**Table 2**).[27] Polymerase chain reaction analyses of myocardial tissue samples from 44 children contributing to the Pediatric Cardiomyopathy Specimen Repository, revealed 2 were positive for Epstein-Barr virus (1 with dilated cardiomyopathy and 1 with hypertrophic cardiomyopathy), and 6 were positive for parvovirus (4 with idiopathic disease and 2 with myocarditis). Tests for adenovirus, cytomegalovirus, and enterovirus, among others, were negative.

INTERNATIONAL CONFERENCE ON PEDIATRIC CARDIOMYOPATHY

In January 2007, PCMR investigators organized the first International Workshop on Idiopathic and Primary Pediatric Cardiomyopathies. Cosponsored by the Children's Cardiomyopathy Foundation and NHLBI, more than 50 researchers, young investigators, and NHLBI staff attended the 2-day conference. The results of the conference were published in 3 issues of the journal, *Progress in Pediatric Cardiology*.[28–62] In addition to the conference results, 2 additional special articles were included in these issues that addressed ethical issues in the care of children with cardiomyopathy and the importance of a comprehensive multidisciplinary approach to this care.[63,64] A second international conference took place in May of 2010, the results of which will be disseminated in dedicated issues of progress in Pediatric Cardiology to be published over the course of the next year.

PCMR: FUTURE DIRECTIONS

By continuously collecting follow-up data from children enrolled in the PCMR, the description of the clinical course of pediatric cardiomyopathy will be made more complete. These data will also allow for risk factors to be examined in more detail, and their long-term utility in diagnosis, prognosis and care to be determined. This type of registry data and their usefulness in guiding clinical decision making is increasingly appreciated by research methodologists and is being made more useful with advances in analytic and statistical theory.[65] The PCMR investigators have proposed using the PCMR to identify the genetic causes of pediatric cardiomyopathy and the usefulness of cardiac biomarkers in the evaluation of these children. The ultimate goal is to identify cause-specific treatment and clinical approaches for these children.

SUMMARY

Currently in its 15th year of funding by the NHLBI, the PCMR contains clinically important information on more than 3500 cases of pediatric cardiomyopathy. Important contributions to date include refined estimates of the incidence and outcomes of pediatric cardiomyopathy, the identification of risk factors and predictors of outcomes for children with several cause-specific forms of cardiomyopathy, the identification of the factors associated with making a causal diagnosis of pediatric cardiomyopathy, and a description of the clinical care being provided to children with dilated cardiomyopathy. The most recent funding period for the PCMR is nearing a successful completion and analyses are already beginning to produce results. As increased follow-up information is acquired and linked with information from blood and tissue specimens, PCMR data are likely to become only more valuable over time.

ACKNOWLEDGMENTS

The work of the PCMR would not be possible without the collaboration of many physicians and other health professionals, scientists, and research staff from the United States and Canada. Special acknowledgment should be given to our current and former PCMR Study group: Jane Messere, RN; Stephanie Ware, MD, PhD; John Lynn Jefferies, MD, MPH; Linda Addonizio, MD; Beth Kaufman, MD; Melanie Everitt, MD; Elfriede Pahl, MD; Paul Kantor, MBBCh; Paulo Rusconi, MD; Robert E. Shaddy, MD; and Paul R. Lurie, MD. We would also like to acknowledge Mrs Lisa Yue and the Children's Cardiomyopathy Foundation for their continuing support of the PCMR. We would like to express our most sincere gratitude to the children with cardiomyopathy and their families whose participation has made the PCMR possible.

REFERENCES

1. Towbin JA, Lowe AM, Colan SD, et al. Incidence, causes, and outcomes of dilated cardiomyopathy in children. JAMA 2006;296:1867–76.

2. Webber SA. New-onset heart failure in children in the absence of structural congenital heart disease. Circulation 2008;117:11–2.

3. Andrews RE, Fenton MJ, Ridout DA, et al. New-onset heart failure due to heart muscle disease in childhood: a prospective study in the United Kingdom and Ireland. Circulation 2008;117:79–84.

4. Massin MM, Astadicko I, Dessy H. Epidemiology of heart failure in a tertiary pediatric center. Clin Cardiol 2008;31:388–91.

5. Grenier MA, Osganian SK, Cox GF, et al. Design and implementation of the North American Pediatric Cardiomyopathy Registry. Am Heart J 2000;139: S86–95.

6. Bione S, D'Adamo P, Maestrini E, et al. A novel X-linked gene, G4.5, is responsible for Barth syndrome. Nat Genet 1996;12:385–9.

7. Schlame M, Towbin JA, Heerdt PM, et al. Deficiency of tetralinoleoyl-cardiolipin in Barth syndrome. Ann Neurol 2002;51:634–7.

8. Lipshultz SE, Sleeper LA, Towbin JA, et al. The incidence of pediatric cardiomyopathy in two regions of the United States. N Engl J Med 2003;348:1647–55.

9. Arola A, Jokinen E, Ruuskanen O, et al. Epidemiology of idiopathic cardiomyopathies in children and adolescents. A nationwide study in Finland. Am J Epidemiol 1997;146:385–93.

10. Nugent AW, Daubeney PEF, Chondros P, et al. The epidemiology of childhood cardiomyopathy in Australia. N Engl J Med 2003;348:1639–46.

11. Colan SD, Lipshultz SE, Lowe AM, et al. Epidemiology and cause specific outcome of hypertrophic cardiomyopathy in children: findings from the Pediatric Cardiomyopathy Registry. Circulation 2007; 115:773–81.

12. Cox GF, Sleeper LA, Lowe AM, et al. Factors associated with establishing a causal diagnosis for children with cardiomyopathy. Pediatrics 2006;118: 1519–31.

13. Harmon WG, Sleeper LA, Cuniberti L, et al. Treating children with idiopathic dilated cardiomyopathy (from the Pediatric Cardiomyopathy Registry). Am J Cardiol 2009;104:281–6.

14. Rosenthal D, Chrisant MR, Edens E, et al. International Society for Heart and Lung Transplantation: practice guidelines for the management of heart failure in children. J Heart Lung Transplant 2004; 23:1313–33.

15. Miller TL, Orav EJ, Wilkinson JD, et al. Nutritional status associated with cardiac outcomes and mortality in children with idiopathic dilated cardiomyopathy. Oral presentation at the 2009 American Heart Association Scientific Sessions [abstract]. Orlando (FL), November 18, 2009.

16. Connuck DM, Sleeper LA, Colan SD, et al. Characteristics and outcomes of cardiomyopathy in children with Duchenne or Becker muscular dystrophy: a comparative study from the Pediatric Cardiomyopathy Registry. Am Heart J 2008;155:998–1005.

17. Cox GF, Colan SD, Towbin JA, et al. Mitochondrial disorders: characteristics and outcomes from the pediatric cardiomyopathy registry [abstract]. In: Proceedings of the 5th World Congress of Paediatric Cardiology and Cardiac Surgery 2009;5:134.

18. Lipshultz SE, Orav EJ, Wilkinson JD, et al. A risk stratification analysis of predictors of death or transplant in children with hypertrophic cardiomyopathy. Circulation 2008;118(Suppl):4956.

19. Wilkinson JD, Lowe AM, Salbert BA, et al. Outcomes in children with Noonan syndrome and cardiomyopathy [abstract]. Circulation 2007;116(Suppl II):513.

20. Jefferies JL, Colan SD, Sleeper LA, et al. Outcome and risk stratification for children with left ventricular noncompaction: findings from the pediatric cardiomyopathy registry [abstract]. Oral presentation at the 2009 American Heart Association Scientific Sessions. Orlando (FL), November 16, 2009.

21. Webber S, Lipshultz SE, Sleeper LA, et al. Phenotypic heterogeneity and outcomes of restrictive cardiomyopathy in childhood: a report from the NHLBI pediatric cardiomyopathy registry [abstract]. Circulation 2008;118(Suppl):6071.

22. Singh TP, Gauvreau K, Thiagarajan R, et al. Racial and ethnic differences in mortality in children awaiting heart transplant in the United States. Am J Transplant 2009;9:1–8.

23. Pietra BA, Kantor PF, Bartlett HL, et al. Clinical factors associated with UNOS status and outcome after listing for heart transplant in children with dilated cardiomyopathy [abstract]. Circulation 2007;116(Suppl II):565.

24. Larsen R, Naftel DC, Rosenthal DN, et al. The impact of heart failure severity at time of listing for cardiac transplantation on short and long term stability with pediatric cardiomyopathy [abstract]. Circulation 2008;118(Suppl):4953.

25. Kelley RI, Cheatham JP, Clark BJ, et al. X-linked dilated cardiomyopathy with neutropenia, growth retardation, and 3-methylglutaconic aciduria. J Pediatr 1991;119:738–47.

26. Sleeper LA, Towbin JA, Colan SD, et al. Functional status is impaired and correlated with clinical status in pediatric cardiomyopathy [abstract]. In: Proceedings of the 5th World Congress of Paediatric Cardiology and Cardiac Surgery 2009;5:134.

27. Towbin JA, Sleeper L, Jefferies JL, et al. Genetic and viral genome analysis of childhood cardiomyopathy: the PCMR/PCSR experience [abstract]. J Am Coll Cardiol 2010;55. A43.E409.

28. Lipshultz SE, Colan SD, Towbin JA, et al. Introduction for "idiopathic and primary cardiomyopathy in children". Prog Pediatr Cardiol 2007;23(1–2):3.

29. Colan SD. Classification of the cardiomyopathies. Prog Pediatr Cardiol 2007;23(1–2):5–15.

30. Weintraub RG, Nugent AW, Daubeney PEF. Pediatric cardiomyopathy: the Australian experience. Prog Pediatr Cardiol 2007;23(1–2):17–24.

31. Alvarez JA, Wilkinson JD, Lipshultz SE. Outcome predictors for pediatric dilated cardiomyopathy: a systematic review. Prog Pediatr Cardiol 2007; 23(1–2):25–32.

32. Chung WK. Predictive genetic testing for cardiomyopathies. Prog Pediatr Cardiol 2007;23(1–2):33–8.

33. Kishnani PS, Burns Wechsler S, Li JS. Enzyme-deficiency metabolic cardiomyopathies and the role of enzyme replacement therapy. Prog Pediatr Cardiol 2007;23(1–2):39–48.

34. Rodrigues CO, Shehadeh LA, Webster KA, et al. Myocyte deficiency as a target in the treatment of cardiomyopathy. Prog Pediatr Cardiol 2007;23(1–2): 49–59.

35. Jefferies JL. Novel medical therapies for pediatric heart failure. Prog Pediatr Cardiol 2007;23(1–2):61–6.

36. Canter CE, Kantor PF. Heart transplant for pediatric cardiomyopathy. Prog Pediatr Cardiol 2007;23(1–2): 67–72.

37. Hsu DT. Age-related factors in child heart transplants. Prog Pediatr Cardiol 2007;23(1–2):73–9.

38. Lipshultz SE, Colan SD, Towbin JA, et al. Idiopathic and primary cardiomyopathies in children. Prog Pediatr Cardiol 2007;24(1):1.

39. Mestroni L, Miyamoto SD, Taylor MRG. Genetics of dilated cardiomyopathy conduction disease. Prog Pediatr Cardiol 2007;24(1):3–13.

40. Cox GF. Diagnostic approaches to pediatric cardiomyopathy of metabolic genetic etiologies and their relation to therapy. Prog Pediatr Cardiol 2007; 24(1):15–25.

41. Sheikh F, Chen J. Mouse models for cardiomyopathy research. Prog Pediatr Cardiol 2007;24(1):27–34.

42. Dellefave LM, McNally EM. Cardiomyopathy in neuromuscular disorders. Prog Pediatr Cardiol 2007;24(1):35–46.

43. Cooper LT Jr. Giant cell myocarditis in children. Prog Pediatr Cardiol 2007;24(1):47–9.

44. Kaufman BD, Shaddy RE. Beta-adrenergic receptor blockade and pediatric dilated cardiomyopathy. Prog Pediatr Cardiol 2007;24(1):51–7.

45. Miller TL, Neri D, Extein J, et al. Nutrition in pediatric cardiomyopathy. Prog Pediatr Cardiol 2007;24(1): 59–71.

46. Alcalai R, Arad M, Depreux F, et al. Hypertrophy, electrical abnormalities, autophagic vacuoles accumulation and cardiac fibrosis in LAMP2 cardiomyopathy mouse model. Prog Pediatr Cardiol 2007;24(1):73–4.

47. Joshi VA, Roberts AE, Kucherlapati RS. Noonan syndrome associated congenital hypertrophic cardiomyopathy and the role of sarcomere gene mutations. Prog Pediatr Cardiol 2007;24(1):75–6.

48. Rossano JW, Dreyer WJ, Kim JJ, et al. Pre-transplant serum creatinine predicts long-term outcome in pediatric heart transplant patients. Prog Pediatr Cardiol 2007;24(1):77–8.

49. Taylor MRG. When echocardiogram screening "is not enough". Prog Pediatr Cardiol 2007; 24(1):79–80.

50. Ratnasamy C, Kinnamon DD, Lipshultz SE, et al. Associations between neurohormonal and

inflammatory activation and heart failure in children. Prog Pediatr Cardiol 2007;24(1):81–2.

51. Lipshultz SE, Colan SD, Towbin JA, et al. Introduction for "idiopathic and primary cardiomyopathy in children". Prog Pediatr Cardiol 2008;25(1):1.

52. Towbin JA. Molecular mechanisms of pediatric cardiomyopathies and new targeted therapies. Prog Pediatr Cardiol 2008;25(3):3–21.

53. Lipshultz SE, Wilkinson JD. Epidemiological and outcomes research in children with pediatric cardiomyopathy. Prog Pediatr Cardiol 2008;25(3):23–5.

54. Colan SD. Clinical issues in the pediatric hypertrophic cardiomyopathies. Prog Pediatr Cardiol 2008;25(3):27–9.

55. Wilkinson JD, Sleeper LA, Alvarez JA, et al. The Pediatric Cardiomyopathy Registry: 1995–2007. Prog Pediatr Cardiol 2008;25(3):31–6.

56. Young K, Hare JM. Stem cells in cardiopulmonary development: implications for novel approaches to therapy for pediatric cardiopulmonary disease. Prog Pediatr Cardiol 2008;25(3):37–49.

57. Negro A, Dodge-Kafka K, Kapiloff MS. Signalosomes as therapeutic targets. Prog Pediatr Cardiol 2008;25(3):51–6.

58. Menon SC, Olson TM, Michels V. Genetics of familial dilated cardiomyopathy. Prog Pediatr Cardiol 2008; 25(3):57–67.

59. Hill KD, Rizwan H, Exil VJ. Pediatric cardiomyopathies related to fatty acid metabolism. Prog Pediatr Cardiol 2008;25(3):69–78.

60. Fisher SD, Pearson GD. Peripartum cardiomyopathy: an update. Prog Pediatr Cardiol 2008;25(3): 79–84.

61. Webber SA. Primary restrictive cardiomyopathy in childhood. Prog Pediatr Cardiol 2008;25(3):85–90.

62. Somarriba G, Extein J, Miller TL. Exercise rehabilitation in pediatric cardiomyopathy. Prog Pediatr Cardiol 2008;25(3):91–102.

63. Sokol KC, Armstrong FD, Rosenkranz ER, et al. Ethical issues in children with cardiomyopathy: making sense of ethical challenges in the clinical setting. Prog Pediatr Cardiol 2007;23(1–2):81–7.

64. Bublik N, Alvarez JA, Lipshultz SE. Pediatric cardiomyopathy as a chronic disease: a look at comprehensive care programs. Prog Pediatr Cardiol 2008; 25:103–11.

65. Dreyer NA, Garner S. Registries for robust evidence. JAMA 2009;302:790–1.

Dilated Cardiomyopathy and Heart Failure in Children

Daphne T. Hsu, MD[a,b,*], Charles E. Canter, MD[c,d]

KEYWORDS

• Pediatric • Heart failure • Cardiomyopathy • Transplantation

Pediatric cardiomyopathies represent the new frontier in pediatric cardiology. During the past decade there has been intense clinical research into their epidemiology, causes, and management. Traditionally, cardiomyopathies have been classified by their gross anatomic and physiologic phenotypes: dilated, hypertrophic, and restrictive.[1] Dilated cardiomyopathy (DCM) is a phenotype that is characterized by an enlarged left ventricular chamber and reduced systolic ejection without an increase in left ventricular wall thickness. This phenotype may be encountered in patients with repaired and unrepaired congenital heart disease and as a secondary phenomenon in multiorgan diseases. This review focuses on dilated cardiomyopathies associated with primary myocardial disease.

DEFINING PEDIATRIC DCM: A PHENOTYPE, NOT A SPECIFIC DISEASE

The original World Health Organization classification of cardiomyopathies published in 1980[1] described dilated, hypertrophic, and restrictive cardiomyopathies, recommending restriction of the term cardiomyopathy to denote heart disease of idiopathic origin. This classification was last revised in 1995 as "diseases of myocardium associated with cardiac dysfunction."[2] Advances in diagnosis, especially in molecular genetics, have exposed weaknesses in this classification of myocardial disease from its gross phenotype. The recognition of new cardiomyopathies, such as arrhythmogenic right ventricular dysplasia and left ventricular noncompaction, which has been labeled as a hypertrophic or a DCM, further weakens this scheme. Recently, the American Heart Association convened a Consensus Panel[3] that redefined primary cardiomyopathies not by phenotype, but by broad causes: genetic, acquired, and mixed. Within these classifications schemes, a cardiomyopathy may have varying phenotypic patterns that may be different in affected individuals and may change during the course of the disease. Thus this system also has its difficulties[4] and, in some instances, continues to classify cardiac phenotypes as distinct diseases.

Although defining cardiomyopathic disease as dilated, hypertrophic, or restrictive has become increasingly problematic, echocardiographic delineation of a dilated, hypertrophic, and even a restrictive phenotype is straightforward, especially in children whose echocardiographic

[a] Department of Pediatrics, Albert Einstein College of Medicine, 3415 Bainbrige Avenue, Bronx, NY 10467, USA
[b] Department of Pediatrics, Pediatric Heart Center, Children's Hospital at Montefiore, 3415 Bainbridge Avenue, Bronx, NY 10467, USA
[c] Department of Pediatrics, Washington University, One Chlidren's Place, NWT Campus, Box 8116, St Louis, MO 63110, USA
[d] Division of Pediatric Cardiology, One Children's Place, NWT Campus Box 8116, St Louis, MO 63110, USA
* Corresponding author. Pediatric Heart Center, Children's Hospital at Montefiore, 3415 Bainbridge Avenue, Bronx, NY 10467.
E-mail address: dhsu@montefiore.org

Heart Failure Clin 6 (2010) 415–432
doi:10.1016/j.hfc.2010.05.003
1551-7136/10/$ – see front matter © 2010 Elsevier Inc. All rights reserved.

windows are superior to those in adults. The ease of echocardiographic identification of these phenotypes has permitted large multicenter registries[5,6] to study the epidemiology and outcomes of pediatric cardiomyopathies. However, pediatric cardiomyopathies, especially those caused by metabolic and mitochondrial disease, often have the mixed phenotype of left ventricular hypertrophy with reduced systolic function, and these phenotypes have been excluded from analyses of the outcome of DCM.[7,8]

These analyses generally mirror how clinicians approach pediatric cardiomyopathies in children. An echocardiographically defined phenotype is identified that leads to phenotypically driven protocols for determining causes and management. The echocardiographic phenotype of the dilated left ventricle with normal wall thickness and reduced systolic function has multiple causes, outcomes after presentation that are identifiably different from other echocardiographic phenotypes, and specific treatment regimens.[5–8] Thus these analyses of pediatric DCM are analyses of the DCM phenotype observed in multiple cardiomyopathic diseases. They differ from older,[9–13] smaller single-center studies of pediatric DCM that focused on patients with a DCM phenotype with no apparent cause: idiopathic DCM.

EPIDEMIOLOGY

The National Australian Childhood Cardiomyopathy Study (NACCS)[6] and the North American Pediatric Cardiomyopathy Registry (PCMR)[5] show striking similarities in the incidence of cardiomyopathy (1.24/100,000 NACCS vs 1.13/100,000 PCMR), high (approximately 50%) prevalence of cases in the first year of life, and incidence of ethnic and gender differences. Cardiomyopathies associated with neuromuscular diseases and metabolic diseases were included in the PCMR but not the NACCS. In both studies, DCM accounted for slightly more than 50% of the total number of cardiomyopathies observed.[7,8] Within the PCMR, the annual incidence of DCM phenotype was 0.57/100,000. Both studies found infants (<1 year of age) to contain the largest proportion of cases (NACCS 65.8%, PCMR 41%) of any age group. A similar proportion of DCM cases had a family history of cardiomyopathy at time of diagnosis (NACCS 14.7%, PCMR 19%). Most cases in the PCMR were male (54%) and most cases in the NACCS were female (56%). The ethnic breakdown of cases in the PCMR was: whites (57%), blacks (20%), and Hispanic (17%). In both studies, most patients had congestive heart failure at presentation (NACCS 89.7%, PCMR 71%).

CAUSES

A DCM phenotype can accompany primary pediatric cardiomyopathies associated with infection (myocarditis), mutations in myocardial proteins, inborn errors of metabolism, and myocardial toxins. Although an increasing number of myocardial protein mutations[14] and metabolic disorders[15] are being associated with a DCM phenotype in children, most cases remain idiopathic. An etiologic diagnosis could not be made in two-thirds of the cases of DCM within the PCMR,[8] followed by myocarditis (16%), neuromuscular disorders (9%), familial DCM (5%), inborn errors of metabolism (4%), and malformation syndrome (1%). Discovering a specific cause for a DCM within the PCMR was associated with older age; lower heart rate; smaller ventricular dimensions, and greater left ventricular shortening fraction at presentation; use of viral serologic testing and endomyocardial biopsy; and a family history of cardiomyopathy.[16] The NACCS and PCMR excluded patients with dilated cardiomyopathies from toxins in their analyses. In children, the DCM associated with chemotherapy for neoplasm is an important cause of heart failure in children. Anthracycline toxicity was responsible for 5/114 cases of new-onset heart failure from pediatric heart muscle disease in the United Kingdom and Ireland in 2003.[17]

MYOCARDITIS

A DCM phenotype is clearly associated with myocarditis.[18–23] Myocarditis has many presentations in children, ranging from sudden death to mimicking myocardial infarction to cardiogenic shock to chronic heart failure. The classic viral prodrome of fever, muscle pain, and nonspecific respiratory and gastrointestinal symptoms appearing in the clinical histories of pediatric patients presenting with echocardiograms with a DCM phenotype often leads to an appropriate clinical diagnosis of myocarditis. The importance of arriving at a diagnosis of myocarditis for children and their families is the better prognosis for survival and eventual recovery with myocarditis compared with other diseases with similar echocardiographic findings. A recent[24] analysis from the PCMR suggests that a clinical diagnosis of myocarditis is associated with a substantially decreased risk for death or heart transplantation and increased chance for recovery than children diagnosed with idiopathic DCM. An echocardiographic picture of reduced systolic function with normal left ventricular wall thickness and chamber size in children[24] and adults[25] diagnosed with myocarditis has a better outcome than a presentation with left ventricular dilatation.

Although myocarditis and idiopathic DCM have differing outcomes, suggesting that they are separate disease entities, an increasing consensus has evolved suggesting that there is a continuum between viral infection of the myocardium and the ultimate development of a chronic DCM.[18,21,23] In this scenario, many cases of idiopathic DCM represent an end stage of previously undiagnosed myocarditis. Thus myocarditis and idiopathic DCM may represent different stages of a disease process that share a common echocardiographic phenotype.

The lack of sensitive and specific tests to make a laboratory diagnosis of myocarditis complicates the distinction between these entities. The use of endomyocardial biopsy to make a pathologic diagnosis of myocarditis is complicated by variability in interpretation, sensitivities dependent on sampling, and low prognostic value.[26] Identification of viral genome within myocardial samples has been reported in myocarditis[27,28] and idiopathic DCM.[29,30] Autoantibodies to myocardial proteins can be observed in patients diagnosed with both diseases. The accumulating experience with cardiac magnetic resonance (CMR) imaging with the use of gadolinium enhancement suggests that different patterns exist in patients with myocarditis[31] compared with idiopathic DCM.[32] CMR studies in pediatric cardiomyopathies are limited, and their true usefulness in the diagnosis of pediatric myocarditis remains to be determined.

FAMILIAL (GENETIC) CARDIOMYOPATHIES

A positive family history of cardiomyopathy suggests the presence of a genetic defect. Initial studies in the 1980s suggested that the number of cases of idiopathic DCM that seemed to have a familial origin was at most 10%.[33,34] When relatives were screened for possible cardiomyopathy with electrocardiograms and echocardiograms, the familial cardiomyopathy rates among patients with idiopathic DCM increased to 35%,[35] 48%,[36] and 65%.[37] No particular clinical or morphologic features within individual patients have distinguished familial from idiopathic disease, emphasizing the need for evaluation of families when a diagnosis of DCM is made.[38,39]

More than 20 genes have been identified as being associated with a DCM phenotype with dominant, X-linked, recessive, and mitochondrial inheritance patterns (**Tables 1** and **2**).[14] The clinical onset of most familial DCM is in adulthood, with only sporadic presentation in infants or children. Penetrance of disease in familial cardiomyopathy has been estimated to be 10% before 20 years of age; 34% between ages 20 and 30 years; 60% between 30 and 40 years; and 90% at 40 years of age.[39]

Table 1 also shows that mutations in the same gene can lead to a DCM or a hypertrophic cardiomyopathy. Mutations in proteins commonly associated with hypertrophic cardiomyopathy, such as β-myosin heavy chain, α-tropomyosin, α-cardiac actin, CTnT, cTnC, and titin also can display a primary DCM phenotype that is distinct from the end-stage dilated phase of hypertrophic cardiomyopathy. LAMP2 mutations (Danon disease) can present with a hypertrophic or DCM in males and a DCM in females of the same family.[40] Differences in the effects of different mutations in the same protein can result in different functionalities that may determine a specific phenotype. Recent functional studies in sarcomeric regulatory proteins show that mutations leading to hypertrophic cardiomyopathy generally increase calcium sensitivity of the cardiac myofilament, whereas mutations in the same protein leading to a DCM phenotype decrease calcium sensitivity.[41]

Dilated cardiomyopathies associated with dystrophin mutations are likely the most common genetic cardiomyopathy encountered by a pediatric cardiologist. A DCM phenotype generally evolves in dystrophin cardiomyopathies in middle to late adolescence. Duchenne muscular dystrophy is usually accompanied by a skeletal myopathy that is as, or more, severe than the cardiomyopathy. In Becker muscular dystrophy, the DCM in adolescents is markedly more severe than the skeletal myopathy, and most patients with Becker muscular dystrophy are ambulatory at the time of presentation with their cardiomyopathy. An adolescent male presenting with a DCM and an increased serum creatine phosphokinase may have previously undiagnosed Becker muscular dystrophy. Dystrophin mutations limited to myocardium may also present as an X-linked adolescent DCM with no evidence of skeletal myopathy.[42] Phenotypic variability apparently exists within specific dystrophin mutations in patients with muscular dystrophy because some mutations are more or less predisposed to be associated with a cardiomyopathy.[43]

Subtle electrocardiographic anomalies are apparent in patients with Duchenne muscular dystrophy years before the development of an overt DCM phenotype.[44] Subtle cardiac dysfunction can also be detected by echocardiographic tissue Doppler imaging[45] and CMR[46] in patients with Duchenne muscular dystrophy with normal left ventricular volumes and ejection fractions.

Table 1
Genetic cardiomyopathies with a dilated phenotype

Gene	Locus	OMIM[a]	Gene Product	Frequency (%)[b]	Allelic Disorders
Autosomal dominant DCM					
LMNA	1q21.2	150,330	Lamin A/C	4–8	Lipodystrophy, Charcot-Marie-Tooth 2B1, Emery-Dreifuss muscular dystrophy, Hutchinson-Gilford progeria syndrome, LGMD 1B
MYH7	14q12	160,760	β-Myosin heavy chain	4–6	Laing distal myopathy, HCM
TNNT2	1q32	191,045	Cardiac troponin T	3	HCM
SCN5A	3p21	600,163	Sodium channel	2–3	Long QT syndrome type 3, Brugada syndrome idiopathic ventricular fibrillation, sick sinus syndrome, cardiac conduction system disease
MYH6	14q12	160,710	α-myosin heavy chain	?2–3	HCM, dominantly inherited atrial septal defect
DES	2q35	125,660	Desmin	<1–1	Desminopathy, myofibrillar myopathy
VCL	10q22.1-23	193,065	Metavinculin	<1–1	HCM
LDB3	10q 22.2-23.3	605,906	LIM domain-binding 3	<1–1	HCM, myofibrillar myopathy
TCAP	17q12	604,488	Titin-cap or telethonin	<1–1	LGMD2G, HCM
PSEN1/PSEN2	14q24.3/1q31-q42	104,311/600,759	Presenilin 1/2	<1–1	Early-onset Alzheimer disease/early- and late-onset Alzheimer disease
ACTC	15q14	102,540	Cardiac actin	<1	HCM
TPM1	15q22.1	191,010	α-Trapomyosin 1	<1	HCM
SGCD	5q33-34	601,411	δ-Sarcoglycan	<1	δ Sarcoglycanopathy (LGMD2F)
CSRP3	11p15.1	600,824	Muscle LIM protein	<1	HCM
ACTN2	1q42-q43	102,573	α-Actinin-2	<1	HCM

ABCC9	12p12.1	601,439	SUR2A	<1	NA
TNNC1	3p21.3-p14.3	191,040	Cardiac troponin C	<1	NA
TTN	2q31	188,840	Titin	?	Udd distal myopathy, HCM, Edstrom myopathy early-onset myopathy with fatal cardiomyopathy
MYBPC3	11p11.2	600,958	Myosin-binding protein C	?	HCM
PLN	6q22.1	172,405	Phospholamban	?	HCM
EYA4	6q23	603,550	Eyes-absent 4	?	NA
TMPO	12q22	188,380	Thymopoietin	?	NA
X-linked FDC					
DMD	Xp21.2	300,377	Dystrophin	?	Dystrophinopathies (Duchenne muscular dystrophy, Becker muscular dystrophy)
TAZ/G4.5	Xq28	300,394	Tafazzin	?	Barth syndrome, endocardial fibroelastosis type 2, familial isolated noncompaction of the left ventricular myocardium
Autosomal recessive DCM					
TNM3	19q13.4	191,044	Cardiac troponin I	<1	HCM, restrictive cardiomyopathy

Abbreviations: HCM, hypertrophic cardiomyopathy; LGMD, limb girdle muscular dystrophy.
[a] OMIM: Online Mendelian Inheritance in Man, URL:http://www.ncbi.nlm.nih.gov/sites/entrez?db=omim, where additional information for each gene can be found.
[b] These estimates have been generated from primary and available secondary reports.
Data from Hershberger RE, Cowan J, Morales A, et al. Progress with genetic cardiomyopathies: screening, counseling, and testing in dilated, hypertrophic, and arrhythmogenic right ventricular dysplasia/cardiomyopathy. Circ Heart Fail 2009;2(3):253–61.

Table 2
Genetic cardiomyopathies in syndromic and multisystem disease with a dilated phenotype

Gene	Locus	OMIM[a]	Gene Product	Associated Syndromes	Inheritance Pattern	Additional Clinical Features
DCM						
HFE	6p21.3	235,200	Hereditary hemochromatosis	Hemochromatosis	AR	Cirrhosis, diabetes, hypermelanotic pigmentation, ↑ serum iron, ferritin
LMNA[b]	1q21.2	150,330	Lamin A/C	EMD2 and EMD3, LGMD 1B	EMD2, AD; EMD3, AR; LGMD1B, AD	EMD: joint contractures (elbow, Achilles tendon, neck), ↑ CK, arrhythmias, childhood muscle weakness, ↑ CK, arrhythmias shoulder/hip-girdle weakness
MYH7[b]	14q12	160,760	β-myosin heavy chain	Laing distal myopathy	AD	Childhood onset weakness of ankles and great toes, followed by the finger extensors, neck flexors, and facial weakness
DSP[b]	6p24	125,647	Desmoplakin	Carvajal syndrome	AR	Woolly hair, keratoderma
DMD[b]	Xp21.2	300,377	Dystrophin	DMD, BMD	XL	DMD: males: ↑ CK, childhood muscle weakness, wheelchair bound by age 12 years, DCM after age 18 years; BMD: ↑ CK, skeletal muscle weakness in 20s or later. Females can be affected with milder phenotype or DCM alone

TAZ/G4.5[b]	Xq28	300,394	Tafazzin	Barth syndrome	XL	Growth retardation, intermittent lactic acidemia, granulocytopenia, recurrent infections
MTTY	mtDNA	590,100	TRNA^{Tyr}	Focal segmental glomerulosclerosis and DCM	Maternal	Focal segmental glomerulosclerosis, migraines
Variable (eg, MTND5, MTND4, MTND3, MTCD3, MTATP6, MTATP8)	mtDNA multigene deletion	530,000	NADH dehydrogenase subunit 3,4, and 5; cytochrome c oxidase subunit 3	Keams-Sayre syndrome	De novo	Progressive external ophthalmoplegia, muscle weakness, cerebellar ataxia, diabetes mellitus

Abbreviations: AD, autosomal dominant; AR, autosomal recessive; BMD, Becker muscular dystrophy; CK, creatine kinase; DMD, Duchenne muscular dystrophy; EMD, Emery-Dreifuss muscular dystrophy; mtDNA, mitochondrial DNA; XL, X-linked.

[a] OMIM is Online Mendelian Inheritance in Man, URL:http://www.ncbi.nlm.nih.gov/sites/entrez?db=omim, where additional information for each gene can be found.

[b] These estimates have been generated from primary and available secondary reports.

Data from Hershberger RE, Cowan J, Morales A, et al. Progress with genetic cardiomyopathies: screening, counseling, and testing in dilated, hypertrophic, and arrhythmogenic right ventricular dysplasia/cardiomyopathy. Circ Heart Fail 2009;2(3):253–61.

These studies in children with preclinical genetic cardiomyopathies may become of clinical importance in determining when to institute therapies to ameliorate or retard progression of cardiac dysfunction, similar to the experience with angiotensin-converting enzyme (ACE) inhibitors in the DCM in Duchenne muscular dystrophy.[47]

CARDIOMYOPATHIES ASSOCIATED WITH INBORN ERRORS OF METABOLISM

Inborn errors of metabolism involving amino and organic acids, fatty acids, glycogen, glycoproteins, lysosomal storage disorders, oxidative phosphorylation, and mitochondria[15,48–50] can have associated cardiomyopathies. Mitochondrial DNA and transfer RNA mutations are generally included in this group (see **Table 2**).[14] These disorders tend to involve multiple organ systems. Subclinical cardiomyopathy may exist in these patients without overt cardiac symptomatology.[50] These disorders are believed to cause cardiomyopathy from a mechanical effect of bulk infiltration of a substrate within the cardiomyocyte, impairment of cardiac energy production, or by the production of metabolites toxic to the myocardium.

Most patients with inborn errors of metabolism will exhibit a hypertrophic cardiomyopathy phenotype or a mixed phenotype of a hypertrophic cardiomyopathy with reduced systolic function. Different cardiomyopathy phenotypes may occur within a given inborn error of metabolism similar to other genetic cardiomyopathies. Phenotypes may change in individual patients with some mitochondrial disorders. **Fig. 1** shows the distribution of inborn errors of metabolism detected in the early retrospective arm of the PCMR from 1990 to 1995.[15] An inborn error of metabolism was

considered to account for only 5% of the cardiomyopathies in this patient cohort. A DCM phenotype was present in only 21% of the cardiomyopathies associated with inborn errors of metabolism and were confined to mucopolysaccharidoses, disorders of oxidative phosphorylation, disorders of fatty acid oxidation/carnitine metabolism, and amino/organic acidurias. Thus, although a DCM phenotype is generally not encountered in these diseases, routine evaluation for its presence in a patient with a DCM is important to determine (1) the feasibility of heart transplantation, and (2) the potential to ameliorate or reverse the cardiomyopathy associated with these rare diseases with diet or use of supplements such as carnitine.[51]

ETIOLOGIC EVALUATION OF NEWLY IDENTIFIED DCM

The first step in the evaluation of a newly encountered DCM phenotype is to exclude secondary cardiomyopathies. Several toxic, nutritional, endocrinologic, or electrolyte abnormalities can be associated with a DCM phenotype.[52] In dark-skinned infants and young children, rickets should be considered because it continues to be recognized as a cause of heart failure with a DCM picture.[53] Careful echocardiography to exclude anomalous coronary artery arising from the pulmonary artery should be performed because the associated cardiomyopathy is reversible with surgery.[54] Electrocardiograms should be scrutinized not only for findings (various degrees of atrioventricular block, Wolff-Parkinson-White pattern) that would provide clues for a specific cardiomyopathy but also to exclude incessant tachyarrhythmias that would result in

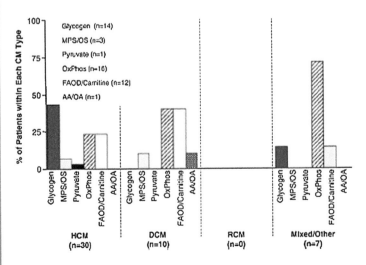

Fig. 1. Distribution of different inborn errors of metabolism associated with different cardiomyopathy phenotypes in the PCMR, 1990 to 1995, N = 916. AA/OA aminoacidopathies/organic acidemias; FAOD/Carnitine, fatty oxidation/carnitine transport defects; Glycogen, glycogen storage diseases; HCM, hypertrophic cardiomyopathy; MPS/OS, muopolysccharidoses/oligosaccharidoses; OxPhos, oxidative phosphorylation defects; RCM, restrictive cardiomyopathy. (*From* Cox GF. Diagnostic approaches to pediatric cardiomyoapthy of metabolic genetic etiologies and their relation to therapy. Prog Pediatr Cardiol 2007; 24:17; with permission.)

a tachycardia-induced cardiomyopathy that is treatable with electrophysiologic ablation.[55]

Many inborn errors of metabolism, especially disorders of fatty acid oxidation, have distinct biochemical profiles that are present acutely, but may disappear with supportive care. Aside from a comprehensive blood chemistry panel and complete blood count, other blood tests would include creatine phosphokinase, aldolase, lipid panel, uric acid, lactate, pyruvate, amino acids, acylcarnitine profile with quantitative carnitine, and urine for organic and amino acids. Depending on the results of these screening tests, detailed protocols have been developed[15,56] to aid in the diagnosis of specific diseases. If myocarditis is clinically suspected, evaluation of nasal swab and stool viruses and blood polymerase chain reaction tests for enterovirus, adenovirus, parvovirus B19, human herpes virus 6, Epstein-Barr virus, and other potential viral pathogens should be considered with or without metabolic disease screening studies.

Expert opinion continues to favor endomyocardial biopsy as a reasonable class IIa indication in unexplained cardiomyopathies in children.[57] Certain genetic and metabolic cardiomyopathies have histopathologic patterns that can lead to a specific diagnosis, as do the rarely encountered giant cell and eosinophilic myocarditis. The limitations of endomyocardial biopsy in the diagnosis of myocarditis are well known, and a negative biopsy does not exclude the disease.[57,58] Furthermore, different viral infections seem to lead to different histologic patterns than the classic lymphocytic infiltration with myocyte necrosis.[27,59] CMR, as previously discussed, has been associated with patterns that distinguish myocarditis from other dilated cardiomyopathies.[31,32] In adult patients, a comprehensive CMR evaluation involving 3 distinct tests of tissue characterization has an estimated diagnostic accuracy for myocarditis of 78% when 2 or more tests are positive.[32]

The first step in the evaluation of potential familial/genetic cardiomyopathies is a careful family history for cardiac disease, extending back at least 3 generations.[33,34] Consultation with a geneticist or a neurologist specializing in muscular dystrophies may be helpful. Many cardiomyopathies can be associated with skeletal muscle findings. A skeletal muscle biopsy may be helpful in infants for whom endomyocardial biopsy may be of higher risk and in pediatric patients with associated abnormalities of skeletal muscle strength or tone. Genetic testing for specific mutations in myocardial protein and mitochondria are clinically available from several laboratories. GeneTests (www.genetests.org) is an NIH-supported web site that lists clinical and research molecular genetic testing laboratories. Such testing is expensive and may not be covered by commercial insurance. Currently the sensitivity of genetic testing in the evaluation of a DCM phenotype is lower than described in hypertrophic cardiomyopathies and its role in the routine evaluation of a DCM phenotype is uncertain.[34]

OUTCOMES OF DCM

DCM has one of the highest mortalities among the congenital and acquired heart diseases that occur in children. Most deaths in children with DCM are caused by progressive heart failure or complications from mechanical support or transplantation.[7,12,60] In contrast with the adult population, the incidence of sudden death is low in children with cardiomyopathy. In a report from the Pediatric Heart Transplant Study group, only 5 of 655 patients (0.7%) with end-stage cardiomyopathy died suddenly while awaiting transplantation.[61]

In the 1980s and early 1990s mortality ranged between 20% and 80% 5 years after diagnosis.[9,11–13,39,62] In the past 2 decades, survival in children with DCM has improved, with some series reporting a 90% 1-year, and 83% 5-year, survival following presentation.[63] This improvement is largely attributed to improved survival following heart transplantation and the availability of ventricular assist devices suitable to successfully bridge the child with intractable heart failure to transplantation.[60,64–66] Although survival has improved, the incidence of heart death has remained surprisingly constant. A recent report from the United Kingdom and Ireland describes a 34% incidence of death or transplant within a year in patients with DCM presenting with congestive heart failure.[17]

Although many children who present with acute decompensated heart failure and DCM have poor outcomes, there is a significant population of children (15%–30%) in whom ventricular function may return to normal, with recovery more likely in children presenting with severe heart failure.[63] This dichotomy of outcomes was found in the multicenter trial of carvedilol in symptomatic children with ventricular dysfunction. In this group of children with chronic heart failure, most of whom were Ross heart failure class II at enrollment, the clinical status of children with DCM improved during the 8-month study period in 62% and worsened in 22%.[67] Although most patients showed a clinical improvement over time, there was a 17% incidence of death or transplant, even in this mildly symptomatic group of children with ventricular dysfunction.

PREDICTORS OF OUTCOME

The presence of such diverse outcomes in children with DCM has led investigators to search for predictors to identify patients likely to improve or at increased risk for death or transplant. Despite these efforts, a risk stratification profile for children has not been developed. In a systematic review of outcome predictors in pediatric DCM, Alvarez and colleagues[68] identified 3 factors that indicated better prognosis across multiple articles: younger age, higher ejection fraction or shortening fraction at presentation, and the presence of myocarditis. Younger age and higher ejection fraction may be surrogates for the presence of myocarditis. In early studies, children less than 2 years of age had a better prognosis,[11,62,69] whereas, in the NACCS and PCMR, age greater than 5 to 6 years was associated with a higher incidence of death or transplantation.[7,8]

Quantitative echocardiography has been extensively studied as a predictor of outcome in children with DCM. In most series, a higher baseline fractional shortening or ejection fraction at presentation is associated with better outcome,[9,63,70] although other small series have been unable to find a relationship between the degree of systolic impairment and worse outcome.[71–74] A lower left ventricular fractional z-score was an independent predictor of death or transplant in the NACCS and PCMR analyses.[7,8] In several studies, serial improvement in systolic ventricular function within 6 months of presentation was associated with a better outcome and lack of improvement was a predictor of death or transplant.[7,75] In general, studies have not shown an association between left ventricular dilatation and survival, although a recent report indicates that, among infants and young children (age <5 years) listed for transplantation, a higher left ventricular end-diastolic dimension z-score is associated with higher mortality.[76] Other echocardiographic measures that have been associated with worse outcome in small studies include moderate-severe mitral regurgitation, larger left atrial dimension, and higher tricuspid Ea velocity.[70,75]

Small series have reported that lower exercise performance and a higher pulmonary capillary wedge pressure have been associated with worse outcome in children with DCM. Cardiopulmonary exercise testing has not been widely applied in the risk stratification of children with DCM; however, a recent report indicates that decreasing exercise time is predictive of death or transplantation.[77] Although invasive hemodynamic assessment is not commonly performed in children with DCM, 2 small series found that a markedly increased pulmonary capillary wedge pressure (>20–25 mm Hg) was associated with a higher mortality.[11,72] Cardiac index measured at cardiac catheterization, chest radiography, and electrocardiography findings have not been found to be predictive of outcome. Congestive heart failure has not been shown to be an independent predictor of worse outcome, perhaps because of the high prevalence of heart failure at presentation.[17] In the PCMR, congestive heart failure was predictive of death or transplant only in infants less than 1 year of age at presentation.[8]

In the adult patient, brain natriuretic peptide (BNP) and N-terminal prohormone BNP (NT pro-BNP) levels are used to detect and risk stratify patients with acute decompensated heart failure, and guidelines have been developed regarding their use in the clinical setting.[78] The adult guidelines for the use of BNP and NT pro-BNP testing are not generalizable to children, because it is apparent that age, gender, and assay method may affect the reference values for these markers.[79] BNP and NT pro-BNP levels are higher in normal neonates, and some studies have found gender differences.[80–85] A few studies have shown that BNP levels can distinguish between cardiac and pulmonary causes of respiratory distress in neonates and children.[86–88] In acute decompensated heart failure caused by cardiomyopathy, small series have shown that BNP levels are increased and related to the degree of symptomatology.[89–94] Price and colleagues[91] found that a BNP level greater than 300 pg/mL was a strong predictor of death, transplantation, or heart failure hospitalization and was more strongly correlated with poor outcome than symptoms or echocardiographic finding.

TREATMENT

In adult patients with heart failure, guidelines have been developed for the evaluation and treatment of patients in 4 stages of heart failure (A–D) that reflect the development and progression of this disease.[95] Stage A includes asymptomatic patients at high risk for heart failure with no evidence of ventricular dysfunction, stage B includes asymptomatic patients with evidence of ventricular dysfunction, stage C includes symptomatic patients with ventricular dysfunction, and stage D includes patients with refractory heart failure and symptoms at rest. In 2004 the International Society for Heart and Lung Transplantation published practice guidelines for the management of heart failure in children. An adaptation of the heart failure stages was proposed for the pediatric patient and can serve as a framework when considering treatment options for children with heart failure (**Table 3**).[96] The practice guidelines were based on expert consensus opinion because of a lack of multicenter outcome studies in the pediatric heart failure population.

General Health

The general health recommendations for adult patients with heart failure are applicable to the pediatric population. These include discouraging smoking, alcohol intake, and illicit drug use; treatment of hypertension; control of the metabolic syndrome; and encouraging exercise. Although potential effects of the increasing incidence of obesity, hypertension, and the metabolic syndrome in children on the incidence of pediatric heart failure are not known, controlling these factors is an important goal of general health maintenance.[97] A 2004 consensus document outlined recommendations for physical activity and recreational sports participation in young patients with genetic cardiovascular diseases, including DCM; however, the main focus of these recommendations was the prevention of sudden death, a rare occurrence in children with DCM.[98] Specific exercise recommendations have not been proposed for children with DCM, but a recent pilot study confirmed the safety of exercise training in children with end-stage heart failure waiting for transplantation; no beneficial effects were shown.[99]

Medical Therapy: Heart Failure Stage A

In children at risk for heart failure, the populations of childhood cancer survivors who received anthracycline therapy and patients with Duchenne muscular dystrophy meet the criteria for heart failure stage A. A multicenter study of ACE inhibitor therapy in childhood cancer survivors found a beneficial effect of enalapril on left ventricular end-systolic wall stress but no effect on exercise performance or left ventricular fractional shortening. Enalapril therapy was complicated by a 32% incidence of dizziness, hypotension, and fatigue, and the study concluded that the prophylactic use of enalapril could not be generally recommended in this population.[100] Data from a small, randomized trial of perindopril in patients with Duchenne muscular dystrophy showed a persistent beneficial effect on ventricular function 5 years after therapy. Other small series have suggested a beneficial effect of combination therapy with β-blockade and ACE inhibition.[43,47,101] Based on these small studies, some pediatric heart failure physicians recommend the use of ACE inhibitor therapy in the patient with Duchenne muscular dystrophy and normal ventricular function.

Medical Therapy: Heart Failure Stages B, C, and D

Adult heart failure guidelines recommend instituting β-blockade in patients with stage B, C, and D heart failure, based on extensive evidence showing a beneficial effect of β-blockade on mortality, morbidity, and ventricular remodeling.[95] The trial of carvedilol in children with ventricular dysfunction is the only multicenter, randomized study of medical therapy that has been performed in children with heart failure.[67,102] The study population included symptomatic patients with

Table 3	
Proposed heart failure staging for infants and children	
Stage	**Interpretation**
A	Patients with increased risk of developing HF, but who have normal cardiac function and no evidence of cardiac chamber volume overload. Examples: previous exposure to cardiotoxic agents, family history of heritable cardiomyopathy, univentricular heart, congenitally corrected transposition of the great arteries
B	Patients with abnormal cardiac morphology or cardiac function, with no symptoms of HF, past or present. Examples: aortic insufficiency with LV enlargement, history of anthracycline with decreased LV systolic function
C	Patients with underlying structural or functional heart disease, and past or current symptoms of HF
D	Patients with end-stage HF requiring continuous infusion of inotropic agents, mechanical circulatory support, cardiac transplantation, or hospice care

Abbreviations: HF, heart failure; LV, left ventricular.

Reprinted from Rosenthal D, Chrisant MR, Edens E, et al. International Society for Heart and Lung Transplantation: practice guidelines for management of heart failure in children. J Heart Lung Transplant 2004;23(12):1313–33; with permission from Elsevier.

ventricular dysfunction caused by cardiomyopathy or congenital heart disease. The proportion of patients who reached the primary end point (worsened clinical status, heart failure hospitalization, death, or transplant) was not different between the placebo and the carvedilol-treated groups. A prespecified analysis showed an interaction effect between the patients with left ventricular dysfunction (primarily caused by DCM) and patients with congenital heart disease and treatment effect. There was a trend toward better ejection fraction and clinical status in the carvedilol group in the children with cardiomyopathy. Thus, although the overall results of this trial failed to show a beneficial effect of carvedilol, most pediatric heart failure physicians recommend therapy in patients with DCM and stage C and D heart failure.

There have been no randomized trials studying the efficacy of ACE inhibitor therapy in children with DCM. There is compelling evidence in the adult literature that ACE inhibitor therapy is beneficial in patients with stages B, C, and D heart failure.[95] Thus, the pediatric guidelines have been extrapolated from the adult data to recommend the use of ACE inhibitor therapy in children with moderate to severe ventricular dysfunction with or without symptoms.[96] No recommendations are given for asymptomatic children with mild ventricular dysfunction, and the use of ACE inhibitor therapy in this population is variable.

Digoxin has been used in the treatment of volume overload and myocardial dysfunction heart failure in children with an excellent safety profile. Data from the adult population failed to show a survival benefit with the use of digoxin,[95] but did report decreased morbidity; thus, many pediatric heart failure physicians continue to advocate the use of digoxin in the setting of DCM.

Medical Therapy: Acute Decompensated Heart Failure

Acute decompensated heart failure is characterized by symptoms of fluid overload, such as pulmonary edema or systemic venous congestion, and, in some cases, low cardiac output with poor peripheral perfusion. In the setting of fluid retention, diuretic therapy is the mainstay of treatment. In patients who are refractory to diuretics, small pediatric series have described a beneficial response to nesiritide infusion.[103–105] The adult heart failure guidelines also recommend the use of vasodilator therapy with nitroprusside or nitroglycerin to promote diuresis in the absence of systemic hypotension.[95] In the adult patient, inotropic agents are not recommended for patients with acute decompensated heart failure

and no evidence of hypotension or low cardiac output. This recommendation has not been widely adopted by the pediatric heart failure community, despite the lack of evidence of efficacy of these agents in children with ventricular dysfunction and no evidence of low cardiac output. Home inotropic therapy in pediatric heart transplant candidates with chronic low cardiac output unresponsive to oral agents has been reported.[106] In a small, nonrandomized series of children with heart failure, the calcium sensitizing agent levosimendan resulted in a decrease in the inotropic dose and improvement in ejection fraction.[107]

IMPLANTABLE CARDIOVERTER DEFIBRILLATOR AND PACEMAKER THERAPY

The AHA/ACC/HRS 2008 guidelines for device-based therapy for cardiac rhythm abnormalities include the recommendations for implantable cardioverter defibrillator (ICD) use in children with heart failure based on expert consensus opinion. In a large multicenter series of children with heart failure awaiting heart transplantation, the incidence of sudden death was 1.3%.[62] This low incidence of sudden death in children compared with adults with heart failure has led to the recommendation that routine implantation of ICD in children with left ventricular dysfunction is not indicated.[108] ICD therapy may be indicated as a bridge to transplantation in the pediatric patient with ventricular arrhythmias.[109]

In most children with DCM, the QRS duration does not meet the adult criteria for resynchronization therapy. There is considerable interest in the use of newer echocardiographic techniques to find evidence of mechanical dyssynchrony as an indication for biventricular pacing.[110,111] Several small case series have reported improvement in functional status with biventricular or multisite pacing in children with heart failure, but no long-term trials have been performed to establish efficacy.[112,113] The use of biventricular pacing has not been widely implemented in the pediatric patient with DCM.

MITRAL VALVE SURGERY

Mitral regurgitation is commonly associated with left ventricular dysfunction and, in the adult population, there is growing interest in the role of mitral valve repair in the management of chronic heart failure. Two small series have reported a combined total of 12 children with DCM who underwent mitral valve surgery. There were no deaths, and most patients had improvement in left ventricular geometry and function. Four children required

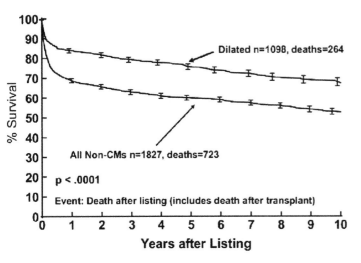

Fig. 2. Kaplan-Meier survival curve for patients with DCM (*CM*) listed for transplantation from the Pediatric Heart Transplant Study Registry data. (*Reprinted from* Kirk R, Naftel D, Hoffman TM, et al. Outcome of pediatric patients with dilated cardiomyopathy listed for transplant: a multi-institutional study. J Heart Lung Transplant 2009;28(12):1322–8; with permission from Elsevier.)

transplantation between 3 weeks and 3.5 years after repair.[114,115] These data are insufficient to determine the role of mitral valve surgery in the management of the child with symptomatic heart failure.

VENTRICULAR ASSIST DEVICES

The use of mechanical assist devices for the treatment of end-stage heart failure in children awaiting transplant has been increasing as improved device design has allowed lower pump volumes. In the older child and adolescent, use of a mechanical assist device results in successful bridging to transplantation in 80% of cases.[66] The options for mechanical support in the infant and young child are more limited. Historically, infants with intractable heart failure have been supported using an extracorporeal membrane oxygenator, with a reported 45% survival to heart transplantation or recovery. Improved outcomes have been reported using a paracorporeal pulsatile ventricular assist device in small children with survival ranging between 60% and 85%.[116,117] Ventricular assist device support has the potential to improve the condition of the child with end-stage heart failure while waiting for a donor organ, but this benefit must be weighed against the significant risk of thromboembolic and bleeding complications.

HEART TRANSPLANTATION

Heart transplantation remains the therapy of choice for end-state heart failure in children refractory to surgical and medical therapy. Current 1-year survival following heart transplantation in children is 85% and overall survival 20 years after transplantation is 40%. Transplantation in children with DCM has the best survival of all the diagnostic groups. An analysis of 1098 children with DCM listed for heart transplantation was recently performed by the Pediatric Heart Transplant Study group.[67] Mortality on the waiting list was 11% and overall survival after listing for transplantation was 72% at 10 years (**Fig. 2**). This survival compares favorably with the high mortality reported in studies of the natural history of DCM in children.[9,11–13,39,63]

SUMMARY

DCM is a disease of the heart muscle characterized by ventricular dilatation and decreased systolic function. The cause of DCM is multifactorial. Although most cases are idiopathic, there is increasing evidence for gene-specific forms of the disease, and other causes include infection (myocarditis), mutations in myocardial proteins, inborn errors of metabolism, and myocardial toxins. The outcome of children with DCM is poor, with a 30% to 50% 5-year survival. Treatments for DCM can be disease-specific or targeted toward reverse remodeling and symptoms. Current pediatric guidelines recommend the use of ACE inhibitor therapy and β-blockade in symptomatic children with ventricular dysfunction. Diuretics are used in the presence of acute or chronic volume overload and inotropic agents are reserved for patients with signs of low cardiac output or hypotension. The efficacy of ICD or biventricular pacing therapy remains unknown. Ventricular assist device support has improved for small children, and heart transplantation has excellent results in children with intractable heart failure.

REFERENCES

1. Report of the WHO/ISFC task force on the definition and classification of cardiomyopathies. Br Heart J 1980;44(6):672–3.
2. Richardson P, McKenna W, Bristow M, et al. Report of the 1995 World Health Organization/International Society and Federation of Cardiology Task Force on the definition and classification of cardiomyopathies. Circulation 1996;93(5):841–2.
3. Maron BJ, Towbin JA, Thiene G, et al. Contemporary definitions and classification of the cardiomyopathies: an American Heart Association Scientific Statement from the Council on Clinical Cardiology, Heart Failure and Transplantation Committee; Quality of Care and Outcomes Research and Functional Genomics and Translational Biology Interdisciplinary Working Groups; and Council on Epidemiology and Prevention. Circulation 2006;113(14):1807–16.
4. Colan SD. Classification of the cardiomyopathies. Prog Pediatr Cardiol 2007;23(1):5–15.
5. Lipshultz SE, Sleeper LA, Towbin JA, et al. The incidence of pediatric cardiomyopathy in two regions of the United States. N Engl J Med 2003;348(17):1647–55.
6. Nugent AW, Daubeney PE, Chondros P, et al. The epidemiology of childhood cardiomyopathy in Australia. N Engl J Med 2003;348(17):1639–46.
7. Daubeney PE, Nugent AW, Chondros P, et al. Clinical features and outcomes of childhood dilated cardiomyopathy: results from a national population-based study. Circulation 2006;114(24):2671–8.
8. Towbin JA, Lowe AM, Colan SD, et al. Incidence, causes, and outcomes of dilated cardiomyopathy in children. JAMA 2006;296(15):1867–76.
9. Akagi T, Benson LN, Lightfoot NE, et al. Natural history of dilated cardiomyopathy in children. Am Heart J 1991;121(5):1502–6.
10. Arola A, Tuominen J, Ruuskanen O, et al. Idiopathic dilated cardiomyopathy in children: prognostic indicators and outcome. Pediatrics 1998;101(3 Pt 1):369–76.
11. Burch M, Siddiqi SA, Celermajer DS, et al. Dilated cardiomyopathy in children: determinants of outcome. Br Heart J 1994;72(3):246–50.
12. Friedman RA, Moak JP, Garson A Jr. Clinical course of idiopathic dilated cardiomyopathy in children. J Am Coll Cardiol 1994;18(1):152–6.
13. Taliercio CP, Seward JB, Driscoll DJ, et al. Idiopathic dilated cardiomyopathy in the young: clinical profile and natural history. J Am Coll Cardiol 1985;6(5):1126–31.
14. Hershberger RE, Cowan J, Morales A, et al. Progress with genetic cardiomyopathies: screening, counseling, and testing in dilated, hypertrophic, and arrhythmogenic right ventricular dysplasia/cardiomyopathy. Circ Heart Fail 2009;2(3):253–61.
15. Cox GF. Diagnostic approaches to pediatric cardiomyopathy of metabolic genetic etiologies and their relation to therapy. Prog Pediatr Cardiol 2007;24(1):15–25.
16. Cox GF, Sleeper LA, Lowe AM, et al. Factors associated with establishing a causal diagnosis for children with cardiomyopathy. Pediatrics 2006;118(4):1519–31.
17. Andrews RE, Fenton MJ, Ridout DA, et al. New-onset heart failure due to heart muscle disease in childhood: a prospective study in the United Kingdom and Ireland. Circulation 2008;117(1):79–84.
18. Cooper LT Jr. Myocarditis. N Engl J Med 2009;360(15):1526–38.
19. Feldman AM, McNamara D. Myocarditis. N Engl J Med 2000;343(19):1388–98.
20. Hufnagel G, Pankuweit S, Richter A, et al. The European Study of Epidemiology and Treatment of Cardiac Inflammatory Diseases (ESETCID). First epidemiological results. Herz 2000;25(3):279–85.
21. Liu PP, Mason JW. Advances in the understanding of myocarditis. Circulation 2001;104(9):1076–82.
22. Magnani JW, Dec GW. Myocarditis: current trends in diagnosis and treatment. Circulation 2006;113(6):876–90.
23. Yajima T, Knowlton KU. Viral myocarditis: from the perspective of the virus. Circulation 2009;119(19):2615–24.
24. Foerster SR, Canter C, Carey A, et al. A comparative analysis of outcome for pediatric patients with biopsy-proven myocarditis, clinical-diagnosed myocarditis and idiopathic dilated cardiomyopathy. Circulation 2007;107(Suppl II):II-565.
25. Felker GM, Boehmer JP, Hruban RH, et al. Echocardiographic findings in fulminant and acute myocarditis. J Am Coll Cardiol 2000;36(1):227–32.
26. Baughman KL. Diagnosis of myocarditis: death of Dallas criteria. Circulation 2006;113(4):593–5.
27. Bowles NE, Ni J, Kearney DL, et al. Detection of viruses in myocardial tissues by polymerase chain reaction. Evidence of adenovirus as a common cause of myocarditis in children and adults. J Am Coll Cardiol 2003;42(3):466–72.
28. Why HJ, Meany BT, Richardson PJ, et al. Clinical and prognostic significance of detection of enteroviral RNA in the myocardium of patients with myocarditis or dilated cardiomyopathy. Circulation 1994;89(6):2582–9.
29. Kuhl U, Pauschinger M, Noutsias M, et al. High prevalence of viral genomes and multiple viral infections in the myocardium of adults with "idiopathic" left ventricular dysfunction. Circulation 2005;111(7):887–93.

30. Pauschinger M, Bowles NE, Fuentes-Garcia FJ, et al. Detection of adenoviral genome in the myocardium of adult patients with idiopathic left ventricular dysfunction. Circulation 1999;99(10): 1348–54.

31. Assomull RG, Prasad SK, Lyne J, et al. Cardiovascular magnetic resonance, fibrosis, and prognosis in dilated cardiomyopathy. J Am Coll Cardiol 2006; 48(10):1977–85.

32. Friedrich MG, Sechtem U, Schulz-Menger J, et al. Cardiovascular magnetic resonance in myocarditis: a JACC white paper. J Am Coll Cardiol 2009;53(17):1475–87.

33. Burkett EL, Hershberger RE. Clinical and genetic issues in familial dilated cardiomyopathy. J Am Coll Cardiol 2005;45(7):969–81.

34. Hershberger RE, Lindenfeld J, Mestroni L, et al. Genetic evaluation of cardiomyopathy–a Heart Failure Society of America practice guideline. J Card Fail 2009;15(2):83–97.

35. Grunig E, Tasman JA, Kucherer H, et al. Frequency and phenotypes of familial dilated cardiomyopathy. J Am Coll Cardiol 1998;31(1):186–94.

36. Baig MK, Goldman JH, Caforio AL, et al. Familial dilated cardiomyopathy: cardiac abnormalities are common in asymptomatic relatives and may represent early disease. J Am Coll Cardiol 1998; 31(1):195–201.

37. Mestroni L, Rocco C, Gregori D, et al. Familial dilated cardiomyopathy: evidence for genetic and phenotypic heterogeneity. Heart Muscle Disease Study Group. J Am Coll Cardiol 1999;34(1):181–90.

38. Kushner JD, Nauman D, Burgess D, et al. Clinical characteristics of 304 kindreds evaluated for familial dilated cardiomyopathy. J Card Fail 2006; 12(6):422–9.

39. Michels VV, Moll PP, Miller FA, et al. The frequency of familial dilated cardiomyopathy in a series of patients with idiopathic dilated cardiomyopathy. N Engl J Med 1992;326(2):77–82.

40. Taylor MR, Ku L, Slavov D, et al. Danon disease presenting with dilated cardiomyopathy and a complex phenotype. J Hum Genet 2007;52(10): 830–5.

41. Morimoto S. Expanded spectrum of gene causing both hypertrophic cardiomyopathy and dilated cardiomyopathy. Circ Res 2009;105(4):313–5.

42. Arbustini E, Diegoli M, Morbini P, et al. Prevalence and characteristics of dystrophin defects in adult male patients with dilated cardiomyopathy. J Am Coll Cardiol 2000;35(7):1760–8.

43. Jefferies JL, Eidem BW, Belmont JW, et al. Genetic predictors and remodeling of dilated cardiomyopathy in muscular dystrophy. Circulation 2005; 112(18):2799–804.

44. Nigro G, Comi LI, Politano L, et al. The incidence and evolution of cardiomyopathy in Duchenne muscular dystrophy. Int J Cardiol 1990;26(3): 271–7.

45. Giatrakos N, Kinali M, Stephens D, et al. Cardiac tissue velocities and strain rate in the early detection of myocardial dysfunction of asymptomatic boys with Duchenne's muscular dystrophy: relationship to clinical outcome. Heart 2006;92(6):840–2.

46. Ashford MW Jr, Liu W, Lin SJ, et al. Occult cardiac contractile dysfunction in dystrophin-deficient children revealed by cardiac magnetic resonance strain imaging. Circulation 2005;112(16):2462–7.

47. Duboc D, Meune C, Lerebours G, et al. Effect of perindopril on the onset and progression of left ventricular dysfunction in Duchenne muscular dystrophy. J Am Coll Cardiol 2005;45(6):855–7.

48. Exil VJ, Summar M, Boles MA, et al. Metabolic basis of pediatric heart disease. Prog Pediatr Cardiol 2005;20(2):143–59.

49. Gilbert-Barness E. Review: metabolic cardiomyopathy and conduction system defects in children. Ann Clin Lab Sci 2004;34(1):15–34.

50. Yaplito-Lee J, Weintraub R, Jamsen K, et al. Cardiac manifestations in oxidative phosphorylation disorders of childhood. J Pediatr 2007; 150(4):407–11.

51. Winter SC, Buist NR. Cardiomyopathy in childhood, mitochondrial dysfunction, and the role of L-carnitine. Am Heart J 2000;139(2 Pt 3):S63–9.

52. Dec GW, Fuster V. Idiopathic dilated cardiomyopathy. N Engl J Med 1994;331(23):1564–75.

53. Maiya S, Sullivan I, Allgrove J, et al. Hypocalcaemia and vitamin D deficiency: an important, but preventable, cause of life-threatening infant heart failure. Heart 2008;94(5):581–4.

54. Cochrane AD, Coleman DM, Davis AM, et al. Excellent long-term functional outcome after an operation for anomalous left coronary artery from the pulmonary artery. J Thorac Cardiovasc Surg 1999;117(2):332–42.

55. Medi C, Kalman JM, Haqqani H, et al. Tachycardia-mediated cardiomyopathy secondary to focal atrial tachycardia: long-term outcome after catheter ablation. J Am Coll Cardiol 2009;53(19):1791–7.

56. Schwartz ML, Cox GF, Lin AE, et al. Clinical approach to genetic cardiomyopathy in children. Circulation 1996;94(8):2021–38.

57. Cooper LT, Baughman KL, Feldman AM, et al. The role of endomyocardial biopsy in the management of cardiovascular disease: a scientific statement from the American Heart Association, the American College of Cardiology, and the European Society of Cardiology. Circulation 2007;116(19):2216–33.

58. Hauck AU, Kearney DL, Edwards WD. Evaluation of postmortem endomyocardial biopsy specimens from 38 patients with lymphocytic myocarditis: implications for role of sampling error. Mayo Clin Proc 1989;64(10):1235–45.

59. Martin AB, Webber S, Fricker FJ, et al. Acute myocarditis. Rapid diagnosis by PCR in children. Circulation 1994;90(1):330–9.

60. McMahon AM, van Doorn C, Burch M, et al. Improved early outcome for end-stage dilated cardiomyopathy in children. J Thorac Cardiovasc Surg 2003;126(6):1781–7.

61. Rhee EK, Canter CE, Basile S, et al. Sudden death prior to pediatric heart transplantation: would implantable defibrillators improve outcome? J Heart Lung Transplant 2007;26(5):447–52.

62. Griffin ML, Hernandez A, Martin TC, et al. Dilated cardiomyopathy in infants and children. J Am Coll Cardiol 1988;11(1):139–44.

63. Tsirka AE, Trinkaus K, Chen SC, et al. Improved outcomes of pediatric dilated cardiomyopathy with utilization of heart transplantation. J Am Coll Cardiol 2004;44(2):391–7.

64. del Nido PJ, Armitage JM, Fricker FJ, et al. Extracorporeal membrane oxygenation support as a bridge to pediatric heart transplantation. Circulation 1994;90(5 Pt 2):II66–9.

65. Blume ED, Naftel DC, Bastardi HJ, et al. Outcomes of children bridged to heart transplantation with ventricular assist devices: a multi-institutional study. Circulation 2006;113(19):2313–9.

66. Kirk R, Naftel D, Hoffman TM, et al. Outcome of pediatric patients with dilated cardiomyopathy listed for transplant: a multi-institutional study. J Heart Lung Transplant 2009;28(12):1322–8.

67. Shaddy RE, Boucek MM, Hsu DT, et al. Carvedilol for children and adolescents with heart failure: a randomized controlled trial. JAMA 2007;298(10):1171–9.

68. Alvarez JA, Wilkinson JD, Lipshultz SE. Outcome predictors for pediatric dilated cardiomyopathy: a systematic review. Prog Pediatr Cardiol 2007;23(1):25–32.

69. Di Filippo S, Bozio A, Normand J, et al. [Idiopathic dilated cardiomyopathies in children. Development and prognostic factors]. Arch Mal Coeur Vaiss 1991;84(5):721–6 [in French].

70. McMahon CJ, Nagueh SF, Eapen RS, et al. Echocardiographic predictors of adverse clinical events in children with dilated cardiomyopathy: a prospective clinical study. Heart 2004;90(8):908–15.

71. Arola A, Jokinen E, Ruuskanen O, et al. Epidemiology of idiopathic cardiomyopathies in children and adolescents. A nationwide study in Finland. Am J Epidemiol 1997;146(5):385–93.

72. Lewis AB, Chabot M. Outcome of infants and children with dilated cardiomyopathy. Am J Cardiol 1991;68(4):365–9.

73. Venugopalan P, Agarwal AK, Akinbami FO, et al. Improved prognosis of heart failure due to idiopathic dilated cardiomyopathy in children. Int J Cardiol 1998;65(2):125–8.

74. Wiles HB, McArthur PD, Taylor AB, et al. Prognostic features of children with idiopathic dilated cardiomyopathy. Am J Cardiol 1991;68(13):1372–6.

75. Azevedo VM, Albanesi Filho FM, Santos MA, et al. How can the echocardiogram be useful for predicting death in children with idiopathic dilated cardiomyopathy? Arq Bras Cardiol 2004;82(6):505–14.

76. Singh TP, Sleeper LA, Lipshultz S, et al. Association of left ventricular dilation at listing for heart transplant with postlisting and early posttransplant mortality in children with dilated cardiomyopathy. Circ Heart Fail 2009;2(6):591–8.

77. Guimaraes GV, d'Avila VM, Camargo PR, et al. Prognostic value of cardiopulmonary exercise testing in children with heart failure secondary to idiopathic dilated cardiomyopathy in a non-beta-blocker therapy setting. Eur J Heart Fail 2008;10(6):560–5.

78. Tang WH, Francis GS, Morrow DA, et al. National Academy of Clinical Biochemistry Laboratory Medicine practice guidelines: clinical utilization of cardiac biomarker testing in heart failure. Circulation 2007;116(5):e99–109.

79. Apple FS, Wu AH, Jaffe AS, et al. National Academy of Clinical Biochemistry and IFCC Committee for Standardization of Markers of Cardiac Damage Laboratory Medicine practice guidelines: analytical issues for biomarkers of heart failure. Circulation 2007;116(5):e95–8.

80. Zhang WL, Du ZD. [Mean values of brain natriuretic peptide in 190 healthy children]. Zhongguo Dang Dai Er Ke Za Zhi 2006;8(3):177–80 [in Chinese].

81. Das BB, Raj S, Solinger R. Natriuretic peptides in cardiovascular diseases of fetus, infants and children. Cardiovasc Hematol Agents Med Chem 2009;7(1):43–51.

82. Albers S, Mir TS, Haddad M, et al. N-Terminal pro-brain natriuretic peptide: normal ranges in the pediatric population including method comparison and interlaboratory variability. Clin Chem Lab Med 2006;44(1):80–5.

83. Koch A, Singer H. Normal values of B type natriuretic peptide in infants, children, and adolescents. Heart 2003;89(8):875–8.

84. Mir TS, Marohn S, Laer S, et al. Plasma concentrations of N-terminal pro-brain natriuretic peptide in control children from the neonatal to adolescent period and in children with congestive heart failure. Pediatrics 2002;110(6):e76.

85. Yoshibayashi M, Kamiya T, Saito Y, et al. Plasma brain natriuretic peptide concentrations in healthy children from birth to adolescence: marked and rapid increase after birth. Eur J Endocrinol 1995;133(2):207–9.

86. Reynolds EW, Ellington JG, Vranicar M, et al. Brain-type natriuretic peptide in the diagnosis and

management of persistent pulmonary hypertension of the newborn. Pediatrics 2004;114(5):1297–304.

87. Nir A, Nasser N. Clinical value of NT-ProBNP and BNP in pediatric cardiology. J Card Fail 2005; 11(Suppl 5):S76–80.

88. Ko HK, Lee JH, Choi BM, et al. Utility of the rapid B-type natriuretic peptide assay for detection of cardiovascular problems in newborn infants with respiratory difficulties. Neonatology 2008;94(1): 16–21.

89. Westerlind A, Wahlander H, Lindstedt G, et al. Clinical signs of heart failure are associated with increased levels of natriuretic peptide types B and A in children with congenital heart defects or cardiomyopathy. Acta Paediatr 2004;93(3):340–5.

90. Soker M, Kervancioglu M. Plasma concentrations of NT-pro-BNP and cardiac troponin-I in relation to doxorubicin-induced cardiomyopathy and cardiac function in childhood malignancy. Saudi Med J 2005;26(8):1197–202.

91. Price JF, Thomas AK, Grenier M, et al. B-type natriuretic peptide predicts adverse cardiovascular events in pediatric outpatients with chronic left ventricular systolic dysfunction. Circulation 2006; 114(10):1063–9.

92. Mori K, Manabe T, Nii M, et al. Plasma levels of natriuretic peptide and echocardiographic parameters in patients with Duchenne's progressive muscular dystrophy. Pediatr Cardiol 2002;23(2): 160–6.

93. Aggarwal S, Pettersen MD, Bhambhani K, et al. B-type natriuretic peptide as a marker for cardiac dysfunction in anthracycline-treated children. Pediatr Blood Cancer 2007;49(6):812–6.

94. Fried I, Bar-Oz B, Perles Z, et al. N-terminal pro-B-type natriuretic peptide levels in acute versus chronic left ventricular dysfunction. J Pediatr 2006;149(1):28–31.

95. Jessup M, Abraham WT, Casey DE, et al. 2009 focused update: ACCF/AHA guidelines for the diagnosis and management of heart failure in adults: a report of the American College of Cardiology Foundation/American Heart Association Task Force on Practice Guidelines: developed in collaboration with the International Society for Heart and Lung Transplantation. Circulation 2009; 119(14):1977–2016.

96. Rosenthal D, Chrisant MR, Edens E, et al. International Society for Heart and Lung Transplantation: practice guidelines for management of heart failure in children. J Heart Lung Transplant 2004;23(12): 1313–33.

97. Johnson WD, Kroon JJ, Greenway FL, et al. Prevalence of risk factors for metabolic syndrome in adolescents: National Health and Nutrition Examination Survey (NHANES), 2001–2006. Arch Pediatr Adolesc Med 2009;163(4):371–7.

98. Maron BJ, Chaitman BR, Ackerman MJ, et al. Recommendations for physical activity and recreational sports participation for young patients with genetic cardiovascular diseases. Circulation 2004;109(22):2807–16.

99. McBride MG, Binder TJ, Paridon SM. Safety and feasibility of inpatient exercise training in pediatric heart failure: a preliminary report. J Cardiopulm Rehabil Prev 2007;27(4):219–22.

100. Silber JH, Cnaan A, Clark BJ, et al. Enalapril to prevent cardiac function decline in long-term survivors of pediatric cancer exposed to anthracyclines. J Clin Oncol 2004;22(5):820–8.

101. Kajimoto H, Ishigaki K, Okumura K, et al. Beta-blocker therapy for cardiac dysfunction in patients with muscular dystrophy. Circ J 2006; 70(8):991–4.

102. Shaddy RE, Curtin EL, Sower B, et al. The Pediatric Randomized Carvedilol Trial in children with heart failure: rationale and design. Am Heart J 2002; 144(3):383–9.

103. Jefferies JL, Denfield SW, Price JF, et al. A prospective evaluation of nesiritide in the treatment of pediatric heart failure. Pediatr Cardiol 2006;27(4):402–7.

104. Jefferies JL, Price JF, Denfield SW, et al. Safety and efficacy of nesiritide in pediatric heart failure. J Card Fail 2007;13(7):541–8.

105. Mahle WT, Cuadrado AR, Kirshbom PM, et al. Nesiritide in infants and children with congestive heart failure. Pediatr Crit Care Med 2005;6(5): 543–6.

106. Berg AM, Snell L, Mahle WT. Home inotropic therapy in children. J Heart Lung Transplant 2007;26(5):453–7.

107. Namachivayam P, Crossland DS, Butt WW, et al. Early experience with Levosimendan in children with ventricular dysfunction. Pediatr Crit Care Med 2006;7(5):445–8.

108. Epstein AE, DiMarco JP, Ellenbogen KA, et al. ACC/AHA/HRS 2008 guidelines for device-based therapy of cardiac rhythm abnormalities: a report of the American College of Cardiology/American Heart Association Task Force on Practice Guidelines (Writing Committee to Revise the ACC/AHA/NASPE 2002 Guideline Update for Implantation of Cardiac Pacemakers and Antiarrhythmia Devices): developed in collaboration with the American Association for Thoracic Surgery and Society of Thoracic Surgeons. Circulation 2008;117(21): e350–408.

109. Dubin AM, Berul CI, Bevilacqua LM, et al. The use of implantable cardioverter-defibrillators in pediatric patients awaiting heart transplantation. J Card Fail 2003;9(5):375–9.

110. Friedberg MK, Roche SL, Balasingam M, et al. Evaluation of mechanical dyssynchrony in children with

idiopathic dilated cardiomyopathy and associated clinical outcomes. Am J Cardiol 2008;101(8):1191–5.

111. Mohammed A, Friedberg MK. Feasibility of a new tissue Doppler based method for comprehensive evaluation of left-ventricular intra-ventricular mechanical dyssynchrony in children with dilated cardiomyopathy. J Am Soc Echocardiogr 2008; 21(9):1062–7.

112. Karpawich PP. Pediatric cardiac resynchronization pacing therapy. Curr Opin Cardiol 2007; 22(2):72–6.

113. Cecchin F, Frangini PA, Brown DW, et al. Cardiac resynchronization therapy (and multisite pacing) in pediatrics and congenital heart disease: five years experience in a single institution. J Cardiovasc Electrophysiol 2008;20(1):58–65.

114. Breinholt JP, Fraser CD, Dreyer WJ, et al. The efficacy of mitral valve surgery in children with dilated cardiomyopathy and severe mitral regurgitation. Pediatr Cardiol 2008;29(1):13–8.

115. Walsh MA, Benson LN, Dipchand AI, et al. Surgical repair of the mitral valve in children with dilated cardiomyopathy and mitral regurgitation. Ann Thorac Surg 2008;85(6):2085–8.

116. Gandhi SK, Huddleston CB, Balzer DT, et al. Biventricular assist devices as a bridge to heart transplantation in small children. Circulation 2008; 118(Suppl 14):S89–93.

117. Rockett SR, Bryant JC, Morrow WR, et al. Preliminary single center North American experience with the Berlin Heart pediatric EXCOR device. ASAIO J 2008;54(5):479–82.

Hypertrophic Cardiomyopathy in Childhood

Steven D. Colan, MD

KEYWORDS

- Cardiomyopathy • Hypertrophic cardiomyopathy
- Sudden death • Pediatrics • Children • Infants

Hypertrophic cardiomyopathy (HCM) is defined as the presence of a hypertrophied, nondilated ventricle in the absence of another disease that creates a hemodynamic disturbance that is capable of producing the existent magnitude of wall thickening (eg, hypertension, aortic valve stenosis, catecholamine secreting tumors, hyperthyroidism, and so forth). HCM accounts for 42% of childhood cardiomyopathy, has an incidence of 0.47 of 100,000 children[1] and represents a heterogeneous group of disorders with a diversity that is more apparent in childhood than at any other age. It is possible to further subdivide these diseases based on several characteristics. A classification is presented in **Box 1** based on groupings of familial, syndromic, neuromuscular, and metabolic (storage disease and mitochondrial) disorders. Other classification schemes are commonly used, including division into primary and secondary forms where the primary form is a familial disorder (familial hypertrophic cardiomyopathy [FHC]) typically devoid of findings outside of the heart and the secondary forms include diseases, such as Friedreich ataxia,[2] where ventricular hypertrophy is common but is not the dominant clinical manifestation, and others, such as glycogenosis type IX,[3] in which a systemic disorder has primarily or exclusively cardiac manifestations.

Most of the available information for HCM derives from studies in adult populations and the implication of these observations for pediatric populations is often uncertain. The purpose of this review is not to attempt to review the vast body of literature that has accumulated about HCM but rather to summarize key findings and to discuss their implications for diagnosis and management of children with HCM.

EPIDEMIOLOGY AND SURVIVAL

The Pediatric Cardiomyopathy Registry is a multicenter observational study of pediatric cardiomyopathies initiated in 1995 that in 2003 reported the sex, age, and race-specific incidence of the several forms of cardiomyopathy based on two geographically diverse sections of the United States.[1] The incidence of HCM was found to be 69% more common in boys, occurred at 10 times the rate in subjects under 1 year of age, and was significantly more common in blacks than in whites or Hispanics. Subsequently, the distribution of etiologies and the etiology-specific survival in 849 children, the largest series to date, was reported.[4] Overall, there was nearly equal distribution between inborn errors of metabolism (IEM, 9%), malformation syndromes (MFS, 9%), and neuromuscular disorders (NMD, 8%), with the remaining 75% represented by the idiopathic patients and patients with FHC. The mean age at diagnosis was under 6 months in the IEM and MFS groups, whereas the other groups were typically older at the time of diagnosis. Survival was found to be etiology and age specific, confirming that survival in infants is much poorer than in older groups but documenting that this can be attributed to the high incidence of IEM and NMD at this age, whereas the survival for patients with NMD and FHC was similar regardless of age at diagnosis (**Fig. 1**). A notable observation was that annual

This work was supported by grant 5 R01 HL53392-09 from the National Institutes of Health.
Department of Cardiology, Children's Hospital Boston, 300 Longwood Avenue, Boston, MA 02115, USA
E-mail address: colan@alum.mit.edu

Heart Failure Clin 6 (2010) 433–444
doi:10.1016/j.hfc.2010.05.004

Box 1
Phenotypically based classification of hypertrophic cardiomyopathy

Familial hypertrophic cardiomyopathy

   Sarcomeric hypertrophic cardiomyopathy

   Maternally inherited hypertrophic cardiomyopathy syndromes

Syndromic hypertrophic cardiomyopathy

   Noonan's syndrome

   Beckwith-Wiedemann syndrome

   Cardio-facial-cutaneous syndrome

   Costello syndrome

   Lentiginosis (LEOPARD syndrome)

Neuromuscular disease

   Friedreich's ataxia

Metabolic disorders

   Anabolic steroid therapy and abuse

   Carnitine deficiency (carnitine palmitoyl transferase II deficiency, carnitine-acylcarnitine translocase deficiency)

   Fucosidosis type 1

   Glycogenosis type 2, 3, and 9 (Pompe disease, Forbes' disease, Phosphorylase kinase deficiency)

   Glycolipid lipidosis (Fabry disease)

   Glycosylation disorders

   I-cell disease

   Infant of diabetic mother

   Lipodystrophy, total

   Lysosomal disorders (Danon's disease)

   Mannosidosis

   Mitochondrial disorders (multiple forms)

   Mucopolysaccharidosis type 1, 2, and 5 (Hurler's syndrome, Hunter's syndrome, Scheie's syndrome)

   Prenatal and postnatal corticosteroid therapy

   Selenium deficiency

Abbreviations: LEOPARD, lentingines, electrocardiographic abnormalities, ocular hypertelorism, pulmonary stenosis, abnormal genitalia, retarded growth, deafness.

---

children that reported much higher annual mortality.

INFANTILE HYPERTROPHIC CARDIOMYOPATHY

The infant with HCM represents a particularly difficult challenge with regard to determining an etiologic diagnosis because of the wide range of disorders for which an association has been reported (see **Box 1**). Successful determination of a specific diagnosis is likely to have significant impact on management and survival because of the differences in etiology-specific survival. Although the pace of advances in genetic and metabolic diagnostics has quickened and the chances that a specific diagnosis can be achieved has improved substantially in recent years, about 50% of HCM cases under the age of 1 year remain idiopathic.[4] Amongst those patients for whom a defined etiology is identified, a few disorders (Pompe disease, Noonan syndrome, and FHC) account for the largest percent and etiologic diagnosis in the remainder is far more difficult. From the cardiac perspective, the association of particular patterns of the cardiac phenotype with specific etiologies has been an area of considerable interest because of the potential to guide the evaluation. For example, the finding of a hypertrophic, hypokinetic left ventricle has been most frequently associated with IEM, and in particular with mitochondrial defects. Biventricular outflow tract obstruction is more common in Noonan syndrome than in other forms of infantile HCM. Asymmetric patterns of hypertrophy are more commonly seen in syndromic and familial HCM than in IEM. Although these sorts of observations can provide some guidance, for most infants with HCM early referral for multispecialty evaluation, including specialists in cardiology, neurology, genetics, and metabolism, is warranted.

FAMILIAL HYPERTROPHIC CARDIOMYOPATHY
Genetics

The genetic transmission of FHC is usually autosomal dominant, with a significant percentage of cases representing apparently new mutations. Maternally inherited mitochondrial pattern of transmission has also been reported,[5] adding to the complexity of the disease. There has been a virtual explosion of information since the early 1990s concerning the genetic abnormalities associated with this disorder. One of the most striking findings has been the sheer number of diverse mutations that manifest clinically as HCM. The results of

mortality in children with FHC was 1.1 per 100 patient-years, which compares favorably with contemporary reports in adults with FHC. This finding contrasted to earlier and smaller series in

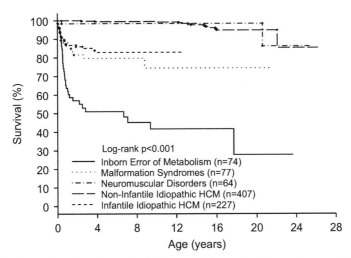

Fig. 1. Percent survival as a function of age in children with hypertrophic cardiomyopathy caused by various classes of etiology.

molecular studies so far have implicated several sarcomeric proteins in the etiology, including beta-myosin heavy chain, alpha-myosin heavy chain, myosin essential light chain, myosin regulatory light chain, cardiac troponin T, cardiac troponin I, alpha-tropomyosin, myosin binding protein C, titin, and actin.[6] These gene mutations display allelic heterogeneity; that is, multiple distinct mutations of each of these genes can cause the disease. The frequent finding of mutations in the sarcomeric proteins resulted in the paradigm of FHC as a disease of the sarcomere,[7] an understanding that has been disrupted by the more recent identification of mutations in genes encoding nonsarcomeric proteins within the z-disc and calcium handling control mechanisms that result in a similar phenotype.[6] There are also familial forms of HCM caused by nonsarcomeric genes, such as those caused by mitochondrial defects, potassium channel,[8] and the gamma subunit of protein kinase A.[9] Although sarcomeric defects appear to be the most common cause of FHC, they are not the only cause. Furthermore, at present the genotype responsible for the HCM phenotype cannot be determined in 30% to 40% of patients.

Commercially available genetic testing for some of the more common mutations causing FHC is a recent event and one that has stimulated considerable discussion concerning who should have this testing performed. Although certain mutations may imply greater or lesser risk, the expectation that genotyping would markedly improve risk stratification and clinical management has been largely undercut by recent data.[10] For example, mutations in troponin T were initially reported to have a consistent phenotype of mild or absent hypertrophy associated with a high incidence of

sudden death,[11] but families have been described with troponin T defects who have a low risk of early death.[12] Other factors, such as the coexistence of mitochondrial DNA mutations in some families,[13] multiple mutations,[14] or the impact of coexistent genetic polymorphisms within the renin-angiotensin system,[15] account for some of the variability in disease expression. It has been argued that detection of gene carriers in FHC may have too little impact on clinical care to justify the cost and the potential for adverse psychological and social consequences.[16]

Implications for pediatrics

For infants, children, and young adults there are several benefits that are not considered in the foregoing analysis. One of the most feared complications of HCM in children and young adults is diagnosis of the disease at the time of sudden death. The potential to avert such events rests on diagnosis of the disease in children who are asymptomatic. Because development of the phenotype can be noted throughout childhood, current practice is to periodically screen offspring of affected individuals throughout childhood. Identification of a familial gene allows children who are genotype negative to avoid longitudinal evaluation for development of hypertrophy, markedly reducing the overall cost of care, in addition to anxiety reduction and elimination of concerns about exercise participation. Those children who carry the gene can be followed more closely for development of disease and they also become eligible for trials of interventions to prevent development of the phenotype. The potential to prevent the onset of hypertrophy remains an unproven hypothesis in humans, although a mouse model of myosin heavy chain HCM treated before the onset of hypertrophy with diltiazem had less hypertrophy, fibrosis, and myocyte disarray than placebo-treated mice,[17] and a clinical trial in phenotype-negative, genotype-positive children and young adults is currently in progress.

The phenomenon of incomplete penetrance (a negative phenotype in genotype-positive adult members of a pedigree) has been well described in familial HCM and appears more common than has been previously thought. One of the implications of this finding is that all children in the pedigree, even offspring of phenotype-negative parents, must be considered at risk and should undergo longitudinal evaluation for development of the phenotype unless the parents can be shown to be genotype negative. As a result, adult members of the pedigree who are found to carry the gene can be advised that they are at risk for transmitting the gene even if they are phenotypically negative. Finally, identification of the gene permits use of the new technique of embryo preselection to allow carriers of the gene to avoid transmission to their offspring.

Diagnosis

The diagnosis of HCM in infants is generally made during evaluation for a murmur or for congestive heart failure. Older children are diagnosed during investigations for murmurs, symptoms (impaired exercise capacity, chest pain, palpitations, or syncope), electrocardiographic abnormalities, and screening of offspring of affected adults. The echocardiogram provides definitive noninvasive assessment of ventricular size, wall thickness, systolic and diastolic function, outflow obstruction, and valvar insufficiency in nearly all children. Diagnosis has typically been based on increased regional or global wall thickness and excess regional variation in thickness. The usual adult criteria for diagnosis are based on an absolute wall thickness more than the normal range (>12 mm), resulting in a significant false-positive rate. Improved longitudinal observations and the advent of more widespread genotyping have improved the ability to refine these echocardiographic criteria. This issue is of particular importance in distinguishing physiologic from pathologic hypertrophies. Cardiac hypertrophy associated with intense athletic participation is well described in both children and young adults.[18] In athletic patients with mild hypertrophy on echocardiography, findings that increase the probability of HCM include unusual patterns of hypertrophy, small left ventricular cavity size, abnormal diastolic function indices, female gender, family history of hypertrophic cardiomyopathy, and evidence of delayed enhancement with gadolinium on cardiac MRI.[19] Findings that increase the probability of physiologic hypertrophy include left ventricular cavity size near or more than the upper limits of normal and elevated peak oxygen consumption on exercise testing. The electrocardiogram is not helpful in making this distinction. Ultimately, if reasonable certainty is not achieved based on these additional criteria, cessation of exercise participation for 6 months can be used to identify patients with HCM, who will not experience a decrement in wall thickness. Unfortunately, obtaining adequate compliance with this recommendation is challenging in most athletes.

Implications for pediatrics

Use of age and body surface area adjusted normal values is necessary in children. The use of z scores (defined as the number of standard deviations from the population mean) has been particularly helpful in this regard.[20] The sensitivity and specificity for specific z-score values relative to diagnosis of HCM in children has not been tested, although in general the range of uncertainty between physiologic and pathologic hypertrophy corresponds to a z score between 2 and 3, with physiologic hypertrophy rarely resulting in a wall thickness relative to body surface area that is more than 3 standard deviations above the population mean. Studies performed in children who are genotypically positive have identified several echocardiographic and electrocardiographic findings that can be abnormal despite the absence of hypertrophy.[21–23] In particular, abnormal, noninvasive diastolic function indices, such as reduced early diastolic tissue velocities, prolonged isovolumic relaxation times, and increased left atrial volume, have been described.[23,24] These findings have important implications concerning the pathophysiology of the disease but the implications concerning diagnosis are more ambiguous. In children with mild hypertrophy, abnormal diastolic function indices make it highly likely that the hypertrophy is not physiologic. However, in the absence of hypertrophy, individuals who are genotypically positive do not meet the definition of hypertrophic cardiomyopathy, are not known to be at increased risk for sudden death, and do not manifest symptoms. Furthermore, it is unclear whether all individuals who are genotype positive and phenotype negative will manifest hypertrophy over time. Although the term *hypertrophic cardiomyopathy without hypertrophy* has been used, the implication that disease status should be based on genetic status rather than phenotype remains unclear. This uncertainty is apparent in the conflicting exercise guidelines issued by the 36th Bethesda Conference and the European Society of Cardiology recommendations for sports participation, with the European but not the American group recommending against participation in individuals who are phenotypically negative and genotypically positive.[25]

Management of Symptoms

The goals of therapy in this disorder are to reduce symptoms and prolong survival. The symptoms of chest pain, dyspnea, and exercise intolerance can often be managed medically, and surgery has been successful in certain patient groups. Digitalis is not helpful and is usually contraindicated unless atrial fibrillation occurs. Although dyspnea is a common symptom, diuretic therapy is usually not beneficial, can increase the outflow gradient because of a reduction in chamber volume, and can reduce cardiac output. Outflow tract obstruction plays an important role with regard to symptom status in HCM. The clinical importance of outflow obstruction has been highly controversial over the years, as recently recounted in some detail by Maron and colleagues.[26] Patients with outflow tract obstruction are at greater risk for symptoms and progression to heart failure and death,[27] and exercise-induced or exacerbated outflow tract obstruction is both common and associated with a higher risk for symptoms.[28] Reduction in outflow tract obstruction is one of the primary targets of therapy for patients who are symptomatic. The gradient can be detected at rest or only with provocation, such as inotropic stimulation, vasodilation, or exercise, and often demonstrates marked spontaneous lability.[29] Although provocation of latent outflow obstruction with maneuvers, such as amyl nitrate, has been recommended, the clinical significance of gradients elicited in this fashion remains uncertain, in part because of the difficulty in standardization.

Beta-blockers

The mainstay of therapy for many years has been beta-adrenergic blockade. Chest pain and dyspnea are often relieved by propranolol, but improved exercise capacity is seen less often. The response appears to be dose dependent, and high dosage levels have often been tried. Side effects, such as fatigue, depression, sleep disorders, and impaired school performance, are often encountered at these high dosage levels, particularly in children and adolescents, and can be intolerable. Despite early improvement, symptoms often recur and may not respond to dose

escalation. Studies of the impact of beta-blocker therapy on survival in adults and children have invariably been uncontrolled but have not identified a measurable effect of propranolol on survival. In a single, uncontrolled study in children, comparison of a small number of pediatric subjects in each of two geographically distinct areas (one of which treated all subjects with HCM with high-dose propranolol) found unusually high mortality (52% 10-year survival) in the untreated cohort with no mortality in the treated cohort.[30] It is difficult to reconcile these findings with the many prior, larger studies that have failed to identify a survival benefit from propranolol and the high mortality in the untreated group is difficult to reconcile with large pediatric studies that have found a 10-year survival of 80% in unselected populations.[4] Differential therapy based solely on geographic location is potentially highly biased because of the potential for genetically similar subjects in each geographic region, and the differences in outcome do not exceed those observed between other studies in small groups of pediatric subjects with HCM.

Calcium channel blockers

Calcium channel blockers in general and verapamil in particular have been used extensively in patients with FHC. Sustained improvement in diastolic relaxation is generally noted in response to verapamil administration with secondary reduction in diastolic pressure and mean left atrial pressure,[31,32] resulting in a reduction in dyspnea and increase in exercise capacity. Improved distribution of subendocardial flow and diminished inducible ischemia have also been noted.[33] Although verapamil may exacerbate congestive heart failure in older patients, pediatric tolerance has been excellent, even in neonates.[34]

Angiotensin converting enzyme inhibitors

Inhibition of the renin-angiotensin system has a favorable impact on ventricular hypertrophy and diastolic function in secondary hypertrophy, but has rarely been used in FHC. Angiotensin-converting enzyme inhibitors given to patients with dynamic left ventricular outflow tract obstruction result in a fall in cavity size and increase in outflow gradient, as well as impaired left ventricular relaxation and compliance.[35] Based on theoretical considerations and data such as these, it is generally believed that these agents and other systemic vasodilators are contraindicated in HCM when left ventricular outflow tract obstruction is present. However, there are also recent data indicating a significant role for aldosterone,[15] and the renin-angiotensin system in general,[36] in modulating the phenotypic manifestations of

HCM, leading to the suggestion that blocking this system might reduce hypertrophy and fibrosis.[37]

Pacemaker therapy

Despite a wave of enthusiasm for asynchronous ventricular pacing for treatment of symptoms in patients with left ventricular outflow tract obstruction, this therapy has largely fallen into disfavor. Results in small cohorts of children with outflow obstruction who were symptomatic despite medical therapy noted symptomatic improvement, reduced outflow obstruction, reduced left ventricular hypertrophy, and improved exercise tolerance.[38–40] Despite early studies,[41] subsequent controlled studies found that only about 60% of subjects improved. Furthermore, in two-thirds of these the benefit appeared to reflect placebo effect and an adverse effect on symptoms was seen in 5%.[42] The significant placebo effect has been seen in other studies,[43] perhaps explaining reports of persistent symptom relief after pacing termination,[44] an effect not confirmed in later studies.[45] Based on current information, dual chamber pacing should at best be considered as an alternative to surgical or transcatheter septal reduction in patients with obstructive FHC who are symptomatic despite maximum medical therapy and are poor candidates for other interventions.

Alcohol septal ablation

Direct transcatheter infusion of absolute alcohol directly into septal coronary perforators can result in tissue infarction, reduction in septal thickness, and relief of left ventricular outflow tract obstruction, with symptomatic improvement and increased exercise tolerance. Toxicity has included a 1% to 2% rate of procedural death; 20% to 50% incidence of transient heart block; and a 10% to 20% incidence of permanent complete heart block,[46,47] peri-procedure ventricular arrhythmias that may require cardioversion, unintended distal infarction caused by inadvertent alcohol infusion into the anterior descending coronary, and late appearance of complete heart block. Success is highest when obstruction is related to basilar septal hypertrophy. Patients with mitral valve abnormalities or obstruction that is more apical are poor candidates. Late outcome is unknown for this new technique, but current results indicate this may represent a reasonable alternative to surgery for relief of outflow tract obstruction in selected patients.[48] Recently, coil occlusion of these vessels has been reported as an alternative method of inducing controlled infarction.[49] Heart block was not seen in this series, the size of the infarction was smaller than with alcohol ablation, and the reduction in outflow gradient was less. The relative advantages to these two techniques remain to be determined.

Surgical myectomy

In symptomatic subaortic stenosis, septal myotomy-myectomy results in symptomatic improvement in nearly all patients and most contemporary studies have documented a high success rate, near zero mortality, and few complications with the procedure in adults.[50–52] Results in children have been similar to those reported in adults.[53,54] Mitral regurgitation often improves in response to myectomy because of improved intraventricular flow patterns, and surgery permits concomitant mitral valve repair in patients with underlying mitral valve abnormalities. Although recurrence of obstruction is rare in older patients (2%[55]), it is more frequent in the neonate and infant.

Implications for children

In the absence of symptoms, medical therapies have no proven benefits. Propranolol or verapamil are the first-line therapy for patients who are symptomatic. If symptoms are unresponsive to medical therapy and outflow tract obstruction is present, particularly if associated with mitral regurgitation, reduction or elimination of the outflow gradient should be considered. The technical feasibility of transcatheter septal reduction in adolescents has been demonstrated, though experience in this age group is at present limited to case series. The higher procedural complication rate compared with myectomy and concerns for potential late risks associated with a large infarction have led most clinicians to await longer-term results before use in children. Younger patients are not considered candidates for this procedure because of the inability to cannulate the smaller coronary feeder vessels in these patients. Therefore, surgical myectomy is generally recommended for management of medically intractable symptoms.

PREVENTION OF SUDDEN DEATH
Exercise Restriction

Avoidance of high-intensity exercise is generally recommended for patients with FHC. The rational for this restriction is based on the observations that sudden death is the usual cause of death in FHC and has a higher-than-expected association with exercise.[56] Nevertheless, the basis for this recommendation has several serious weaknesses.[57] The true incidence of FHC in athletes who experience sudden death is uncertain because genetic confirmation was not available and diagnosis was based on morphologic criteria that cannot unequivocally differentiate FHC from physiologic hypertrophy. It is clear that some patients with FHC tolerate intense, competitive athletic participation without symptoms or sudden death.[58] Population studies have documented the apparent paradox that although there is a transient increase in the risk for sudden death during intense exercise in patients with coronary artery disease who regularly participate in low- and high-level exertion, these individuals experience an overall reduction in the risk for sudden death.[59,60] Additionally, individuals who do not exercise regularly have an exaggerated risk of sudden death during exercise.[61] In fact, it is precisely those individuals with cardiovascular risk factors who derive the largest risk reduction from regular participation in moderate to intense exercise.[61] Several population studies have now documented that exercise and sports participation during childhood are predictive of activity level in adults.[62] Detraining and social stigmatization are particularly difficult problems for the adolescent who is excluded from the usual school activities and peer interactions. Competitive team sports elicit an emotional overlay that appears to increase the risk associated with the sport itself, in addition to demanding more intense exercise, and can therefore be justifiably proscribed. Certain activities, such as weight lifting, are associated with high levels of circulating catecholamines that can predispose to arrhythmias and elicit a marked stimulus to concentric cardiac hypertrophy. However, in patients who do not manifest high-grade arrhythmias or exercise-induced arrhythmias or hypotension, there is little evidence to indicate that moderate aerobic-type exercise represents a significant risk and it does provide measurable hemodynamic and psychological benefits.

Antiarrhythmics

Although most instances of sudden death in FHC are arrhythmic events, antiarrhythmic therapy has not been effective.[63] Amiodarone was initially reported to reduce the incidence of sudden death in certain high-risk subgroups, but subsequent studies indicated an increased risk for sudden death.[64] Furthermore, the pediatric experience with amiodarone therapy for FHC is limited because of the toxicity associated with chronic therapy. The promising early experience with implantable cardioverter defibrillators (ICD) has resulted in a shift to recommending an ICD for patients with ventricular tachycardia on Holter monitor or resuscitated cardiac arrest.[65]

Implantable Cardioverter Defibrillators Implantation

The incidence of sudden death in HCM is less than 1% per year in both adults and children and ICDs are not without hazard, including reduced quality of life, depression, anxiety, and inappropriate discharges that can at times be fatal. Optimization of the risk/benefit for ICD use is therefore dependent on the ability to identify individuals at high risk for sudden death. Several risk factors for sudden death in adults with HCM have been proposed (**Box 2**), and it is worth noting that this list continues to evolve with the introduction of newly proposed risk factors in addition to both the promotion and demotion of those previously proposed.[66,67] Few series have been focused on children, with severity of hypertrophy (wall thickness z-score >6) and an abnormal blood pressure response to exercise having been confirmed as risk factors in young patients.[68,69] The understanding of several of the proposed risk factors in **Box 2** has changed based on recent data and these newer findings are worth specific discussion.

Arrhythmias

Ventricular arrhythmias, including ventricular tachycardia and fibrillation, are common and are the presumed mechanism of sudden death in most cases. Despite this, there are conflicting data concerning the prognostic implications of nonsustained ventricular tachycardia (NSVT) found on Holter monitor recording in patients

---

Box 2
Risk factors for sudden death in HCM

Generally agreed

    Aborted sudden death

    Nonsustained ventricular tachycardia

    Family history of sudden death

    Syncope

    Extreme hypertrophy

    Abnormal blood pressure response to exercise

Conflicting or insufficient data

    Left ventricular outflow tract obstruction

    Late hyper-enhancement on MRI

    Specific, high-risk mutations

    Atrial fibrillation

    Myocardial bridging

with FHC. The presence of asymptomatic NSVT on Holter monitoring has been reported as a risk factor in some series [70] but not in others.[71,72] These differences may relate to age distribution included in each study because NSVT is generally associated with a low incremental risk (relative risk 2.0–2.5), which appears to be higher in adults younger than 30 years of age (22% vs 5% 5-year risk of sudden death).[70] Similarly, in children NSVT on Holter monitoring is less frequent than in adults,[73] but when present appears to be associated with a higher annual risk for sudden death.

Extreme Hypertrophy

Several recent reports have evaluated the impact of the severity of left ventricular hypertrophy on survival and risk for sudden death. Extreme wall thickness, in particular, has been suggested as an important risk factor[74] and therefore as a potential indication for an implantable cardioverter-defibrillator.[75] Other reports have not confirmed this association.[76–78] These conflicting data may in part be related to the observation that the increase in risk is primarily incurred in patients presenting younger than 30 years of age.[79] Further supporting this concept, severity of hypertrophy has also been found to be a risk factor in children.[68]

Outflow Tract Obstruction

The clinical importance of outflow obstruction has been highly controversial over the years, as recently recounted in some detail by Maron and colleagues.[26] The reduced survival in patients with outflow tract obstruction has been primarily related to death caused by congestive heart failure[27] with, at most, a small increase in risk for sudden death. Most studies have failed to identify any relationship to sudden death.[80] Surgical or pharmacologic reduction in the outflow gradient in patients who are symptomatic is usually associated with a reduction in symptoms and possibly improved overall survival, although there are no data to suggest that the incidence of sudden death is reduced. In patients with an ICD, a reduction in appropriate discharges after myectomy has been documented and has been proposed as a surrogate for a reduction in sudden death.[81] However, the accuracy of this surrogate is questionable because appropriate discharges occur at a far higher rate than the expected rate of sudden death. Based on current data, intervention based on gradient alone or for the purpose of averting sudden death cannot be recommended.

Myocardial Bridging

Muscle bands overlying epicardial coronary arteries (myocardial bridges) are congenital and sufficiently common that they are considered an anatomic variant rather than a congenital anomaly, having been observed in 20% to 66% of hearts.[82] In a provocative report of a relationship between sudden death and the presence of myocardial bridging in children with FHC,[83] Yetman and colleagues[83] suggest that surgical unroofing of the coronary can prevent sudden death. It is unclear why myocardial bridges would have a greater impact on children than has been described in adults, where bridging is extremely common and does not appear to represent a risk for sudden death.[84] Perhaps more troubling is the observation in this report that patients with bridges were older than the patients without, and the overall incidence (28%) was identical to the frequency described in adults (30%[85]) in contrast to the diminishing prevalence that would be anticipated in a congenital disorder that represents a risk for sudden death. Thus, although surgical intervention is possible,[86] further confirmation is required before myocardial bridging can be accepted as an adverse risk factor worthy of surgical intervention.

Syncope

Unexplained syncope (that is, excluding neurally mediated syncope) has been identified as a risk factor for sudden death in an adult series, but the relative risk was only 1.8[87]; however, the risk was much higher in patients younger than 18 years of age (hazard ratio 8), although the limited number of children and adolescents in this series limits the strength of the conclusion. Recurrent episodes did not appear to increase this risk.

Delayed Hyper-Enhancement on MRI

Delayed hyper-enhancement on MRI (DHE-MRI) has been identified as a sensitive imaging technique for myocardial scar, correlating with histologically proven myocardial fibrosis.[88] Myocardial scar is a known risk factor for ventricular arrhythmias and DHE-MRI is noted more frequently in patients with HCM who manifest NSVT than those who do not.[89,90] Based on current data, the increase in 5-year risk for sudden death in adults with DHE-MRI has been estimated at 1.6.[91]

Implications for Children

With the exception of aborted sudden death, the various clinical parameters associated with increased risk for sudden cardiac death have low positive predictive value. The presence of multiple risk factors incurs higher risk, leading to the recommendation that ICD use should be limited to patients who manifest multiple risk factors.[78] Nevertheless, current methods for risk stratification remain inadequate to the extent that, based on current ICD use rates after implantation in high-risk subjects and an anticipated device lifespan of 5 years, 83% of devices will be not be used before replacement.[92] This dilemma is further compounded in children, for whom the risk-benefit ratio for the use of ICD is less favorable than in adults. In a recent review, 28% of children experienced appropriate, potentially life-saving ICD discharges, 25% experienced inappropriate discharges, and there was a 21% incidence of lead failure.[93] Children are also at higher risk for device-related infections and adverse psychosocial impact than adults. Therefore, although potentially life-saving, pediatric-specific implantation indications must be developed and tested before this technology will achieve its full potential in children. At present, the author's institution has adopted an age-adjusted management approach. Aborted sudden death is considered an indication for ICD regardless of age. An ICD is recommended for adolescents with 2 or more of the other accepted risk factors. For preadolescents, additional evidence of risk is required before primary prevention is considered.

SUMMARY

This review emphasizes the recent data concerning the etiology, natural history, management, and outcome in the diverse set of diseases that fall within the clinical phenotype of hypertrophic cardiomyopathy. Changes in the understanding of the genetics of familial hypertrophic cardiomyopathy and the escalating clinical utility of genotyping, particularly in children, are discussed. There is a large body of observational literature concerning familial hypertrophic cardiomyopathy in adults with a much smaller body of data in children. This review summarizes those situations in which the findings in children have been found to be different from the information available from adult cohorts and emphasizes how certain management recommendations must be modified when applied to pediatric patients.

REFERENCES

1. Lipshultz SE, Sleeper LA, Towbin JA, et al. The incidence of pediatric cardiomyopathy in two regions of the United States. N Engl J Med 2003;348(17):1647–55.

2. Dutka DP, Donnelly JE, Nihoyannopoulos P, et al. Marked variation in the cardiomyopathy associated with Friedreich's ataxia. Heart 1999;81(2):141–7.

3. Regalado JJ, Rodriguez MM, Ferrer PL. Infantile hypertrophic cardiomyopathy of glycogenosis Type IX: isolated cardiac phosphorylase kinase deficiency. Pediatr Cardiol 1999;20(4):304–7.

4. Colan SD, Lipshultz SE, Lowe AM, et al. Epidemiology and cause-specific outcome of hypertrophic cardiomyopathy in children: findings from the Pediatric Cardiomyopathy Registry. Circulation 2007; 115(6):773–81.

5. Geier C, Perrot A, Özcelik C, et al. Mutations in the human muscle LIM protein gene in families with hypertrophic cardiomyopathy. Circulation 2003; 107(10):1390–5.

6. Bos JM, Towbin JA, Ackerman MJ. Diagnostic, prognostic, and therapeutic implications of genetic testing for hypertrophic cardiomyopathy. J Am Coll Cardiol 2009;54(3):201–11.

7. Nakaura H, Morimoto S, Yanaga F, et al. Functional changes in troponin T by a splice donor site mutation that causes hypertrophic cardiomyopathy. Am J Physiol Cell Physiol 1999;277(2):C225–32.

8. Marian AJ, Roberts R. The molecular genetic basis for hypertrophic cardiomyopathy. J Mol Cell Cardiol 2001;33(4):655–70.

9. Arad M, Benson DW, Perez-Atayde AR, et al. Constitutively active AMP kinase mutations cause glycogen storage disease mimicking hypertrophic cardiomyopathy. J Clin Invest 2002;109(3): 357–62.

10. Mogensen J, Murphy RT, Shaw T, et al. Severe disease expression of cardiac troponin C and T mutations in patients with idiopathic dilated cardiomyopathy. J Am Coll Cardiol 2004;44(10):2033–40.

11. Moolman JC, Corfield VA, Posen B, et al. Sudden death due to troponin T mutations. J Am Coll Cardiol 1997;29(3):549–55.

12. Anan R, Shono H, Kisanuki A, et al. Patients with familial hypertrophic cardiomyopathy caused by a Phe110Ile missense mutation in the cardiac troponin T gene have variable cardiac morphologies and a favorable prognosis. Circulation 1998;98(5):391–7.

13. Arbustini E, Fasani R, Morbini P, et al. Coexistence of mitochondrial DNA and β myosin heavy chain mutations in hypertrophic cardiomyopathy with late congestive heart failure. Heart 1998;80(6):548–58.

14. Van Driest SL, Vasile VC, Ommen SR, et al. Myosin binding protein C mutations and compound heterozygosity in hypertrophic cardiomyopathy. J Am Coll Cardiol 2004;44(9):1903–10.

15. Ortlepp JR, Vosberg HP, Reith S, et al. Genetic polymorphisms in the renin-angiotensin-aldosterone system associated with expression of left ventricular hypertrophy in hypertrophic cardiomyopathy: a study of five polymorphic genes in a family with

a disease causing mutation in the myosin binding protein C gene. Heart 2002;87(3):270–5.

16. Burn J, Camm J, Davies MJ, et al. The phenotype/genotype relation and the current status of genetic screening in hypertrophic cardiomyopathy, Marfan syndrome, and the long QT syndrome. Heart 1997; 78(2):110–6.

17. Semsarian C, Ahmad I, Giewat M, et al. The L-type calcium channel inhibitor diltiazem prevents cardiomyopathy in a mouse model. J Clin Invest 2002; 109(8):1013–20.

18. Colan SD, Sanders SP, Borow KM. Physiologic hypertrophy: effects on left ventricular systolic mechanics in athletes. J Am Coll Cardiol 1987; 9(4):776–83.

19. Maron BJ. Distinguishing hypertrophic cardiomyopathy from athlete's heart physiological remodelling: clinical significance, diagnostic strategies and implications for preparticipation screening. Br J Sports Med 2009;43(9):649–56.

20. Sluysmans T, Colan SD. Theoretical and empirical derivation of cardiovascular allometric relationships in children. J Appl Physiol 2005;99(2):445–57.

21. Charron P, Dubourg O, Desnos M, et al. Diagnostic value of electrocardiography and echocardiography for familial hypertrophic cardiomyopathy in genotyped children. Eur Heart J 1998;19(9):1377–82.

22. Nagueh SF, McFalls J, Meyer D, et al. Tissue Doppler imaging predicts the development of hypertrophic cardiomyopathy in subjects with subclinical disease. Circulation 2003;108(4):395–8.

23. Poutanen T, Tikanoja T, Jaaskelainen P, et al. Diastolic dysfunction without left ventricular hypertrophy is an early finding in children with hypertrophic cardiomyopathy-causing mutations in the beta-myosin heavy chain, alpha-tropomyosin, and myosin-binding protein C genes. Am Heart J 2006;151(3):725.

24. McTaggart DR. Tissue doppler imaging in hypertrophic cardiomyopathy without left ventricular hypertrophy. Heart Lung Circ 2002;11(2):92–4.

25. Pelliccia A, Zipes DP, Maron BJ. Bethesda Conference #36 and the European Society of Cardiology Consensus Recommendations revisited a comparison of U.S. and European criteria for eligibility and disqualification of competitive athletes with cardiovascular abnormalities. J Am Coll Cardiol 2008; 52(24):1990–6.

26. Maron BJ, Maron MS, Wigle ED, et al. The 50-year history, controversy, and clinical implications of left ventricular outflow tract obstruction in hypertrophic cardiomyopathy from idiopathic hypertrophic subaortic stenosis to hypertrophic cardiomyopathy: from idiopathic hypertrophic subaortic stenosis to hypertrophic cardiomyopathy. J Am Coll Cardiol 2009;54(3):191–200.

27. Maron MS, Olivotto I, Betocchi S, et al. Effect of left ventricular outflow tract obstruction on clinical outcome in hypertrophic cardiomyopathy. N Engl J Med 2003;348(4):295–303.

28. Shah JS, Esteban MT, Thaman R, et al. Prevalence of exercise-induced left ventricular outflow tract obstruction in symptomatic patients with non-obstructive hypertrophic cardiomyopathy. Heart 2008;94(10):1288–94.

29. Kizilbash AM, Heinle SK, Grayburn PA. Spontaneous variability of left ventricular outflow tract gradient in hypertrophic obstructive cardiomyopathy. Circulation 1998;97(5):461–6.

30. Ostman-Smith I, Wettrell G, Riesenfeld T. A cohort study of childhood hypertrophic cardiomyopathy: improved survival following high-dose beta-adrenoceptor antagonist treatment. J Am Coll Cardiol 1999;34(6):1813–22.

31. Posma JL, Blanksma PK, Van der Wall E, et al. Acute intravenous versus chronic oral drug effects of verapamil on left ventricular diastolic function in patients with hypertrophic cardiomyopathy. J Cardiovasc Pharmacol 1994;24(6):969–73.

32. Hartmann A, Schnell J, Hopf R, et al. Persisting effect of Ca(2+)-channel blockers on left ventricular function in hypertrophic cardiomyopathy after 14 years' treatment. Angiology 1996;47(8):765–73.

33. Gistri R, Cecchi F, Choudhury L, et al. Effect of verapamil on absolute myocardial blood flow in hypertrophic cardiomyopathy. Am J Cardiol 1994; 74(4):363–8.

34. Moran AM, Colan SD. Verapamil therapy in infants with hypertrophic cardiomyopathy. Cardiol Young 1998;8(3):310–9.

35. Kyriakidis M, Triposkiadis F, Dernellis J, et al. Effects of cardiac versus circulatory angiotensin-converting enzyme inhibition on left ventricular diastolic function and coronary blood flow in hypertrophic obstructive cardiomyopathy. Circulation 1998; 97(14):1342–7.

36. Tsybouleva N, Zhang LF, Chen SN, et al. Aldosterone, through novel signaling proteins, is a fundamental molecular bridge between the genetic defect and the cardiac phenotype of hypertrophic cardiomyopathy. Circulation 2004;109(10): 1284–91.

37. Yamazaki T, Suzuki J, Shimamoto R, et al. A new therapeutic strategy for hypertrophic nonobstructive cardiomyopathy in humans. A randomized and prospective study with an Angiotensin II receptor blocker. Int Heart J 2007;48(6):715–24.

38. Alday LE, Bruno E, Moreyra E, et al. Mid-term results of dual-chamber pacing in children with hypertrophic obstructive cardiomyopathy. Echocardiography 1998;15(3):289–95.

39. Rishi F, Hulse JE, Auld DO, et al. Effects of dual-chamber pacing for pediatric patients with hypertrophic obstructive cardiomyopathy. J Am Coll Cardiol 1997;29(4):734–40.

40. Dimitrow PP, Podolec P, Grodecki J, et al. Comparison of dual-chamber pacing with nonsurgical septal reduction effect in patients with hypertrophic obstructive cardiomyopathy. Int J Cardiol 2004;94(1):31–4.

41. Fananapazir L, Epstein ND, Curiel RV, et al. Long-term results of dual-chamber (DDD) pacing in obstructive hypertrophic cardiomyopathy: evidence for progressive symptomatic and hemodynamic improvement and reduction of left ventricular hypertrophy. Circulation 1994;90(6):2731–42.

42. Nishimura RA, Trusty JM, Hayes DL, et al. Dual-chamber pacing for hypertrophic cardiomyopathy: a randomized, double-blind, crossover trial. J Am Coll Cardiol 1997;29(2):435–41.

43. Linde C, Gadler F, Kappenberger L, et al. Placebo effect of pacemaker implantation in obstructive hypertrophic cardiomyopathy. Am J Cardiol 1999;83(6):903–7.

44. Fananapazir L, Cannon RO III, Tripodi D, et al. Impact of dual-chamber permanent pacing in patients with obstructive hypertrophic cardiomyopathy with symptoms refractory to verapamil and β-adrenergic blocker therapy. Circulation 1992; 85(6):2149–61.

45. Gadler F, Linde C, Rydén L. Rapid return of left ventricular outflow tract obstruction and symptoms following cessation of long-term atrioventricular synchronous pacing for obstructive hypertrophic cardiomyopathy. Am J Cardiol 1999;83(4):553–7.

46. Togni M, Billinger M, Cook S, et al. Septal myectomy: cut, coil, or boil? Eur Heart J 2008;29(3):296–8.

47. Sorajja P, Valeti U, Nishimura RA, et al. Outcome of alcohol septal ablation for obstructive hypertrophic cardiomyopathy. Circulation 2008;118(2):131–9.

48. Kimmelstiel CD, Maron BJ. Role of percutaneous septal ablation in hypertrophic obstructive cardiomyopathy. Circulation 2004;109(4):452–6.

49. Durand E, Mousseaux E, Coste P, et al. Nonsurgical septal myocardial reduction by coil embolization for hypertrophic obstructive cardiomyopathy: early and 6 months follow-up. Eur Heart J 2008;29(3):348–55.

50. Woo A, Williams WG, Choi R, et al. Clinical and echocardiographic determinants of long-term survival after surgical myectomy in obstructive hypertrophic cardiomyopathy. Circulation 2005; 111(16):2033–41.

51. Nishimura RA, Holmes DR Jr. Hypertrophic obstructive cardiomyopathy. N Engl J Med 2004;350(13): 1320–7.

52. Smedira NG, Lytle BW, Lever HM, et al. Current effectiveness and risks of isolated septal myectomy for hypertrophic obstructive cardiomyopathy. Ann Thorac Surg 2008;85(1):127–33.

53. Minakata K, Dearani JA, O'Leary PW, et al. Septal myectomy for obstructive hypertrophic cardiomyopathy in pediatric patients: early and late results. Ann Thorac Surg 2005;80(4):1424–9.

54. Menon SC, Ackerman MJ, Ommen SR, et al. Impact of septal myectomy on left atrial volume and left ventricular diastolic filling patterns: an echocardiographic study of young patients with obstructive hypertrophic cardiomyopathy. J Am Soc Echocardiogr 2008;21(6):684–8.

55. Minakata K, Dearani JA, Schaff HV, et al. Mechanisms for recurrent left ventricular outflow tract obstruction after septal myectomy for obstructive hypertrophic cardiomyopathy. Ann Thorac Surg 2005;80(3):851–6.

56. Semsarian C, Richmond DR. Sudden cardiac death in familial hypertrophic cardiomyopathy: an Australian experience. Aust N Z J Med 1999;29(3):368–70.

57. Shephard RJ. The athlete's heart: is big beautiful? Br J Sports Med 1996;30(1):5–10.

58. Maron BJ, Klues HG. Surviving competitive athletics with hypertrophic cardiomyopathy. Am J Cardiol 1994;73(15):1098–104.

59. Friedewald VE Jr, Spence DW. Sudden cardiac death associated with exercise: the risk- benefit issue. Am J Cardiol 1990;66(2):183–8.

60. Kohl HW, Powell KE, Gordon NF, et al. Physical activity, physical fitness, and sudden cardiac death. Epidemiol Rev 1992;14(1):37–58.

61. Richardson CR, Kriska AM, Lantz PM, et al. Physical activity and mortality across cardiovascular disease risk groups. Med Sci Sports Exerc 2004;36(11): 1923–9.

62. Beunen GP, Lefevre J, Philippaerts RM, et al. Adolescent correlates of adult physical activity: a 26-year follow-up. Med Sci Sports Exerc 2004; 36(11):1930–6.

63. Tung R, Zimetbaum P, Josephson ME. A critical appraisal of implantable cardioverter-defibrillator therapy for the prevention of sudden cardiac death. J Am Coll Cardiol 2008;52(14):1111–21.

64. Fananapazir L, Leon MB, Bonow RO, et al. Sudden death during empiric amiodarone therapy in symptomatic hypertrophic cardiomyopathy. Am J Cardiol 1991;67(2):169–74.

65. Melacini P, Maron BJ, Bobbo F, et al. Evidence that pharmacological strategies lack efficacy for the prevention of sudden death in hypertrophic cardiomyopathy. Heart 2007;93(6):708–10.

66. Maron BJ, McKenna WJ, Danielson GK, et al. American College of Cardiology/European Society of Cardiology clinical expert consensus document on hypertrophic cardiomyopathy. A report of the American College of Cardiology Foundation Task Force on Clinical Expert Consensus Documents and the European Society of Cardiology Committee for Practice Guidelines. J Am Coll Cardiol 2003;42(9):1687–713.

67. Elliott P, Spirito P. Prevention of hypertrophic cardiomyopathy-related deaths: theory and practice. Heart 2008;94(10):1269–75.

68. Decker JA, Rossano JW, Smith EO, et al. Risk factors and mode of death in isolated hypertrophic cardiomyopathy in children. J Am Coll Cardiol 2009;54(3):250–4.

69. Ostman-Smith I, Wettrell G, Keeton B, et al. Echocardiographic and electrocardiographic identification of those children with hypertrophic cardiomyopathy who should be considered at high-risk of dying suddenly. Cardiol Young 2005;15(6):632–42.

70. Monserrat L, Elliott PM, Gimeno JR, et al. Non-sustained ventricular tachycardia in hypertrophic cardiomyopathy: an independent marker of sudden death risk in young patients. J Am Coll Cardiol 2003; 42(5):873–9.

71. Cecchi F, Olivotto I, Montereggi A, et al. Prognostic value of non-sustained ventricular tachycardia and the potential role of amiodarone treatment in hypertrophic cardiomyopathy: assessment in an unselected non-referral based patient population. Heart 1998;79(4):331–6.

72. Kofflard MJM, ten Cate FJ, Van Der Lee C, et al. Hypertrophic cardiomyopathy in a large community-based population: clinical outcome and identification of risk factors for sudden cardiac death and clinical deterioration. J Am Coll Cardiol 2003;41(6):987–93.

73. McKenna WJ, Franklin RC, Nihoyannopoulos P, et al. Arrhythmia and prognosis in infants, children and adolescents with hypertrophic cardiomyopathy. J Am Coll Cardiol 1988;11(1):147–53.

74. Spirito P, Maron BJ. Relation between extent of left ventricular hypertrophy and occurrence of sudden cardiac death in hypertrophic cardiomyopathy. J Am Coll Cardiol 1990;15(7):1521–6.

75. Spirito P, Bellone P, Harris KM, et al. Magnitude of left ventricular hypertrophy and risk of sudden death in hypertrophic cardiomyopathy. N Engl J Med 2000; 342(24):1778–85.

76. Cecchi F, Olivotto I, Montereggi A, et al. Hypertrophic cardiomyopathy in Tuscany: clinical course and outcome in an unselected regional population. J Am Coll Cardiol 1995;26(6):1529–36.

77. Maron BJ, Olivotto I, Spirito P, et al. Epidemiology of hypertrophic cardiomyopathy-related death – revisited in a large non-referral-based patient population. Circulation 2000;102(8):858–64.

78. Elliott PM, Blanes JRG, Mahon NG, et al. Relation between severity of left-ventricular hypertrophy and prognosis in patients with hypertrophic cardiomyopathy. Lancet 2001;357(9254):420–4.

79. Sorajja P, Nishimura RA, Ommen SR, et al. Use of echocardiography in patients with hypertrophic cardiomyopathy: clinical implications of massive hypertrophy. J Am Soc Echocardiogr 2006;19(6): 788–95.

80. Efthimiadis GK, Parcharidou DG, Giannakoulas G, et al. Left ventricular outflow tract obstruction as a risk factor for sudden cardiac death in hypertrophic cardiomyopathy. Am J Cardiol 2009; 104(5):695–9.

81. McLeod CJ, Ommen SR, Ackerman MJ, et al. Surgical septal myectomy decreases the risk for appropriate implantable cardioverter defibrillator discharge in obstructive hypertrophic cardiomyopathy. Eur Heart J 2007;28(21):2583–8.

82. Yamaguchi M, Tangkawattana P, Hamlin RL. Myocardial bridging as a factor in heart disorders: critical review and hypothesis. Acta Anat (Basel) 1996; 157(3):248–60.

83. Yetman AT, McCrindle BW, MacDonald C, et al. Myocardial bridging in children with hypertrophic cardiomyopathy – a risk factor for sudden death. N Engl J Med 1998;339(17):1201–9.

84. Basso C, Thiene G, Mackey-Bojack S, et al. Myocardial bridging, a frequent component of the hypertrophic cardiomyopathy phenotype, lacks systematic association with sudden cardiac death. Eur Heart J 2009;30(13):1627–34.

85. Miller GL. Functional assessment of coronary stenoses. J Am Coll Cardiol 1998;32(4):1134.

86. Hillman ND, Mavroudis C, Backer CL, et al. Supraarterial decompression myotomy for myocardial bridging in a child. Ann Thorac Surg 1999;68(1): 244–6.

87. Spirito P, Autore C, Rapezzi C, et al. Syncope and risk of sudden death in hypertrophic cardiomyopathy. Circulation 2009;119(13):1703–10.

88. Moon JC, Reed E, Sheppard MN, et al. The histologic basis of late gadolinium enhancement cardiovascular magnetic resonance in hypertrophic cardiomyopathy. J Am Coll Cardiol 2004;43(12):2260–4.

89. Dimitrow PP, Klimeczek P, Vliegenthart R, et al. Late hyperenhancement in gadolinium-enhanced magnetic resonance imaging: comparison of hypertrophic cardiomyopathy patients with and without nonsustained ventricular tachycardia. Int J Cardiovasc Imaging 2008;24(1):77–83.

90. Kwon DH, Smedira NG, Rodriguez ER, et al. Cardiac magnetic resonance detection of myocardial scarring in hypertrophic cardiomyopathy: correlation with histopathology and prevalence of ventricular tachycardia. J Am Coll Cardiol 2009; 54(3):242–9.

91. Nazarian S, Lima JA. Cardiovascular magnetic resonance for risk stratification of arrhythmia in hypertrophic cardiomyopathy. J Am Coll Cardiol 2008; 51(14):1375–6.

92. Maron BJ, Spirito P, Shen WK, et al. Implantable cardioverter-defibrillators and prevention of sudden cardiac death in hypertrophic cardiomyopathy. J Am Med Assoc 2007;298(4):405–12.

93. Alexander ME, Cecchin F, Walsh EP, et al. Implications of implantable cardioverter defibrillator therapy in congenital heart disease and pediatrics. J Cardiovasc Electrophysiol 2004;15(1):72–6.

Restrictive Cardiomyopathy in Childhood

Susan W. Denfield, MD[a],*,
Steven A. Webber, MBChB, MRCP[b,c,d,e]

KEYWORDS

- Restrictive cardiomyopathy • Children
- Causes • Outcomes

Restrictive cardiomyopathy (RCM) defines a phenotype that may be primary or secondary to another disease. Depending on the part of the world one lives in, it is either one of the rarest forms of cardiomyopathy in childhood, with no cause usually identified,[1–4] or it is secondary to a poorly understood disease, endomyocardial fibrosis (EMF), that is endemic in some populations, with a prevalence as high as 20%.[5] Regardless of underlying cause, outcome is poor by the time most cases become clinically apparent.[3–5]

Primary and secondary RCMs and restrictive physiology in children have received increased recognition recently, yet little progress has been made in understanding the origins of this condition, the identification of risk factors for adverse prognosis, or the development of new therapies. Renewed interest in research on pediatric cardiomyopathies has developed over the past 10 to 15 years, driven largely by the Pediatric Cardiomyopathy Registry (PCMR) funded by the National Heart, Lung, and Blood Institute of the National Institutes of Health.[6] However, the least progress has been made in understanding of RCM compared with other cardiomyopathies, partly because of the rarity of this disorder in developed countries. This article reviews the definitions, epidemiology, etiologies, genetics, "overlap" phenotypes, clinical presentation, diagnostic evaluation, outcome, and management of pediatric patients with RCM, and summarizes the discussion with more questions than answers.

DEFINITIONS OF RCM

The 1995 World Health Organization/International Society and Federation of Cardiology Task Force on the Definition and Classification of Cardiomyopathies defined RCM as a condition "characterized by restrictive filling and reduced diastolic volume of either or both ventricles with normal or near normal systolic function and wall thickness."[7] It was further stated that increased interstitial fibrosis may be present and that the disorder may be idiopathic or associated with other disease (eg, amyloidosis).

In 2006, a consensus panel organized by the American Heart Association (AHA) drew attention to the rapid advancement of molecular genetics in cardiology, and thought that a need existed to develop "Contemporary Definitions and Classification of the Cardiomyopathies."[8] The AHA

[a] Lillie Frank Abercrombie Division of Pediatric Cardiology, Texas Children's Hospital, Baylor College of Medicine, 6621 Fannin MC-19345C, Houston, TX 77030, USA
[b] Department of Pediatrics, University of Pittsburgh School of Medicine, 4401 Penn Avenue, Pittsburgh, PA 15224, USA
[c] Division of Cardiology, Children's Hospital of Pittsburgh of UPMC, 4401 Penn Avenue, Pittsburgh, PA 15224, USA
[d] Heart Center, Children's Hospital of Pittsburgh, 4401 Penn Avenue, Pittsburgh, PA 15224, USA
[e] Pediatric Heart-Lung Transplantation, Children's Hospital of Pittsburgh, 4401 Penn Avenue, Pittsburgh, PA 15224, USA
* Corresponding author.
E-mail address: swdenfie@texaschildrenshospital.org

Heart Failure Clin 6 (2010) 445–452
doi:10.1016/j.hfc.2010.05.005

consensus statement defined primary RCM as a rare form of heart disease characterized by "normal or decreased volume of both ventricles associated with biatrial enlargement, normal left ventricular wall thickness and atrioventricular valves, impaired ventricular filling with restrictive physiology, and normal (or near normal) systolic function."[8] The panel placed RCM in a "mixed" category, as opposed to genetic or acquired, because the diseases were believed to be predominantly nongenetic. As more is learned about RCM, a shift in categorization is likely as genetic and acquired causes are recognized.

EPIDEMIOLOGY

In children in the United States and Australia, RCM accounts for 2.5% to 5% of the diagnosed cardiomyopathies, with most having no specific cause identified.[1,2,4,9] Three different single-institution studies reported 5%, which may have been because of referral bias.[4,9,10] In the Australian-based study by Nugent and colleagues,[2] RCM accounted for 2.5% of the cardiomyopathies diagnosed in children younger than 10 years. This finding is similar to a United States study of two geographic regions, in which Lipshultz and colleagues[1] reported that RCM or other specified types (not dilated or hypertrophic) accounted for 3% of the cardiomyopathies in children younger than 18 years. The estimated annual incidence in the United States and Australia is 0.04 and 0.03 per 100,000 children, respectively.

Sporadic and familial cases of RCM are reported. Of the published cases not secondary to EMF, approximately 30% of patients, in whom family history was reported, had a positive family history.

The most common origin of RCM worldwide is secondary to EMF. EMF is estimated to affect 10 million people worldwide, occurring most often in children and adolescents.[5,11] Familial occurrence, and in some countries a high incidence in some ethnic groups, suggests a possible genetic predisposition.[5,11] In a rural area of Mozambique, the overall prevalence of disease was 20% in the population, but increased to 28% when two family members were affected, and 39% when three or more were affected.[5]

ETIOLOGY, GENETICS, AND OVERLAPPING PHENOTYPES

Outside of the tropics, a specific cause of childhood RCM is rarely found. Infiltrative and storage disorders are very rare in children, and the diagnoses of amyloidosis, sarcoidosis, and hemachromatosis are almost never made. Endomyocardial biopsy usually shows nonspecific changes, such as interstitial fibrosis of varying severity and variable myocyte hypertrophy. Histopathologic changes may be unimpressive. **Box 1** uses a format similar to the AHA consensus statement[8] on primary cardiomyopathies, listing the known causes of RCM. The application of the tools of molecular cardiology to this disorder is in its infancy, but reports of specific gene mutations are increasing in frequency in children.[12–17]

Box 1
Causes of RCM

Genetic

Sarcomeric mutations

    Troponin I

    Troponin T

    Alpha cardiac actin

    Myosin-binding protein C

    Beta myosin heavy chain

    Myosin light chain

Nonsarcomeric mutations

    Desmin

    RSK2 (Coffin-Lowry)

    Lamin A/C (Emery-Dreifuss)

    Transthyretin (amyloidosis)

Mixed

Amyloidosis

Endocardial fiboelastosis

Acquired

EMF

Myocarditis

Cardiac transplant

Pseudoxanthoma elasticum

Diabetic cardiomyopathy

Sarcoidosis

Hemochromatosis

Loffler syndrome

Scleroderma

Carcinoid

Metastatic cancers

Radiation

Drugs

Fatty infiltration

Sarcomeric Protein Gene Defects

RCM has been associated with abnormalities of sarcomeric proteins in children and adults.[12–16] Mogensen and colleagues[12] identified a novel missense mutation of troponin I in a large family with multiple members exhibiting hypertrophic cardiomyopathy (HCM) or RCM. Nine additional cases of RCM were also studied (all nonrelated), and six of these also showed various troponin I mutations. The proband in the large family presented as an 11-year-old boy with heart failure. Family members labeled as having HCM had only mild to moderate hypertrophy, with most having large atria and evidence of restrictive ventricular filling. This family highlights the dilemma of establishing genotypic–phenotypic relationships: should patients with some hypertrophy be labeled as having "atypical RCM with hypertrophy" or should they be considered to have "HCM with restrictive physiology"?

In a follow-up study to the one reported by Mogensen and colleagues,[12] Kubo and colleagues[18] studied a group of adults with HCM and restrictive phenotype. Of 15 patients, 8 had identifiable mutations of sarcomeric genes: 4 in the beta myosin heavy chain gene and 4 in troponin I.[18] This group of patients had a poor prognosis.

In a small series of pediatric patients with RCM, Kaski and colleagues[16] reported that 4 of the 12 patients had a positive family history of cardiomyopathy, but the phenotypes varied and included restrictive, dilated, and left ventricular noncompaction forms. Gene mutations were found in troponin I (TNNI3), troponin T (TNNT2), and alpha cardiac actin (ACTC). In another report, an infant presenting with malignant arrhythmias and RCM was identified as having a de novo mutation of cardiac troponin T.[13] The diversity of the phenotypic expression of troponin (and other) mutations in families suggests that additional genetic and environmental factors, or both, play a role in disease expression.

Ware and colleagues[14] described a mutation in a beta myosin heavy chain gene in an infant with RCM who underwent cardiac transplantation. In adults, mutations in the beta myosin heavy chain account for approximately 40% of mutations found in HCM.[19]

The overlapping genotypic–phenotypic correlations are also evident in a report by Olson and colleagues.[15] A myosin light chain mutation resulted in a cardiomyopathy with mid-cavitary hypertrophy and restrictive physiology that was inherited in an autosomal recessive manner. The proband was a child with two older brothers who had cardiomyopathy with dilated atria, both of whom died of causes related to thrombotic complications: one from a thromboembolic event and the other after surgery to remove a thrombus from the left ventricle. Clinically unaffected family members were either heterozygotes or lacked the mutant allele.

Other mutations in genes encoding sarcomeric proteins have been reported in association with RCM, and others are likely to be forthcoming in the future. It is apparent (as it is for hypertrophic and dilated cardiomyopathies) that many genetic abnormalities can lead to the phenotype of RCM. Furthermore, some of the identified genotypes for RCM can cause hypertrophic and dilated phenotypes in some family members. Evidence also exists of phenotypic overlap between RCM and noncompaction cardiomyopathy.[20–22] Thus, genetic abnormalities identified in noncompaction forms of cardiomyopathy in childhood should also be sought in cases of idiopathic RCM.

Nonsarcomeric Protein Gene Defects

Several mutations of the desmin gene have been found in association with cardiomyopathy, including those of restrictive phenotype.[17,23–25] Desmin is the chief intermediate filament of skeletal and cardiac muscle. It plays an important role in maintaining the structural and functional integrity of the myofibrils. Most desmin mutations seem to be inherited in an autosomal dominant fashion and are associated with skeletal myopathy and cardiomyopathy. Sporadic mutations have also been identified.[23] Conduction abnormalities, including high-grade atrioventricular block, are often present.[17,23] In one large kindred with desmin-associated RCM spanning four generations, no skeletal myopathy was apparent.[24]

Another family has been described in whom five of nine living children had RCM with skeletal and muscle abnormalities.[26] The parents and four siblings were unaffected, suggesting an autosomal recessive inheritance pattern. In this family, desmin accumulation was not seen on endomyocardial biopsy, nor was multicore myopathy on skeletal muscle biopsy. Genetic testing did not show an origin, suggesting that additional genes may result in musculoskeletal abnormalities associated with RCM in children. However, desmin mutations have not been sought in a large cohort of patients with RCM presenting in childhood, and therefore their role in childhood onset disease is not well established.

Several genetic variants of the plasma protein transthyretin (prealbumin) may cause inherited forms of amyloidosis associated with RCM.[27,28] Most seem to be autosomal dominant and may occur with or without peripheral neuropathy. Almost all cases seem to present in adulthood, and these inherited abnormalities have not been reported to be a cause of pediatric RCM.

Coffin-Lowry syndrome is an X-linked disorder caused by mutations in the *RSK2* gene on chromosome Xp22.2.[29] It is characterized by developmental delays, short stature, facial dysmorphism, and progressive skeletal deformities. Cardiac anomalies are reported in approximately 14% of affected men, with cardiomyopathy being one of the rare but reported cardiac abnormalities, including one patient with a restrictive phenotype.[30]

Emery-Dreifuss muscular dystrophy was first described as an X-linked disorder caused by mutations in the gene encoding for emerin on chromosome Xq28.[31] However, it can also be an autosomal disorder caused by mutations in the gene encoding for lamin A and C on chromosome 1q21.2–q21.3.[31] Both variants of the disease can cause cardiac abnormalities, including dilated cardiomyopathy, atrial and ventricular arrhythmias, conduction abnormalities, and sudden death.

Sanna and colleagues[31] reported on the cardiac features of Emery-Dreifuss caused by lamin A/C gene mutations, including one adult patient with a restrictive phenotype. The RCM phenotype has not been reported in children with Emery-Dreifuss.

Overlapping Genotypes/Phenotypes

These reports show that a given gene mutation may have different phenotypic expression, even within the same family, and that phenotypes may overlap with the recognition of patients with mixed features of HCM and RCM. It is of more than semantic interest to correctly identify patients as having overlapping phenotypes. For example, Webber and the PCMR study group[32] evaluated the outcomes of children with a "pure" restrictive phenotype versus those with a mixed RCM/HCM phenotype versus "pure" HCM phenotype. Although both the pure RCM group and the RCM/HCM group fared significantly worse than the pure HCM group, the RCM/HCM group had significantly better event-free survival (freedom from death or transplant) than the pure RCM group. This finding is very important in planning management strategies, because transplantation may be able to be deferred for longer periods in the subgroups with better prognosis. Anecdotally, the authors at their respective institutions have also seen patients with a mixed dilated cardiomyopathy/restrictive phenotype and left ventricular noncompaction with restrictive features. Outcomes of these subtypes await further elucidation.

EMF

EMF was first described by Davies[33] in 1948. It occurs most frequently in tropical and subtropical Africa, particularly Uganda and Nigeria. However, it is found in tropical and subtropical regions throughout the world. It is occasionally seen in temperate climates, usually in individuals who previously lived in tropical areas. The origin or origins remain unknown. Hypereosinophilia, likely related to parasitic infections, has occurred in some patients. However parasitic infections do not seem to have an increased prevalence in patients with EMF. Autoimmunity, genetic, dietary, and environmental chemical factors have all been implicated in the development of EMF.[11]

The histology of EMF is characterized by fibrosis of the endocardium of variable thickness. Histologic changes occur in predominantly three areas: the left ventricular apex, the mitral valve apparatus, and the right ventricular apex, which may extend to the supporting structures of the tricuspid valve. In severe cases, the process may extend to the outflow tracts. Small patches of fibroelastosis may occur in the outflow tracts, but the elastin component is thought to be secondary and not a primary part of the process.

The symptom complex varies with the site or sites of involvement. Symptoms from pulmonary venous congestion and pulmonary hypertension are caused by left-sided disease, whereas right-sided disease results in signs and symptoms from systemic venous congestion. When present, ascites is usually disproportionate to the amount of pedal edema. Involvement of the mitral or tricuspid valve apparatus can result in significant valvular regurgitation. Medical and surgical therapy is palliative.

Mocumbi and colleagues[5] designed a community-based study performed in the costal district of Inharrime, Mozambique to determine the prevalence of the disease and describe its severity and mode of presentation. In their cohort, prevalence was highest among 10- to 19-year-olds, and disease was more common in men than in women and was most commonly biventricular. Most affected subjects had mild to moderate structural and functional echocardiographic abnormalities, but only 23% were symptomatic. These findings are different from those of most studies of RCM, of any origin, because most reports are from hospital referral–based populations, in which most patients are symptomatic.

As Mocumbi and co-authors[5] point out, their large population of affected subjects offers a unique opportunity to study the mechanisms and progression of the disease and to try to develop strategies for prevention and treatment. This research could help promote an understanding of the RCM phenotype, regardless of origin.

CLINICAL PRESENTATION AND DIAGNOSTIC STUDIES

Children with RCM frequently present with respiratory complaints, dyspnea on exertion, "asthma and recurrent lower respiratory tract infections," and exercise intolerance.[34] Abnormal physical examination findings are common, including abnormal heart sounds, such as gallop, loud P2, or murmur; hepatomegaly; and sometimes ascites. Chest pain, syncope, and sudden death have also been presenting signs/symptoms.[35,36]

The electrocardiogram is abnormal approximately 98% of the time.[34] The most common abnormalities are right or left atrial enlargement; however, ST segment depression and ST-T wave abnormalities are frequently present. Right or left ventricular hypertrophy and conduction abnormalities can also be seen.

Holter and event monitors are useful to evaluate for rhythm disturbances, conduction abnormalities, and evidence of ischemia based on ST segment analysis.[35] Arrhythmias have been reported in approximately 15% of pediatric patients and include atrial flutter, high-grade second- and third-degree atrioventricular block, atrial fibrillation, atrial tachycardias, Wolff-Parkinson-White syndrome with supraventricular and ventricular tachycardia, and torsades. Symptomatic sinus bradycardia requiring pacing has also been reported.[35]

On chest radiograph, the most common abnormalities are cardiomegaly, especially atrial enlargement, and pulmonary venous congestion. The chest radiograph is a useful test because it is usually abnormal.[34]

RCM can usually be diagnosed with echocardiogram based on the markedly dilated atria in the absence of significant atrioventricular valve regurgitation. In children, findings consistent with restrictive filling and increased left ventricular end diastolic pressure include elevated mitral valve doppler E/A ratios, short mitral deceleration times, increased pulmonary vein atrial reversal velocity and duration and pulmonary vein atrial reversal duration greater than mitral A duration.[37-39] Systolic function is typically preserved, although some degree of systolic dysfunction has been seen in some patients at presentation, and deterioration of systolic function over time has also been reported in children.[4,38,40,41] Ventricular hypertrophy (by definition) is not prominent, but some degree of concentric increase in septal and left ventricular posterior wall thickness is seen in a significant proportion of patients fulfilling all other criteria for RCM.

Cardiac catheterization is an important part of the evaluation in patients with RCM and should be performed at diagnosis. Pulmonary hypertension is frequently present at initial catheterization, in addition to elevated left or right ventricular end diastolic pressures.[4,38,39,41-43] The pulmonary vasculature may remain reactive, with some studies suggesting the best response to nitric oxide.[42] However, in the study by Weller and colleagues,[41] 40% were precluded from orthotopic heart transplant because of an elevated and nonreactive pulmonary vascular resistance when they were evaluated for cardiac transplantation. None of the studies predicted when, or in whom, fixed pulmonary vascular resistance would develop. Endomyocardial biopsy specimens are usually nondiagnostic, and the procedure is not risk-free in these tenuous patients.[4,44]

MANAGEMENT

No medical therapies clearly improve outcomes in children with RCM. Therapies are predominantly symptom-based. Children with signs and symptoms of pulmonary or systemic venous congestion can benefit symptomatically from the cautious use of diuretics. Care must be taken to avoid excessive diuresis, because these patients are preload-dependent for maintenance of cardiac output.

Children with RCM are at increased risk of thromboembolic events.[4,9,37,38,40,41] Therefore, some form of anticoagulation is warranted in all patients who have no specific contraindications.

As the disease progresses, systolic dysfunction may develop. Use of angiotensin converting enzyme (ACE) inhibitors may be considered. However, vasodilation in patients with minimal to no ability to augment their stroke volume may result in hypotension without augmentation of cardiac output. This phenomenon was observed during acute testing in the cardiac catheterization laboratory in one small series.[45]

β-blockers have been suggested for children who have evidence of ischemia at higher heart rates based on ST-segment analysis on electrocardiogram or Holter.[35] Caution must be used with these agents, because an increase in heart rate may be the only way to augment cardiac output in patients with a relatively fixed stroke volume. If β-blockers are to be used, a careful assessment for evidence of sinus node dysfunction or atrioventricular block should be undertaken before, and after, their institution. Implantable cardiac defibrillators may be considered in patients with evidence of ischemia, unexplained syncope, or ventricular tachycardia. In-hospital monitoring is prudent at the initiation of β-blocker therapy or ACE inhibitors.

Heart transplantation is the definitive treatment for RCM. When comparing survival after RCM diagnosis with survival after cardiac transplantation, cardiac transplantation clearly results in longer survival when considering the population as a whole.[41] Contemporary outcomes from transplantation far exceed the natural history of this disease, which has led some groups to recommend listing for transplantation at presentation, even in asymptomatic patients.[46] Experts widely agree that progressive elevation in pulmonary vascular resistance should lead to early consideration of transplantation.[41,43,47] Elevated pulmonary vascular resistance usually normalizes after transplantation.[43]

Controversy exists over management of patients with few, if any, symptoms and low pulmonary vascular resistance at presentation. However, even these patients have poor transplant-free survival, and this may be the only group of children in whom heart transplantation should be considered in the absence of severe symptoms (the usual criteria for listing for transplantation).[46] Children surviving for 10 years after diagnosis have been reported, but these are a minority and no well-defined predictors exist for determining who these children are prospectively.

OUTCOMES AND THEIR PREDICTION

The prognosis in children with RCM is poor.[4,10,35,37,40,42] Half of the children die or undergo transplantation within 3 years of diagnosis.[3] Sudden cardiac death has been reported to be a common form of death in children with RCM.[35,36] Patients who seem to be at greater risk for sudden death include those who present with signs and symptoms of ischemia, such as syncope and chest pain.[35] However, heart failure–related deaths are the most common. Data from the PCMR showed an increased risk of death or transplant in children who had congestive heart failure at diagnosis.[32] Lower fractional shortening Z score also conferred an incremental increase in risk per unit decrease of fractional shortening Z score.

In some studies, poor prognostic factors for death from heart failure included cardiomegaly and pulmonary venous congestion on chest radiograph, age younger than 5 years, thromboembolism, and elevated pulmonary vascular resistance index.[37,38,41] Children with heart failure are also at risk from ischemic complications.[35] However, in a study by Russo and Webber,[3] age and presence or absence of heart failure symptoms at presentation were not associated with clinical course. The investigators found that right and left ventricular end diastolic pressures and ratio of left atrial to aortic root dimensions (LA:Ao) at presentation had a significantly negative correlation with survival time after diagnosis. Currently, no consistent risk factors have been identified, and early listing for transplantation complicates understanding of the natural history.

FUTURE DIRECTIONS

Improved methods of risk stratification are needed to identify patients with RCM at greatest risk for thromboembolism, rapid progression of elevated pulmonary vascular resistance, heart failure, and sudden death. Longitudinal studies of large asymptomatic populations with EMF could greatly improve understanding of the progression of RCM pathophysiology. Because patients with a mixed RCM/HCM phenotype have a better prognosis than those with pure RCM phenotypes, this is another population that deserves further study to enable a better understanding of the evolution of the phenotype.

The identification of specific genetic mutations, and analysis of their protein products, is leading to mechanistic studies that may unravel the molecular pathology of restrictive disorders. This research may then lead to new therapies that will hopefully delay or reduce the need for cardiac transplantation.

REFERENCES

1. Lipshultz SE, Sleeper LA, Towbin JA, et al. The incidence of pediatric cardiomyopathy in two regions of the United States. N Engl J Med 2003;348:1647–55.
2. Nugent AW, Daubeney P, Chondros P, et al. The epidemiology of childhood cardiomyopathy in Australia. N Engl J Med 2003;348:1639–46.
3. Russo LM, Webber SA. Idiopathic restrictive cardiomyopathy in children. Heart 2005;91:1199–202.
4. Denfield SW, Rosenthal G, Gajarski RJ, et al. Restrictive cardiomyopathies in childhood etiologies and natural history. Tex Heart Inst J 1997; 24:38–44.
5. Mocumbi AO, Ferreira MB, Sidi D, et al. A population study of endomyocardial fibrosis in a rural area of Mozambique. N Engl J Med 2008;359:43–9.
6. Grenier MA, Osganian SK, Cox GF, et al. Design and implementation of the North American

Pediatric Cardiomyopathy Registry. Am Heart J 2000;139:S86–95.

7. Richardson P, McKenna W, Bristow M, et al. Report of the 1995 World Health Organization/International Society and Federation of Cardiology Task Force on the definition and classification of cardiomyopathies. Circulation 1996;93:841–2.

8. Maron BJ, Towbin JA, Thiene G, et al. Contemporary definitions and classification of the cardiomyopathies: an American Heart Association scientific statement. Circulation 2006;1113:1807–16.

9. Lewis AB. Clinical profile and outcome of restrictive cardiomyopathy in children. Am Heart J 1992;123:1589–93.

10. Malčić I, Jelušić M, Kneiwald H, et al. Epidemiology of cardiomyopathies in children and adolescents: a retrospective study over the last 10 years. Cardiol Young 2002;12:253–9.

11. Mocumbi AO, Yacoub S, Yacoub MH. Neglected tropical cardiomyopathies: II. Heart 2008;94:384–90.

12. Mogensen J, Kubo T, Duque M, et al. Idiopathic restrictive cardiomyopathy is part of the clinical expression of cardiac troponin I mutations. J Clin Invest 2003;111(2):209–16.

13. Peddy SB, Vricella LA, Crosson JE, et al. Infantile restrictive cardiomyopathy resulting from a mutation in the cardiac troponin T gene. Pediatrics 2006;117:1830–3.

14. Ware SM, Quinn ME, Ballard ET, et al. Pediatric restrictive cardiomyopathy associated with a mutation in beta-myosin heavy chain. Clin Genet 2008;73:165–70.

15. Olson TM, Karst ML, Whitby FG, et al. Myosin light chain mutation causes autosomal recessive cardiomyopathy with mid-cavitary hypertrophy and restrictive physiology. Circulation 2002;105:2337–40.

16. Kaski JP, Syrris P, Burch M, et al. Idiopathic restrictive cardiomyopathy in children is caused by gene mutations in cardiac sarcomere protein genes. Heart 2008;94:1478–84.

17. Arbustini E, Pasotti M, Pilotto A, et al. Desmin accumulation restrictive cardiomyopathy and atrioventricular block associated with desmin gene defects. Eur J Heart Fail 2006;8:477–83.

18. Kubo T, Gimeno JR, Bahl A, et al. Prevalence, clinical significance, and genetic basis of hypertrophic cardiomyopathy with restrictive phenotype. J Am Coll Cardiol 2007;49:2419–26.

19. Richard P, Charron P, Carrier L, et al. Hypertrophic cardiomyopathy: distribution of disease genes, spectrum of mutations, and implications for molecular diagnosis strategy. Circulation 2003;107:2227–32.

20. Hook S, Ratliff NB, Rosenkranz E, et al. Isolated noncompaction of the ventricular myocardium. Pediatr Cardiol 1996;17:43–5.

21. Ozkutlu S, Hascelik S, Yalnizoglu D, et al. Familial isolated non-compaction of myocardium presenting as restrictive cardiomyopathy. Pediatr Int 2007;49:536–9.

22. Biagini E, Ragni L, Ferlito M, et al. Different types of cardiomyopathy associated with isolated ventricular noncompaction. Am J Cardiol 2006;98:821–4.

23. Dalakas MC, Park KY, Semino-Mora C, et al. Desmin myopathy, a skeletal myopathy with cardiomyopathy caused by mutations in the desmin gene. N Engl J Med 2000;342:770–80.

24. Zhang J, Kumar A, Stalker HJ, et al. Clinical and molecular studies of a large family with desmin-associated restrictive cardiomyopathy. Clin Genet 2001;59:248–56.

25. Goldfarb LG, Park KY, CerveneKova L, et al. Missense mutations in desmin associated with familial cardiac and skeletal myopathy. Nat Genet 1998;19:402–3.

26. Schwartz ML, Colan SD. Familial restrictive cardiomyopathy with skeletal abnormalities. Am J Cardiol 2003;92:636–9.

27. Kushwaha SS, Fallon JT, Fuster V. Restrictive cardiomyopathy. N Engl J Med 1997;336:267–76.

28. Jacobson R, Ittmann M, Buxbaum JN, et al. Transthyretin ile 122 and cardiac amyloidosis in African-Americans: 2 case reports. Tex Heart Inst J 1997;24:45–52.

29. Delaunoy J, Abidi F, Zeniou M, et al. Mutations in the x-linked RSK 2 gene (RPS6KA3) in patients with Coffin–Lowry Syndrome. Hum Mutat 2001;17(2):103–16.

30. Facher JJ, Regier EJ, Jacobs GH, et al. Cardiomyopathy in Coffin–Lowry syndrome. Am J Med Genet A 2004;128:176–8.

31. Sanna T, Dello Russo A, Toniolo D, et al. Cardiac features of Emery-Dreifuss muscular dystrophy caused by lamin A/C gene mutations. Eur Heart J 2003;24:2227–36.

32. Webber S, Lipshultz SE, Sleeper LA, et al. Phenotypic heterogeneity and outcomes of restrictive cardiomyopathy in childhood – a report from the NHLBI Pediatric Cardiomyopathy Registry. Circulation 2008;118(S2):S1055.

33. Davies JN. Endocardial fibrosis in Africans. East Afr Med J 1948;25:10.

34. Denfield SW. Sudden death in children with restrictive cardiomyopathy. Card Electrophysiol Rev 2002;6:163–7.

35. Rivenes SM, Kearney DL, Smith EO, et al. Sudden death and cardiovascular collapse in children with restrictive cardiomyopathy. Circulation 2000;102:876–82.

36. Fitzpatrick AP, Shapiro LM, Rickards AF, et al. Familial restrictive cardiomyopathy with atrioventricular block and skeletal myopathy. Br Heart J 1990;63:114–8.

37. Cetta F, O'Leary PW, Seward JB, et al. Idiopathic restrictive cardiomyopathy in childhood: diagnostic features and clinical course. Mayo Clin Proc 1995; 70:634–40.

38. Chen S, Balfour IC, Jureidini S. Clinical spectrum of restrictive cardiomyopathy in children. J Heart Lung Transplant 2001;20:90–2.

39. Neudorf U, Bolte A, Lang D, et al. Diagnostic findings and outcome in children with primary restrictive cardiomyopathy. Cardiol Young 1996;6:44–7.

40. Gewillig M, Mertens L, Moerman P, et al. Idiopathic restrictive cardiomyopathy in childhood. A diastolic disorder characterized by delayed relaxation. Eur Heart J 1996;17:1413–20.

41. Weller RJ, Weintraub R, Addonizo LJ, et al. Outcome of idiopathic restrictive cardiomyopathy in children. Am J Cardiol 2002;90:501–6.

42. Hughes ML, Kleinert S, Keogh A, et al. Pulmonary vascular resistance and reactivity in children with end-stage cardiomyopathy. J Heart Lung Transplant 2000;19:701–94.

43. Kimberling MT, Balzer DT, Hirsch R, et al. Cardiac transplantation for pediatric restrictive cardiomyopathy: presentation, evaluation and short term outcome. J Heart Lung Transplant 2002;21:455–9.

44. Maki T, Niimura I, Nishikawa T, et al. An atypical case of cardiomyopathy in a child: hypertrophic or restrictive. Heart Vessels Suppl 1990;5:84–7.

45. Bengur AR, Beekman RH, Rocchini AP, et al. Acute hemodynamic effects of Captopril in children with a congestive or restrictive cardiomyopathy. Circulation 1991;83:523–7.

46. Denfield SW. Restrictive cardiomyopathy and constrictive pericarditis. In: Chang AC, Towbin JA, editors. Heart failure in children and young adults: from molecular mechanisms to medical and surgical strategies. Philadelphia: Elsevier; 2006. p. 264–77.

47. Fenton MJ, Chubb H, McMahon AM, et al. Heart and heart-lung transplantation for idiopathic restrictive cardiomyopathy in children. Heart 2006;92:85–9.

Left Ventricular Noncompaction: A New Form of Heart Failure

Jeffrey A. Towbin, MD

KEYWORDS

- Left ventricular noncompaction • LVNC • Heart failure
- Cardiomyopathy • Cardiac genetics • Sarcomere

Left ventricular noncompaction (LVNC), characterized by excessive and unusual trabeculation of the mature left ventricle (LV), has been considered to be a developmental failure of the heart to form fully the compact myocardium during the later stages of cardiac development. Clinically and pathologically, LVNC is characterized by a spongy morphologic appearance of the myocardium, occurring primarily in the LV with the abnormal trabeculations typically being most evident in the apical portion of the LV.[1,2] LVNC is commonly identified by imaging studies as having deep recesses within the thickened apex, and these sinusoids communicate with the ventricular cavity. During heart development, the myocardium is initially trabeculated during a period before coronary artery development, and this has been believed to be an adaptation to provide blood flow to the developing myocardium. Coronary vasculature development is temporally associated with the loss of trabeculae and the full maturation of the compact myocardium. In the normal embryo, the trabeculae regress between embryonic weeks 5 and 8, as the compact myocardium develops from base to apex. In 2006, the American Heart Association scientific statement on classification of cardiomyopathies formally classified LVNC as its own disease entity.[3]

LVNC: OVERVIEW

This disorder has been considered to be a rare disease and has been identified by a variety of names including spongy myocardium, fetal myocardium, noncompaction of the left ventricular myocardium, hypertrabeculation syndrome, and LVNC.[2,4–7] As noted earlier, the abnormality is believed to represent an arrest in the normal process of myocardial compaction, the final stage of myocardial morphogenesis, resulting in persistence of multiple prominent ventricular trabeculations and deep intertrabecular recesses. This cardiomyopathy is difficult to diagnose unless the physician has a high level of suspicion during echocardiographic evaluation. On careful review of echocardiograms and other clinical data, it seems that LVNC is common in children and is also seen in adults.[4,8]

Multiple forms of LVNC occur, including a primary myocardial form of noncompaction, a form associated with electrophysiologic abnormalities and arrhythmias, and noncompaction associated with congenital heart disease (CHD) such as septal defects (ventricular septal defect [VSD] and/or atrial septal defect [ASD]), pulmonic stenosis (PS), and hypoplastic left heart syndrome (HLHS).[4–7,9] In all forms, metabolic derangements may be notable.[5,10]

Funding Support: Dr Towbin is funded, in part, by the National Institutes of Health, National Heart, Lung and Blood Institute (R01 HL53392, and R01 HL087000, the Pediatric Cardiomyopathy Registry and Pediatric Cardiomyopathy Specimen Repository, respectively), and the Cincinnati Children's Kindervelt-Samuel Kaplan Chair in Cardiology.
The Heart Institute, Pediatric Cardiology, Heart Failure, Cardiomyopathy & Heart Transplant Service, Cincinnati Children's Hospital Medical Center, 3333 Burnet Avenue, Cincinnati, OH 45229, USA
E-mail address: jeffrey.towbin@cchmc.org

HISTORICAL DELINEATION OF LVNC

LVNC was first described by Grant[11] in 1926 and, in the past 75 years, has been identified in association with a variety of congenital heart malformations affecting the coronary arteries, left and right ventricular outflow tracts, and interventricular and interatrial septa.[11–16] In the past 20 years, isolated LVNC (ie, not associated with CHD) has also been described, albeit more rarely.[17–29]

NORMAL CARDIAC STRUCTURE

Cardiac muscle fibers comprise separate cellular units (myocytes) connected in series.[30] In contrast to skeletal muscle fibers, cardiac fibers do not assemble in parallel arrays but bifurcate and recombine to form a complex three-dimensional network. Cardiac myocytes are joined at each end to adjacent myocytes at the intercalated disc, the specialized area of interdigitating cell membrane (**Fig. 1**). The intercalated disc contains gap junctions (containing connexins), mechanical junctions, consisting of adherens junctions (containing N-cadherin, catenins, and vinculin), and desmosomes (containing desmin, desmoplakin, desmocollin, and desmoglein). Cardiac myocytes are surrounded by a thin membrane (sarcolemma), and the interior of each myocyte contains bundles of longitudinally arranged myofibrils. The myofibrils are formed by repeating sarcomeres, the basic contractile units of cardiac muscle consisting of interdigitating thin (actin) and thick (myosin) filaments (see **Fig. 1**), which give the muscle its characteristic striated appearance.[31,32] The thick filaments are composed primarily of myosin but additionally contain myosin-binding proteins C, H, and X. The thin filaments are composed of cardiac actin, α-tropomyosin (α-TM), and troponins T, I, and C (cTnT, cTnI, cTnC). In addition, myofibrils contain a third filament formed by the giant filamentous protein, titin, which extends from the Z disc to the M line and acts as a molecular template for the layout of the sarcomere. The Z disc at the borders of the sarcomere is formed by a lattice of interdigitating proteins that maintain myofilament organization by cross-linking antiparallel titin and thin filaments from adjacent sarcomeres. Other proteins in the Z disc include α-actinin, nebulette, telethonin/T-cap, capZ, muscle LIM protein (MLP), myopalladin, myotilin, Cypher/ZASP, filamin, and FATZ.[31–33]

The extrasarcomeric cytoskeleton, a complex network of proteins linking the sarcomere with the sarcolemma and the extracellular matrix (ECM), provides structural support for subcellular structures and transmits mechanical and chemical signals within and between cells. The extrasarcomeric cytoskeleton has intermyofibrillar and subsarcolemmal components, with the intermyofibrillar cytoskeleton composed of intermediate filaments (IFs), microfilaments, and microtubules.[34,35] Desmin IFs form a three-dimensional scaffold throughout the extrasarcomeric cytoskeleton with desmin filaments surrounding the Z disc, allowing for longitudinal connections to adjacent Z discs and lateral connections to subsarcolemmal costameres.[35] Microfilaments composed of nonsarcomeric actin (mainly γ-actin) also form complex networks linking the sarcomere (via α-actinin) to various components of the costameres. Costameres are subsarcolemmal domains located in a periodic, gridlike pattern, flanking the Z discs and overlying the I bands, along the cytoplasmic side of the sarcolemma. These costameres are sites of interconnection between various cytoskeletal networks linking sarcomere and sarcolemma, and are believed to function as anchor sites for stabilization of the sarcolemma and for integration of pathways involved in mechanical force transduction. Costameres contain 3 principal components: the focal adhesion-type complex, the spectrin-based complex, and the dystrophin/dystrophin-associated protein complex (DAPC).[36,37] The focal adhesion-type complex, comprising cytoplasmic proteins (ie, vinculin, talin, tensin, paxillin, zyxin), connect with cytoskeletal actin filaments and with the transmembrane proteins α-, β-dystroglycan, α-, β-, γ-, δ-sarcoglycans, dystrobrevin, and syntrophin. Several actin-associated proteins are located at sites of attachment of cytoskeletal actin filaments with costameric complexes, including α-actinin and MLP. The C-terminus of dystrophin binds β-dystroglycan (see **Fig. 1**), which in turn interacts with α-dystroglycan to link to the ECM (via α-2-laminin). The N-terminus of dystrophin interacts with actin. Voltage-gated sodium channels colocalize with dystrophin, β-spectrin, ankyrin, and syntrophins whereas potassium channels interact with the sarcomeric Z disc and intercalated discs.[38,39] Because arrhythmias and conduction system diseases are common in children and adults with dilated cardiomyopathy (DCM), this could play an important role. Hence, disruption of the links from the sarcolemma to ECM at the dystrophin C-terminus and those to the sarcomere and nucleus via N-terminal dystrophin interactions could lead to a domino effect disruption of systolic function and development of arrhythmias.

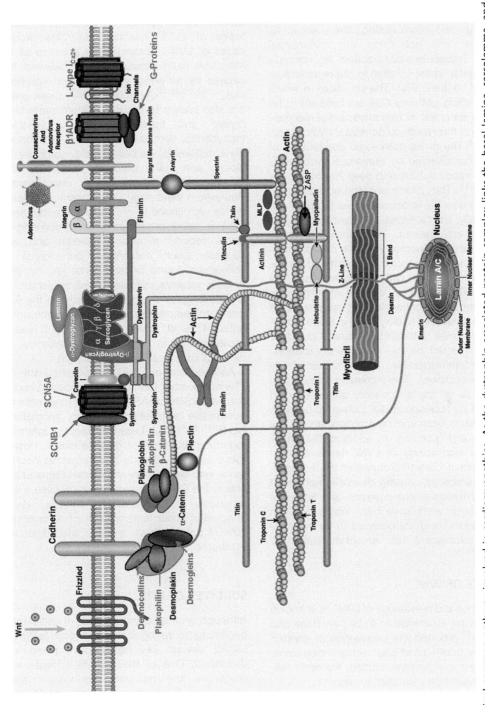

Fig. 1. The final common pathway involved in cardiomyopathies. As the dystrophin-associated protein complex links the basal lamina, sarcolemma, and sarcomere, mutant proteins cause dilated, hypertrophic, or a combined cardiomyopathy.

PATHOLOGY OF LVNC

In the early embryo, the heart is a loose interwoven mesh of muscle fibers.[16] The developing myocardium gradually condenses, and the large spaces within the trabecular meshwork disappear, condensing and compacting the ventricular myocardium and solidifying the endocardial surfaces. Trabecular compaction is normally more complete in the LV than in the myocardium of the right ventricle (RV). The situations in which this compacting pathway fails are believed to be caused by an arrest in endomyocardial morphogenesis, and this results in postnatal LV noncompaction.[4,16] The gross pathologic appearance of LVNC is characterized by numerous excessively prominent trabeculations and deep intertrabecular recesses.[4,17] The prominent trabeculations of LVNC resemble RV endomyocardial morphology. Histologically, the recesses and their troughs are lined with endothelium, indicating that these recesses are not sinusoids. In some cases, zones of fibrous and elastic tissue are scattered on the endocardial surfaces with extension into the recesses. The coronary arterial circulation is usually normal and extramural myocardial blood supply is not believed to play a role in these abnormalities. However, intramural perfusion could be adversely affected by the prominent trabeculations and intertrabecular recesses, particularly the subendocardium. The increased fibrous and elastic tissue on the endocardial surfaces could be caused by subendocardial ischemia, perhaps in response to isometric contraction among the trabeculae and recesses. In addition, the endomyocardial morphology of LVNC lends itself to development of mural thrombi within the recesses, which can embolize, causing clinical symptoms of stroke.[4] Arrhythmias are common and zones of thin ventricular walls have been noted by Chin and colleagues[4] and are believed to be morphologically reminiscent of arrhythmogenic RV dysplasia.[40–42]

INCIDENCE OF LVNC

The incidence and prevalence of LVNC is unknown but the disease is considered to be rare. Ritter and colleagues[17] reported the prevalence of isolated LVNC to be 0.05% of all adult echocardiographic examinations in a large institution. No other reliable data have been reported to date.

CLINICAL FEATURES AND DIAGNOSIS OF LVNC

LVNC commonly presents in infancy with signs and symptoms of congestive heart failure (CHF).[4,7] Echocardiographically, this disorder is characterized by systolic dysfunction associated with a dilated, hypertrophic LV. The characteristic deep trabeculations are typically noted in the LV apex and lateral wall; regional wall motion abnormalities are common. Multiple forms of LVNC are reported. One group of cases of LVNC occurs in the absence of other structural heart disease and is believed to be caused by an arrest of myocardial morphogenesis.[4,7,17–29,43,44] As noted earlier, these patients are also known to develop systemic arterial embolism and severe arrhythmias (ventricular tachycardia, ventricular fibrillation) or conduction abnormalities (sinus bradycardia, complete heart block), and many succumb in infancy. Wolff-Parkinson-White syndrome is also common.[7] However, others may not present until later in life (ie, adulthood.)[17,18] These patients seem to have a good prognosis when presenting late. Some reports in young children and adults suggest poor outcomes, but Ichida and colleagues[7] found better survival and symptoms in their patients, all diagnosed in Japan. Chin and colleagues[4] reported 3 deaths in the 8 children studied, whereas Ritter and colleagues[17] noted 47% of adults dying within 6 years of presentation. In symptomatic patients, 75% died within 6 years of presentation.

Another form of LVNC is associated with CHD. This nonisolated form of LVNC occurs in conjunction with VSDs, or ASDs, PS and other right heart obstructive and pulmonary artery anomalies, or HLHS.[11–14,43,44] Less clinical information regarding this form of disease exists. However, these patients seem to have a similar course to those with the primary myocardial forms of LVNC unless the CHD is severe, in which case a worse prognosis is apparent. The RV may also be affected in either form of LVNC.[29] Approximately 10% of patients have an associated dysmorphic syndrome.

SUBTYPES OF LVNC

Although an increasing number of clinicians are beginning to recognize the clinical features of LVNC, several key points have failed to be described. One of the important issues in the diagnosis and outcomes of these patients, particularly in childhood, is the specific LVNC phenotype that exists in any 1 patient. There are at least 7 different phenotypes of LVNC and these different phenotypes have different outcomes (**Fig. 2**). The subtypes include the following:

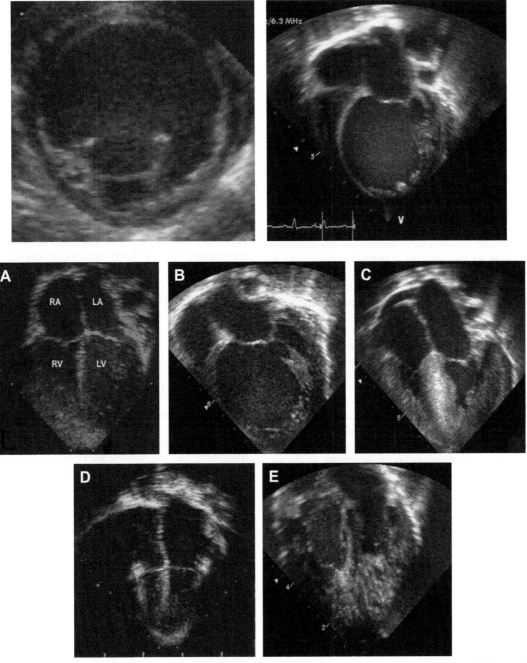

Fig. 2. Echocardiographic image of heterogeneous forms of LV noncompaction. (*Top panel*) Parasternal short-axis view of a dilated form of LVNC. The apical trabeculations are noted at the apex. An apical 4-chamber view at the right side of the figure demonstrates the same findings. (*Lower panel*) Heterogeneous phenotypes associated with LVNC. (*A*) LVNC with normal LV size, thickness, and function. (*B*) Dilated form of LVNC. (*C*) Hypertrophic form of LVNC. (*D*) Restrictive form of LVNC. (*E*) Biventricular LVNC.

Isolated LVNC

In this subtype, there is normal LV size, thickness, and function with no evidence of arrhythmias. Clinically, this subgroup seems to be benign during childhood and approximates 25% of all patients. The authors typically follow this subgroup yearly in the outpatient clinic, do not treat with medication, and do not restrict from activities.

Isolated LVNC with Arrhythmias

This is an uncommon group in which there is normal LV size, thickness, and function on echocardiography but has predominant arrhythmias, most typically runs of tachyarrhythmias. These patients seem to have an increased risk of sudden events and require closer follow-up and therapeutic intervention, either with medication or implantable defibrillator, depending on the specific arrhythmia and associated symptoms.

Dilated Form of LVNC

This patient subgroup clinically mimics DCM and likely has similar outcomes. The follow-up of these patients is similar to those with pure DCM. An important differentiating feature is the potential for this to become an undulating phenotype in which the heart changes its appearance to either a hypertrophic form or one with normal LV size, thickness, and function on echocardiography but later reverts back to the DCM-like phenotype. The electrocardiograms (ECGs) of these patients, particular young children, may include pre-excitation with or without severe increase in voltage, particularly in the midprecordium.

Hypertrophic Form of LVNC

This subgroup mimics hypertrophic cardiomyopathy (HCM) and likely has similar outcomes. The follow-up of these patients is similar to those with pure HCM. An important differentiating feature is the potential for this to become an undulating phenotype in which the heart changes its appearance to either a dilated form or one with normal LV size, thickness, and function on echocardiography but later reverts back to the HCM-like phenotype. The ECGs of these patients, particular young children, may include pre-excitation with or without severe increase in voltage, particularly in the midprecordium.

Hypertrophic and Dilated Form of LVNC

This subgroup seems to be the worst form of LVNC clinically and, in many cases, is associated with neuromuscular disease and hypotonia. These young children, particularly infants, may succumb, especially if they have metabolic derangement. The ECGs of these patients, particular young children, may include pre-excitation with or without severe increase in voltage, particularly in the midprecordium. An important differentiating feature is the potential for this to become an undulating phenotype in which the heart changes its appearance to either a dilated or hypertrophic form on echocardiography but later reverts back to the HCM-dilated phenotype.

Restrictive Form of LVNC

This rare form of LVNC is also clinically challenging as it mimics the clinical behavior of restrictive cardiomyopathy (RCM). Like the children with RCM, patients in this subgroup typically are considered transplant candidates early after diagnosis.

LVNC with CHD

In this subgroup, any form of CHD can occur in conjunction with LVNC. The most common simple forms of CHD include septal defects and/or PS. However, LVNC has been identified in patients with severe forms of CHD including single ventricles and heterotaxy syndrome. Outcomes depend on the specific CHD but may be worse than the postoperative outcomes of the same CHD without LVNC. In this case, the surgeon, cardiac anesthesiologist, and cardiac intensivist must pay close attention to the myocardial function and treat it expectantly.

IMAGING OF LVNC

Echocardiography has been used to diagnose and describe LVNC. Recently, Punn and Silverman[45] investigated LVNC using the 16-segment model described by the American Heart Association and the American Society of Echocardiography in 44 children with LVNC. Using the ratio of noncompaction to compaction, the investigators analyzed the 16 segments and determined whether severity was correlated with poor outcomes in these affected children. The 16-segment noncompaction/compaction ratio, shortening fraction (SF), and ejection fraction (EF) were measured retrospectively in all children with LVNC. Forty-four patients had LVNC, which was consistent with an incidence of 0.3% of admissions. Twenty-eight patients (64%) who remained alive were in one group, and 16 patients (36%) who either died or were transplanted constituted the other group. This latter group had a substantial number of patients with significant associated CHD, compared with the other group that survived (50% vs 18%, $P<.05$). Similar regions of involvement in the 16-segment model was notable, with sparing of basal segments and involvement of the midpapillary and apical regions ($P<.001$); however, patients in the group with a high percentage of death and transplant were noted to have more segments involved (6 vs 4, $P<.05$), lower SFs (16% vs 29%, $P<.001$), and lower EFs

(24% vs 47%, P<.001). The EF was inversely related to the number of segments (r = −0.63, P<.01), suggesting that more noncompaction portends a worse outcome. In the younger patients with noncompaction, poor outcomes, such as low EFs, death, and transplantation, were found to be related to the number of LV segments involved. There was more associated CHD in the pediatric population, and this carried a poorer prognosis than the disease reported in adult populations.

Cardiac magnetic resonance (CMR) imaging is another imaging modality that has been used to evaluate and diagnose LVNC. Thuny and colleagues[46] compared two-dimensional echocardiography images obtained at end diastole and end systole with CMR images obtained at end diastole to validate the diagnosis of LVNC. Sixteen patients (48 ± 17 years) with LVNC underwent echocardiography and CMR within the same week. Echocardiography images obtained at end diastole and end systole were compared in a blinded fashion with those obtained by CMR at end diastole to assess noncompaction in 17 anatomic segments. All segments were analyzed by CMR, whereas only 238 (87.5%) and 237 (87.1%) could be analyzed by echocardiography at end diastole and end systole, respectively (P = .002). Among the analyzable segments, a 2-layered structure was observed in 54% by CMR, 43% by echocardiography at end diastole, and 41% by echocardiography at end systole (P = .006). Similar distribution patterns were observed with echocardiography. However, compared with echocardiography, CMR identified a higher rate of 2-layered structures in the anterior,

anterolateral, inferolateral, and inferior segments. Echocardiography at end systole underestimated the end diastole noncompaction/compaction maximum ratio compared with CMR (P = .04) and echocardiography at end diastole (P = .003). No significant difference was observed between CMR and echocardiography at end diastole (P = .83). Interobserver reproducibility of the non-compaction/compaction maximum ratio was similar between CMR and echocardiography. Therefore, CMR was considered to be superior to standard echocardiography in assessing the extent of noncompaction and provide supplemental morphologic information beyond that obtained with conventional echocardiography. However, in children, this has not been validated.

Irrespective of the imaging modality selected, the specific subtype of LVNC must be characterized in detail. The authors tend to focus a significant amount of effort on the apical 4-chamber view for trabeculations, particular in the apex where a filled-in appearance is commonly notable. Parasternal long- and short-axis views commonly demonstrate a thicker-than-expected apex and free wall, particularly in those with a dilated phenotype.

ELECTROCARDIOGRAPHY IN LVNC

The ECG in patients with LVNC is typically abnormal and commonly has giant voltages (**Fig. 3**).[2,7] These patients, particularly the childhood forms of LVNC, may be associated with pre-excitation. In approximately 30% of patients with LVNC, particularly children, there is extreme mid-precordial voltages that mimic the ECG seen in

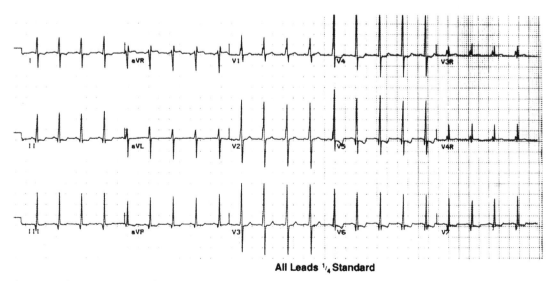

All Leads ¹/₄ Standard

Fig. 3. ECG in LV noncompaction.

Pompe disease. Arrhythmias, including supraventricular tachycardia and ventricular tachycardia, are common and dangerous accompaniments to all subtypes of LVNC.

CLINICAL GENETICS OF LVNC

LVNC most commonly has X-linked recessive or autosomal dominant inheritance.[7,8] In X-linked LVNC, female carriers have not been found to develop frank clinical disease, and are echocardiographically normal. Consistent with X-linked inheritance, no male-to-male transmission of the disease occurs.[19] In some cases of LVNC without CHD, and most, if not all, cases of the form associated with CHD, autosomal dominant inheritance is seen in familial cases.[7,8] When LVNC is associated with CHD, the congenital cardiac defect may be heterogeneous in families but is transmitted as an autosomal dominant trait along with the myocardial abnormality. In some families with autosomal dominant LVNC associated with CHD, affected members may be identified in whom no CHD can be identified at the time of evaluation because the cardiac defects include minor forms of CHD, such as small VSDs, ASDs, or patent ductus arteriosus, which have spontaneously closed, along with other individuals with severe CHD, such as HLHS. Penetrance may be reduced in some families. Ichida and colleagues[7] reported that 44% of her LVNC patients had inherited LVNC, with 70% having autosomal dominant and 30% X-linked inheritance.

MOLECULAR GENETICS OF LVNC

A genetic cause of isolated LVNC was initially described by Bleyl and colleagues[19] when they identified mutations in the gene G4.5/TAZ in patients and carrier women. This gene, known as G4.5 or tafazzin (TAZ), encodes a novel protein family (tafazzins) with unclear function, and is also responsible for Barth syndrome (BTS)[47] and other forms of infantile cardiomyopathies.[48,49] BTS is a clinical association of myocardial dysfunction, neutropenia, skeletal myopathy, abnormal mitochondria, organic aciduria (primarily 3-methylglutaconic aciduria), growth retardation, and cholesterol abnormalities.[50–53] It is an X-linked disorder and has been believed to be allelic to several phenotypically different disorders on Xq28,[54,55] such as LVNC and DCM. Congenital heart defects have not been associated with BTS or other G4.5-associated disease. The genetic basis of autosomal dominant LVNC has also been studied and multiple genes have been identified. In children and young adults with LVNC, with or without CHD, Ichida and colleagues[9]

identified mutations in α-dystrophobrevin as causative. In addition, mutations in the Z-line protein encoding ZASP, located on chromosome 10q22, have been identified in isolated noncompaction.[56] Subsequently, mutations in sarcomere-encoding genes were identified. Klaassen and colleagues[57] demonstrated that mutations in β-myosin heavy chain (MYH7), α-cardiac actin, and cTnT. In addition to sarcomere-encoding genes and the cytoskeleton, mutations in the sodium channel gene, SCN5A, have been shown by Shan and colleagues[58] to cause LVNC and rhythm disturbance. Another cytoskeletal protein that has been associated with LVNC is dystrophin in boys with Duchenne muscular dystrophy (DMD) and Becker muscular dystrophy (BMD).[59] Skeletal muscle biopsy has, in some patients, identified mitochondrial abnormalities, suggesting a nuclear import protein as the primary abnormality. In addition, mutation analysis of the mitochondrial genome has recently identified mutations.[60] Consideration of other potential genetic causes need to take into account the known molecular defects resulting in congenital heart anomalies, as well as those molecular abnormalities resulting in diseases of the myocardium itself.

POTENTIAL MECHANISMS OF LVNC
Final Common Pathway Hypothesis

To put the mechanisms responsible for cardiovascular disorders into perspective, a unifying hypothesis has been developed that helps to predict the central targets and interacting, modifying cascades that, when disordered, result in a specific phenotype. For instance, familial hypertrophic cardiomyopathy (FHC) is a genetically heterogeneous disease in which 17 genes have been identified to cause this phenotype when mutated.[61] As previously noted, the mutated gene most commonly encodes a sarcomeric protein, suggesting that FHC is a disease of the sarcomere (ie, sarcomyopathy).[61,62] In some cases, genes encoding for mitochondrial or other metabolic proteins are causative, and many of these are required for proper sarcomere function because of the need of the sarcomere for ATP. Mild differences in the clinical phenotype may occur but, in general, mutations disrupting proteins of the thick filament (β-myosin heavy chain, myosin-binding protein-C, essential and regulatory myosin light chains), thin filament (actin, troponin T and I, tropomyosin), or support (titin) result in a similar phenotype. Hence, the primary target in FHC is the sarcomere (ie, the final common pathway to hypertrophy). Clinical outcomes may differ depending on the gene mutated, the specific mutation within the gene, or changes within modifying cascades, such as mitochondrial function, the angiotensin-converting enzyme (ACE) gene, calcineurin pathway, or use of medications such as cyclosporine or FK506.[63] Similarly, primary ventricular arrhythmias have been shown by our group and others to occur when the central target, ion channels, is disrupted.[64] In long QT syndrome (LQTS), at least 12 genetic loci have been identified that encode ion channels or protein-binding partners that, when mutated, disturb the proper function of the channel. Mutations in either α subunits of the potassium channels (KVLQT1, HERG) or their associated β subunits (minK, MiRP1) result in ventricular arrhythmias.[65] The β subunit of the sodium channel has also been implicated. Mutations in the ion channel genes result in significant clinical heterogeneity, not dissimilar to that seen in FHC, albeit more severe. For instance, heterozygous mutations show incomplete penetrance, whereas homozygous mutations not only result in severe phenotype and poor prognosis but also result in associated deafness. Mutations in the sodium channel gene SCN5A result in multiple different forms of rhythm disorders including LQTS, idiopathic ventricular fibrillation/Brugada syndrome (short QT interval, ST-segment increase in leads V1-V3, and ventricular fibrillation), and progressive conduction system disease (Lev/Lenegre disease), all different phenotypes. In addition, mutations in SCN5A can cause DCM.

In DCM, the cytoskeleton or sarcolemma seem to be the central targets (see **Fig. 1**).[66,67] Dystrophin has been shown by our laboratory to cause X-linked DCM[68,69] and is also mutated in DMD/BMD, in which skeletal myopathy and associated DCM are notable. Actin, which binds to the N-terminus of dystrophin, thus linking the sarcolemma and sarcomere, also causes DCM when mutated at the dystrophin-binding domain. Desmin, vinculin, lamin A/C, and proteins comprising the DAPC all result in DCM (with or without skeletal myopathy) when mutated.[70] In most cases, these genes play a major role in the integrity of the sarcolemma/cytoskeleton and link with the sarcomere. Similar to that seen with FHC, mitochondrial dysfunction further modifies the clinical phenotype, as does calcineurin, the adrenergic nervous system, and mechanical stress.

This hypothesis can be extended to include vascular disease. Aortic root dilatation and mitral valve prolapse (MVP) are associated with mutations in the collagen vascular system.[71] In Marfan syndrome (MFS), fibrillin mutations result in a pleiotropic, clinically heterogeneous disorder with dilated aortic root and MVP commonly noted.

Other forme frustes of MFS, typically with aortic root and mitral valve disease, also result from fibrillin mutations or mutations in pathways that disrupt the function of fibrillin or members of its pathway (transforming growth factor [TGF]-β). In a high percentage of cases, disruption in the TGF-β pathway seems to be the culprit.[72]

This final common pathway hypothesis is useful in the identification of the central targets and modifying cascades for all cardiovascular phenotypes. Understanding the genetic basis of the disease in any patient could translate into improved survival and better treatment options.

ANIMAL MODELS OF LVNC

A significant number of mouse models with cardiomyopathy have been described in the past several years. However, few have a clear phenotype similar to LVNC, although several have had a hypertrophic, dilated heart with systolic dysfunction. One of the best models of LVNC to date is the FKBP12-deficient mouse, but others exist.[73,74] Models deficient in the sarcoglycan complex and its associated proteins (ie, sarcospan, syntrophin) have commonly been shown to develop a hypertrophic, dilated heart.[75–83] The cardiomyopathic hamster, a naturally occurring model with this type of phenotype, has been shown to be caused by a δ-sarcoglycan deletion.[84–86] Mutations in this and other members of the dystrophin-DAPC complex, have been found to cause DCM with or without skeletal myopathy in humans.

Cypher/ZASP Knockout Mouse

Cypher/ZASP is a cytoskeletal protein localized in the sarcomeric Z line. Mutations in its encoding gene have been identified in patients with LVNC, DCM, and HCM. This gene is known as cypher in the mouse and ZASP or LIM domain–binding protein-3 (LBD3) in the human. Ju Chen and colleagues[87–90] have developed a variety of cypher mutant models including a cardiac-specific cypher knockout mouse which developed a severe form of DCM with disrupted cardiomyocyte ultrastructure and decreased cardiac function. These mice typically died before 23 weeks of age. A similar phenotype was observed by this group in inducible cardiac-specific knockout mice in which cypher was specifically ablated in the adult myocardium. In both cardiac-specific models, ERK and Stat3 signaling pathways were augmented. In addition, they were able to demonstrate the specific binding of the PDZ domain of cypher to the C-terminal region of both calsarcin-1 and myotilin within the Z line.[91] These studies suggest that cypher plays a pivotal role in maintaining adult cardiac structure and cardiac function through protein-protein interactions with other Z-line proteins. Myocardial ablation of cypher resulted in DCM with premature death, and showed that specific signaling pathways participate in cypher mutant–mediated dysfunction of the heart, facilitating the progression to heart failure.

FKBP12 Null Mutation

FKBP12, a *cis-trans* prolyl isomerase that binds the immunosuppressants FK506 and rapamycin, is a ubiquitously expressed protein that interacts with proteins in several intracellular signal transduction systems.[92] FKBP12 interacts with the cytoplasmic domains of type I receptors of the TGF-β superfamily[93–95] as well as with multiple intracellular calcium release channels including the tetrameric skeletal muscle ryanodine receptor (RyR).[96,97] Because exons 3 and 4 of FKBP12 encode functional domains involved in FK506 and rapamycin binding,[98] *cis-trans* prolyl isomerase activity,[98] and TGF-β family type I receptor binding,[92,93] Shou and colleagues[73] developed a mouse model in which this region was deleted, using embryonic stem cell technology to generate a null mutation by targeted deletion (fkbp12[ml]/+) of these key exons. Heterozygous mice (fkbp12^{ml}/+) were viable and fertile and were intercrossed to obtain FKBP12-deficient (fkbp12^{ml}/fkbp12^{ml}) mice. At weaning, 8 viable FKBP12-deficient mice were observed; the remainder died between embryonic stage E14.5 and birth because of severe LVNC with VSD. Anatomically, the hearts had greatly increased weight compared with the wild type (WT), the ventricular walls were of roughly equal thickness and highly trabeculated with deep intertrabecular recesses, and VSD was consistently identified. In addition, the liver had centrolobular necrosis similar to that seen in passive congestion associated with CHF. Echocardiographically, severe reduction in systolic function was noted with SF less than 20% (WT SF = 42%) and EF of approximately 35% (WT EF = 65%). Analysis of RyR1 and RyR2 function in skeletal muscles of affected animals showed increased probability of opening compared with WT mice, as well as increased frequency of substrate channel openings. The investigators suggested that FKBP12 is actively involved in the cooperative interactions between subunits of the RyR tetramer and that the cardiac-specific phenotype (ie, no evidence of skeletal muscle disease) was caused by differences in gating properties between cardiac calcium release channels (which are activated by

Ca^{2+} influx) and skeletal muscle channels (which are regulated by the T-tubule voltage sensor), which reduce the calcium leak from the sarcoplasmic reticuluum in skeletal muscle versus heart. Thus, changes in resting cytosolic calcium in cardiac tissue could contribute to the cardiac functional abnormalities seen in these animals. However, the development of CHD was not clearly defined mechanistically; TGF-β–mediated signaling was not different between WT and mutant animals. FKBP12 (and related proteins) will be a major focus of the mutation screening studies.

NF-ATc Mutant

In lymphocytes, the expression of early immune response genes is regulated by NF-AT transcription factors[99,100] that translocate to the nucleus after dephosphorylation by the Ca^{2+}-dependent phosphatase calcineurin.[101] Mice bearing a disruption of the NF-ATc gene were reported by de la Pompa and colleagues[102] to have abnormal cardiac valves and septa and to die of circulatory failure by embryonic day 14.5. Because NF-ATc is first expressed in the heart at day 7.5 and is restricted to endocardium, disruption is likely to lead to significant defects in the valves, septum, and endocardium, all of which are dependent on normal endocardial development. Within endocardium, specific inductive events activate NF-ATc. FK506 treatment inhibits calcineurin and prevents nuclear localization of NF-ATc, suggesting that Ca^{2+}/calcineurin/NF-ATc signaling pathway is important in normal valve/septal morphogenesis. The mutant mice confirm this because they develop cardiac abnormalities by E12.5. In 40% of mutants, the ventricular walls were hypertrophic and small with LV outflow tract narrowing. The semilunar valves were stenotic and the atrioventricular valves were dysplastic. An ASD was also notable, as was a trabeculated LV. This gene will also be a focus of the candidate gene screening process.

THERAPY AND OUTCOME

The specific therapy depends on the clinical and echocardiographic findings. In patients with systolic dysfunction and heart failure, anticongestive therapy identical to those used in patients with DCM is appropriate. In particular, ACE inhibitors such as captopril and enalapril are useful, as well as β-adrenergic blocking agents such as metoprolol or carvedilol. Diuretics may also be needed. However, in those patients exhibiting findings more consistent with an HCM or diastolic dysfunction physiologic phenotype, β-blocker therapy alone with propranolol or atenolol is more appropriate. In patients with either of these forms of noncompaction with associated mitochondrial or metabolic dysfunction some investigators add a vitamin cocktail to the cardiac therapy with coenzyme Q10, carnitine, riboflavin, and thiamine commonly used alone or in combination.

In patients having associated CHD, appropriate therapeutic approaches may include simple pharmacologic therapy with diuretics for volume overload associated with left-to-right shunts, more complex pharmacologic therapy for patients with restrictive physiology and pulmonary hypertension, or invasive therapy with catheter intervention or surgical repairs, depending on the lesions. Intimate understanding of the cardiac function abnormalities, evidence of thrombi (which should be treated with anticoagulation), and the metabolic status of the patient must be attended to by the interventional cardiologist, cardiac anesthesiologist, and surgeon in approaching these patients invasively. In addition, cardiac rhythm disturbances need to be identified and therapies such as pacemakers, implantable defibrillators, and intracardiac ablations considered.

The clinical outcome of patients with noncompaction has been reported to be poor, with death occurring because of heart failure or sudden death presumably arrhythmia related or stroke related because of embolization of left ventricular thrombi.[7] However, Pignatelli and colleagues[2] found a 5-year survival rate of 86%; when transplanted patients were added, the 5-year survival free of death or transplantation was 75%.

SYSTEMIC DISEASES ASSOCIATED WITH LV NONCOMPACTION
BTS

Initially described as X-linked cardioskeletal myopathy with abnormal mitochondria and neutropenia by Neustein and colleagues[51] and Barth and colleagues,[50] this disorder typically presents in male infants as CHF associated with neutropenia (cyclic) and 3-methylglutaconic aciduria.[52] Mitochondrial dysfunction is noted on electron microscopy and electron transport chain biochemical analysis. In addition, abnormalities in cardiolipin have been noted.[103] Echocardiographically these infants typically have left ventricular dysfunction with left ventricular dilation, endocardial fibroelastosis, or a dilated hypertrophic LV. In some cases, these infants succumb because of CHF/sudden death, ventricular thrombi/ventricular fibrillation, or sepsis caused by leukocyte dysfunction. Most of these children survive past infancy and do well clinically, although DCM

usually persists. In some cases, cardiac transplantation has been performed. Histopathologic evaluation typically demonstrates the features of DCM, although endocardial fibroelastosis may be prominent and the mitochondria are abnormal in shape and abundance.

The genetic basis of BTS was first described by Bione and colleagues,[47] who cloned the disease-causing gene, G4.5. This gene encodes a novel protein called tafazzin, whose gene product is an acyltransferase and results in cardiolipin abnormalities.[103] Mutations in G4.5 result in a wide clinical spectrum, which includes apparently classic DCM, hypertrophic DCM, endocardial fibroelastosis, or LVNC.[8,19]

Energy-dependent Forms of LVNC

Mitochondrial cardiomyopathies
The human mitochondrial genome[103] is a small, circular DNA molecule that is maternally inherited. Mitochondrial DNA (mtDNA) encodes 13 of the 69 proteins required for oxidative metabolism, 22 transfer RNAs (tRNAs), and 2 ribosomal RNAs (rRNAs) required for their translation. Because mtDNA has less redundancy than the nuclear genome (in which essentially identical information is received from both parents), and tRNAs and rRNAs are present in multiple copies, the mitochondrial genome is an excellent target for mutations producing human disease.[104–106] Mitochondria have a symbiotic relationship with the cell. These subcellular organelles are dependent on nucleocytoplasmic mechanisms for most structural components, but do contribute vital peptides that are central to cellular respiration. Mitochondria contain a permeable outer membrane and a highly restrictive inner membrane that guards the chemical microenvironment of the matrix compartment. Adaptive mechanisms exist for the passage of large and small molecules across the inner membrane. Translocases shuttle monocarboxylic acids, amino acids, acylcarnitine conjugates, small ions, and other metabolites in and out of the mitochondrial matrix. Energy is required for importation of proteins into the mitochondria because the nuclear gene-synthesized mitochondrial proteins are precursor molecules that require presequence cleavage. The 13 mtDNA genes are located in the respiratory chain[106–108] and include 7 complex I subunits (ND1, 2, 3, 4L, 4, 5, and 6); 1 complex III subunit (cytochorome b); 3 complex IV subunits (COI, II, III); and 2 complex V subunits (ATPase 6 and 8). Coordination must exist between nuclear and mitochondrial genomes to permit assembly of the complex holoenzymes. Each cell contains numerous mitochondria and

each mitochondrion contains multiple copies of mtDNA. This genetic material derives exclusively from the female gamete and any mutation must be passed from female parent to all progeny, male and female. The replicative segregation of mutant mtDNA copies within the cell determines whether this biologic disadvantage is expressed. In most mitochondrial disorders, patients carry a mix of mutant and normal mitochondria, a condition known as heteroplasmy, with the proportions varying from tissue to tissue and individual to individual within a pedigree in a manner correlating with severity of phenotype.[105,106]

Mitochondrial diseases often produce disturbances of brain and muscle function, presumably because these organs are so metabolically active, and therefore the metabolic demand is high during growth and development.[109] Cardiac disease is most commonly associated with respiratory chain defects.[110,111] Ragged red fibers are present in muscle biopsy specimens almost invariably when the molecular defect involves mtDNA (except in infants).[104] These defects represent the genetics of ATP production. The diverse clinical syndromes associated with various respiratory chain complexes are believed to result from involvement of tissue-nonspecific (generalized) subunits in other cases, and the residual enzyme activity in affected tissues.[112] The cardiac diseases associated with mitochondrial defects include both HCM and DCM, and LV noncompaction.[113] No theory has been advanced to explain the cause of these phenotypically different cardiac abnormalities. However, it is possible that the dilated form occurs after an initial hypertrophic response (ie, it is a burned-out dilated form of HCM).

Recently, Tang and colleagues[60] investigated the mitochondrial genome for mtDNA mutations to determine whether mtDNA mutations can serve as a primary cause for LVNC. Complete nucleotide sequences of mitochondrial genomes from 20 patients with LVNC were determined by Illumina parallel sequencing technology and it was found that substitutions of a highly conserved Met31 in ND1 caused by rare mitochondrial single nucleotide polymorphisms (mtSNP) A3397G and T3398C occurred in 2 of the patients. Previously, T3398C was reported in another patient with LVNC, indicating that mutations in Met31 in ND1 and resultant defects in complex I can be associated with LVNC. In addition, 3 mtSNPs in protein-coding genes, 7 variants in rRNA genes, and 2 transitions in tRNA genes were unrelated to the haplogroup and infrequent in the general population, suggesting that these mtSNPs could also be pathogenic, and that some mtSNPs could represent pathogenic mutations, lead to compromised mitochondrial function, and be associated with LVNC.

Kearns-Sayre syndrome

This mitochondrial myopathy is characterized by ptosis, chronic progressive external ophthalmoplegia, abnormal retinal pigmentation, and cardiac conduction defects, as well as DCM. Channer and colleagues[114] reported a case of rapidly developing progressive CHF and DCM requiring transplantation in a patient with Kearns-Sayre syndrome. Approximately 20% of patients with Kearns-Sayre syndrome have cardiac involvement, and most have conduction defects causing progressive heart block. These patients generally have large, heterogeneous deletions in the mitochondrial chromosome. Poulton and colleagues[115] showed germline deletions of mtDNA in a family with Kearns-Sayre syndrome using polymerase chain reaction (PCR) to amplify across the deletion, with primers flanking these deletions. The patient was shown to have a deletion in muscle mtDNA and at low levels in blood that was identical to that found in the mother and sister. However, the probands had more deleted DNA, correlating with more severe symptoms. Other mutations have also been described.[116,117]

Myoclonic epilepsy with ragged red muscle fibers syndrome

Myoclonic epilepsy with ragged red muscle fibers (MERRF) syndrome is characterized by and caused by a single nucleotide substitution in tRNA LYS that apparently interferes with mitochondrial translation.[118,119] Shoffner and colleagues[120] showed an A to G transition mutation as the cause of the disease associated with defects in complexes I and IV. This abnormality causes decline in ATP-generating capacity, with onset of disease that includes cardiomyopathy. Other reports outline various disease-causing mutations.[121–123]

Muscle is Muscle: Cardiomyopathy and Skeletal Myopathy Genes Overlap

Nearly all of the genes identified for inherited DCM are also known to cause skeletal myopathy in humans and/or mouse models. In the case of dystrophin, mutations cause DMD and BMD, whereas δ-sarcoglycan mutations cause limb girdle muscular dystrophy (LGMD) 2F. Lamin A/C has been shown to cause autosomal dominant Emery-Dreifuss muscular dystrophy and LGMD1B, whereas actin mutations are associated with nemaline myopathy. Desmin, G4.5, α-dystrobrevin, Cypher/ZASP, MLP, α-actinin-2, titin, and δ-sarcoglycan mutations also have associated skeletal myopathy, suggesting that cardiac and skeletal muscle function is interrelated and possibly that the skeletal muscle fatigue seen in patients with DCM with and without CHF may be caused by primary skeletal muscle disease, and not only related to the cardiac dysfunction. It also suggests that the function of these muscles has a final common pathway and that both cardiologists and neurologists should consider evaluation of both sets of muscles.

Further support for this concept comes from studies of animal models. Mutations in δ-sarcoglycan in hamsters results in cardiomyopathy, whereas mutations in all sarcoglycan subcomplex genes in mice cause skeletal and cardiac muscle disease. Mutations in other DAPC genes, as well as dystrophin in murine models, also consistently demonstrate abnormalities of skeletal and cardiac muscle function. Murine mutations in titin, cypher, α-dystrobrevin, desmin, and others all demonstrate cardiac and skeletal muscle disease.

REFERENCES

1. Engberding R, Yelbuz TM, Breithardt G. Isolated noncompaction of the left ventricular myocardium: a review of the literature two decades after the initial case description. Clin Res Cardiol 2007;96: 481–8.
2. Pignatelli RH, McMahon CJ, Dreyer WJ, et al. Clinical characterization of left ventricular noncompaction in children. A relatively common form of cardiomyopathy. Circulation 2003;108:2672–8.
3. Maron BJ, Towbin JA, Thiene G, et al. Contemporary definitions and classification of the cardiomyopathies: an American Heart Association Scientific Statement from the Council on Clinical Cardiology, Heart Failure and Transplantation Committee; Quality of Care and Outcomes Research and Functional Genomics and Translational Biology Interdisciplinary Working Groups; and Council on Epidemiology and Prevention. Circulation 2006;113:1807–16.
4. Chin TK, Perloff JK, Williams RG, et al. Isolated noncompaction of left ventricular myocardium. A study of eight cases. Circulation 1990;82:507–13.
5. Stollberger C, Finsterer J, Blazek G. Left ventricular hypertrabeculation/noncompaction and association with additional cardiac abnormalities and neuromuscular disorders. Am J Cardiol 2002;90: 899–902.
6. Stollberger C, Finsterer J. Left ventricular hypertrabeculation/noncompaction. J Am Soc Echocardiogr 2004;17:91–100.
7. Ichida F, Hamamichi Y, Miyawaki T, et al. Clinical features of isolated noncompaction of the ventricular myocardium: long-term clinical course, hemodynamic properties and genetic background. J Am Coll Cardiol 1999;34:233–40.
8. Towbin JA, Bowles NE. The failing heart. Nature 2002;415:227–33.
9. Ichida F, Tsubata S, Bowles KR, et al. Novel gene mutations in patients with left ventricular noncompaction or Barth syndrome. Circulation 2001;103: 1256–63.
10. Scaglia F, Towbin JA, Craigen WJ, et al. Clinical spectrum, morbidity, and mortality in 113 pediatric patients with mitochondrial disease. Pediatrics 2004;114:925–31.
11. Grant RT. An unusual anomaly of the coronary vessels in the malformed heart of a child. Heart 1926;13:273–83.
12. Freedom RM, Patel RG, Bloom KR, et al. Congenital absence of the pulmonary valve associated with imperforate membrane type of tricuspid atresia, right ventricular tensor apparatus and intact ventricular septum: a curious developmental complex. Eur J Cardiol 1979;10:171–96.
13. Feldt RH, Rahimtoola SH, Davis GD, et al. Anomalous ventricular myocardial pattern in a child with complex congenital heart disease. Am J Cardiol 1969;23:732–4.
14. Bellet S, Gouley BA. Congenital heart disease with multiple cardiac anomalies: report of a case showing aortic atresia, fibrous scar in myocardium and embryonal sinusoidal remains. Am J Med Sci 1932;183:458–65.
15. Elliott LP, Adams PJ, Edwards JE. Pulmonary atresia with intact ventricular septum. Br Heart J 1963;25:489–501.
16. Pepper MS. Transforming growth factor-β: vasculogenesis, angiogenesis, and vessel wall integrity. Cytokine Growth Factor Rev 1997;8:21–43.
17. Ritter M, Oechslin E, Sutsch G, et al. Isolated noncompaction of the myocardium in adults. Mayo Clin Proc 1997;72:26–31.
18. Oechslin E, Ritter M, Sutsch G, et al. Isolated noncompaction of ventricular myocardium: a rare disorder. Circulation 1993;8:551–2.
19. Bleyl SB, Mumford BR, Thompson V, et al. Neonatal lethal noncompaction of the ventricular myocardium is allelic with Barth syndrome. Am J Hum Genet 1997;61:868–72.
20. Bleyl SB, Mumford BR, Brown-Harrison MC, et al. Xq28-linked noncompaction of the left ventricular myocardium: prenatal diagnosis and pathologic analysis of affected individuals. Am J Med Genet 1997;72:257–65.
21. Dusek J, Bohuslav O, Dushova M. Prenatal persistence of spongy myocardium with embryonic blood supply. Arch Pathol 1975;99:312–7.
22. Engberding R, Bender F. Identification of a rare congenital anomaly of the myocardium by two-dimensional echocardiography: persistence of

isolated myocardial sinusoids. Am J Cardiol 1984; 53:1733–4.

23. Conces DJ Jr, Ryan T, Tarver RD. Noncompaction of ventricular myocardium: CT appearance. Am J Roentgenol 1991;156:717–8.

24. Reynen K, Bachmann K, Singer H. Spongy myocardium. Cardiology 1997;88:601–2.

25. Allenby PA, Gould NS, Schwartz MF, et al. Dysplastic cardiac development presenting as cardiomyopathy. Arch Pathol Lab Med 1988; 112:1255–88.

26. Kohl T, Villegas M, Silverman N. Isolated noncompaction of ventricular myocardium: detection during fetal life. Cardiol Young 1995;5:187–9.

27. Hook S, Ratliff NB, Rosenkranz E, et al. Isolated noncompaction of the ventricular myocardium. Pediatr Cardiol 1996;17:43–5.

28. Robida A, Hajar HA. Ventricular conduction defect in isolated noncompaction of the ventricular myocardium. Pediatr Cardiol 1996;17:189–91.

29. Matsuoka Y, Kawaguchi K, Okishima T, et al. An infant with suspected right ventricular dysplasia presenting unique ventriculograms. Clin Cardiol 1988;11:55–8.

30. Schwartz SM, Duffy JY, Pearl JM, et al. Cellular and molecular aspects of myocardial dysfunction. Crit Care Med 2001;29:S214–9.

31. Gregorio CC, Antin PB. To the heart of myofibril assembly. Trends Cell Biol 2000;10:355–62.

32. Clark KA, McElhinny AS, Beckerle MC, et al. Striated muscle cytoarchitecture: an intricate web of form and function. Annu Rev Cell Dev Biol 2002; 18:637–706.

33. Vigoreaux JO. The muscle Z band: lessons in stress management. J Muscle Res Cell Motil 1994;15:237–55.

34. Barth AL, Nathke IS, Nelson WJ. Cadherins, catenins and APC protein; interplay between cytoskeletal complexes and signaling pathways. Curr Opin Cell Biol 1997;9:683–90.

35. Capetanaki Y. Desmin cytoskeleton: a potential regulator of muscle mitochondrial behaviour and function. Trends Cardiovasc Med 2002;12: 339–48.

36. Sharp WW, Simpson DG, Borg TK, et al. Mechanical forces regulate focal adhesion and costamere assembly in cardiac myocytes. Am J Physiol 1997;273:H546–56.

37. Straub V, Campbell KP. Muscular dystrophies and the dystrophin-glycoprotein complex. Curr Opin Neurol 1997;10:168–75.

38. Furukawa T, Ono Y, Tsuchiya H, et al. Specific interaction of the potassium channel beta-subunit iph with the sarcomeric protein T-cap suggests a T-tubule-myofibril linking system. J Mol Biol 2001; 313:775–84.

39. Kucera JP, Rohr S, Rudy Y. Localization of sodium channels in intercalated disks modulates cardiac conduction. Circ Res 2002;91:1176–82.

40. Marcus FI, Fontaine GH, Guiraudon G. Right ventricular dysplasia: a report of 24 adult cases. Circulation 1982;65:383–98.

41. Pinamonti B, Singara G, Salvi A, et al. Left ventricular involvement in right ventricular dysplasia. Am Heart J 1992;123:711–24.

42. Fontaine G, Fontaltaliran F. About the histology of arrhythmogenic right ventricular dysplasia. Circulation 1997;96:2089–90.

43. Jenni R, Goebel N, Tartini R, et al. Persisting myocardial sinusoids of both ventricles as an isolated anomaly: echocardiographic, angiographic, and pathologic anatomical findings. Cardiovasc Intervent Radiol 1986;9:127–31.

44. Chenard J, Samson M, Beaulieu M. Embryonal sinusoids in the myocardium. Report of a case successfully treated surgically. Can Med Assoc J 1965;92:1356–7.

45. Punn R, Silverman NH. Cardiac segmental analysis in left ventricular noncompaction: experience in a pediatric population. J Am Soc Echocardiogr 2010;23(1):46–53.

46. Thuny F, Jacquier A, Jop B, et al. Assessment of left ventricular non-compaction in adults: side-by-side comparison of cardiac magnetic resonance imaging with echocardiography. Arch Cardiovasc Dis 2010;103(3):150–9.

47. Bione S, D'Adamo P, Maestrini E, et al. A novel X-linked gene, G4.5 is responsible for Barth syndrome. Nat Genet 1996;12:385–9.

48. D'Adamo P, Fassone L, Gedeon A, et al. The X-linked gene G4.5 is responsible for different infantile dilated cardiomyopathies. Am J Hum Genet 1997;61:862–7.

49. Johnston J, Kelley RI, Fergenbaum A, et al. Mutation characterization and genotype-phenotype correlation in Barth syndrome. Am J Hum Genet 1997;61:1053–8.

50. Barth PG, Scholte HR, Berden JA, et al. An X-linked mitochondrial disease affecting cardiac muscle, skeletal muscle and neutrophil leukocytes. J Neurol Sci 1983;62:327–55.

51. Neustein HR, Lurie PR, Dahms B, et al. An X-linked recessive cardiomyopathy with abnormal mitochondria. Pediatrics 1979;64:24–9.

52. Kelley RI, Cheatham JP, Clark BJ, et al. X-linked dilated cardiomyopathy with neutropenia, growth retardation and 3-methylglutaconic aciduria. J Pediatr 1991;119:738–47.

53. Ino T, Sherwood WG, Cutz E, et al. Dilated cardiomyopathy with neutropenia, short stature, and abnormal carnitine metabolism. J Pediatr 1988; 113:511–4.

54. Bolhuis PA, Hensels GW, Hulsebos TJM, et al. Mapping of the locus for X-linked cardioskeletal myopathy with neutropenia and abnormal mitochondria (Barth syndrome) to Xq28. Am J Hum Genet 1991;48:481–5.

55. Gedeon AK, Wilson MJ, Colley AC, et al. X-linked fatal infantile cardiomyopathy maps to Xq28 and is possibly allelic to Barth syndrome. J Med Genet 1995;32:383–8.

56. Vatta M, Mohapatra B, Jimenez S, et al. Mutations in Cypher/ZASP in patients with dilated cardiomyopathy and left ventricular non-compaction. J Am Coll Cardiol 2003;42:2014–27.

57. Klaassen S, Probst S, Oechslin E, et al. Mutations in sarcomere protein genes in left ventricular non-compaction. Circulation 2008;117(22):2893–901.

58. Shan L, Makita N, Xing Y, et al. SCN5A variants in Japanese patients with left ventricular noncompaction and arrhythmia. Mol Genet Metab 2008;93(4):468–74.

59. Finsterer J, Stöllberger C. Primary myopathies and the heart. Scand Cardiovasc J 2008;42(1):9–24.

60. Tang S, Batra A, Zhang Y, et al. Left ventricular noncompaction is associated with mutations in the mitochondrial genome. Mitochondrion 2010;10:350–7.

61. Seidman CE, Seidman JG. Gene mutations that cause familial hypertrophic cardiomyopathy. In: Haber E, editor. Molecular cardiovascular medicine. New York: Scientific American; 1995. p. 193–209.

62. Thierfelder L, Watkins H, MacRae C, et al. α-Tropomyosin and cardiac troponin T mutations cause familial hypertrophic cardiomyopathy: a disease of the sarcomere. Cell 1994;77:701–12.

63. Choudhary R, Sastry BK, Subramanyam C. Positive correlations between serum calcineurin activity and left ventricular hypertrophy. Int J Cardiol 2005;105(3):327–31.

64. Towbin JA. Cardiac arrhythmias: the genetic connection. J Cardiovasc Electrophysiol 2000;11:601–2.

65. Hedley PL, Jørgensen P, Schlamowitz S, et al. The genetic basis of long QT and short QT syndromes: a mutation update. Hum Mutat 2009;30(11):1486–511.

66. Bowles NE, Bowles KR, Towbin JA. The "final common pathway" hypothesis and inherited cardiovascular disease: the role of cytoskeletal proteins in dilated cardiomyopathy. Herz 2000;25:168–75.

67. Towbin JA, Bowles KR, Bowles NE. Etiologies of cardiomyopathy and heart failure. Evidence for a final common pathway for disorders of the myocardium. Nat Med 1999;5:226–67.

68. Towbin JA, Hejtmancik JF, Brink P, et al. X-linked dilated cardiomyopathy. Molecular genetic evidence of linkage to the Duchenne muscular dystrophy (dystrophin) gene at the Xp21 locus. Circulation 1993;87:1854–65.

69. Ortiz-Lopez R, Su J, Goytia V, et al. Evidence for dystrophin missense mutation as a cause of X-linked dilated cardiomyopathy (XLCM). Circulation 1997;95:2434–40.

70. Fatkin D, Otway R, Richmond Z. Genetics of dilated cardiomyopathy. Heart Fail Clin 2010;6(2):129–40.

71. Towbin JA. Toward an understanding of the cause of mitral valve prolapse. Am J Hum Genet 1999;65(5):1238–41.

72. Mizuguchi T, Matsumoto N. Recent progress in genetics of Marfan syndrome and Marfan-associated disorders. J Hum Genet 2007;52(1):1–12.

73. Shou W, Aghdasi B, Armstrong DL, et al. Cardiac defects and altered ryanodine receptor function in mice lacking FKBP12. Nature 1998;391:489–92.

74. Chen H, Zhang W, Li D, et al. Analysis of ventricular hypertrabeculation and noncompaction using genetically engineered mouse models. Pediatr Cardiol 2009;30(5):626–34.

75. Coral-Vazquez R, Cohn RD, Moore SA, et al. Disruption of the sarcoglycan-sarcospan complex in vascular smooth muscle: a novel mechanism in the pathogenesis of cardiomyopathy and muscular dystrophy. Cell 1999;98:465–74.

76. Hack AA, Ly CT, Jiang F, et al. γ-Sarcoglycan deficiency leads to muscle membrane defects and apoptosis independent of dystrophin. J Cell Biol 1998;142:1279–87.

77. Deconinck AE, Rafael JA, Skinner SC, et al. Utrophin-dystrophin-deficient mice as a model for Duchenne muscular dystrophy. Cell 1997;90:717–27.

78. Grady RM, Teng H, Nichol JC, et al. Skeletal and cardiac myopathies in mice lacking utrophin and dystrophin: a model for Duchenne muscular dystrophy. Cell 1997;90:729–38.

79. Araishi K, Sassaoka T, Imamura M, et al. Loss of the sarcoglycan complex and sarcospan leads to muscular dystrophy in β-sarcoglycan-deficient mice. Hum Mol Genet 1999;8:1589–98.

80. Cote PD, Moukhles H, Lindenbaum M, et al. Chimeric mice deficient in dystroglycans develop muscular dystrophy and have disrupted myoneural synapses. Nat Genet 1999;23:338–42.

81. Straub V, Rafael JA, Chamberlain JS, et al. Animal models for muscular dystrophy show different patterns of sarcolemmal disruption. J Cell Biol 1997;139:375–85.

82. Grady RM, Grange RW, Lau KS, et al. Role for α-dystrobrevin in the pathogenesis of dystrophin-dependent muscular dystrophies. Nat Cell Biol 1999;1:215–20.

83. Vainzof M, Ayub-Guerrieri D, Onofre PC, et al. Animal models for genetic neuromuscular diseases. J Mol Neurosci 2008;34(3):241–8.

84. Nigro V, Okazaki Y, Belsito A, et al. Identification of the Syrian hamster cardiomyopathy gene. Hum Mol Genet 1997;6:601–7.

85. Sakamoto A, Abe M, Masaki T. Delineation of genomic deletion in cardiomyopathic hamster. FEBS Lett 1999;447:124–8.

86. Sakamoto A, Ono K, Abe M, et al. Both hypertrophic and dilated cardiomyopathies are caused by mutation of the same gene, δ-sarcoglycan, in hamster: an animal model of dystrophin-associated glycoprotein complex. Proc Natl Acad Sci U S A 1997;94:13873–8.

87. Huang C, Zhou Q, Liang P, et al. Characterization and in vivo functional analysis of splice variants of Cypher. J Biol Chem 2003;278:7360–5.

88. Sheikh F, Bang ML, Lange S, et al. "Z"eroing in on the role of Cypher in striated muscle function, signaling, and human disease. Trends Cardiovasc Med 2007;17:258–62.

89. Zhou Q, Ruiz-Lozano P, Martone ME, et al. Cypher, a striated muscle-restricted PDZ and LIM domain-containing protein, binds to alpha-actinin-2 and protein kinase C. J Biol Chem 1999;274:19807–13.

90. Zhou Q, Chu PH, Huang C, et al. Ablation of Cypher, a PDZ-LIM domain Z-line protein, causes a severe form of congenital myopathy. J Cell Biol 2001;155:605–12.

91. Zheng M, Cheng H, Li X, et al. Cardiac-specific ablation of Cypher leads to a severe form of dilated cardiomyopathy with premature death. Hum Mol Genet 2009;18(4):701–13.

92. Snyder SH, Sabatini DM. Immunophilins and the nervous system. Nat Med 1995;1:32–7.

93. Wang T, Li B-Y, Danielson PD, et al. The immunophilin FKBP12 functions as a common inhibitor of the TGF-β family type I receptors. Cell 1996;86: 435–44.

94. Chen Y-G, Liu F, Massagué J. Mechanisms of TGF-β receptor inhibition by FKBP12. EMBO J 1997;13:3866–76.

95. Okadome T, Oeda E, Saitoh M, et al. Characterization of the interaction of FKBP12 with the transforming growth factor-β type I receptor in vivo. J Biol Chem 1996;271:21687–90.

96. Jayaraman T, Brillantes A-M, Timerman AP, et al. FK506-binding protein associated with the calcium release channel (ryanodine receptor). J Biol Chem 1992;267:9474–7.

97. Timermann AP, Onoue H, Xin H-B, et al. Selective binding of FKBP12.6 by the cardiac ryanodine receptor. J Biol Chem 1996;271: 20385–91.

98. Van Duyne GD, Standaert RF, Karplus PA, et al. Atomic structure of FKBP-FK506, an immunophilin-immunosuppressant complex. Science 1991;252: 839–42.

99. McCaffrey PG, Luo C, Kerppolla TK, et al. Isolation of the cyclosporine-sensitive T cell transcription factor NFATp. Science 1993;262:750–4.

100. Rao A, Luo C, Hogan PG. Transcription-factors of the NFAT family: regulation and function. Annu Rev Immunol 1997;15:707–47.

101. Clapstone NA, Crabtree GR. Identification of calcineurin as a key signaling enzyme in T-lymphocyte activation. Nature 1992;357:695–7.

102. de la Pompa J, Timmerman LA, Takimoto H, et al. Role of the NF-ATc transcription factor in morphogenesis of cardiac valves and septum. Nature 1998;392:182–90.

103. Attardi G. The elucidation of the human mitochondrial genome: a historical perspective. Bioessays 1996;5:34–9.

104. Wallace DC, Zheng X, Lott MT, et al. Familial mitochondrial encephalomyopathy (MERRF): genetic, pathophysiological, and biochemical characterization of a mitochondrial DNA disease. Cell 1988;55: 601–10.

105. Wallace DC. Mitochondrial DNA mutation and neuromuscular disease. Trends Genet 1989;5: 9–13.

106. Clarke A. Mitochondrial genome: defects, disease, and evolution. J Med Genet 1990;27:451–6.

107. Grivell LA. Small, beautiful and essential. Nature 1989;341:569–71.

108. Anderson S, Banker AT, Barrell BG. Sequence and organization of the human mitochondrial genome. Nature 1981;290:457–65.

109. Petty RKH, Harding AE, Morgan-Hughes JA. The clinical features of mitochondrial myopathy. Brain 1986;109:915–38.

110. Mariotti C, Tiranti V, Carrara F, et al. Defective respiratory capacity and mitochondrial protein synthesis in transformant cybrids harboring the tRNA$^{Leu(UUR)}$ mutation associated with maternally inherited myopathy and cardiomyopathy. J Clin Invest 1994;93:1102–7.

111. Vogel H. Mitochondrial myopathies and the role of the pathologist in the molecular era. J Neuropathol Exp Neurol 2001;60:217–27.

112. Capaldi RA, Halphen DG, Zhang YZ, et al. Complexity and tissue specificity of the mitochondrial respiratory chain. J Bioenerg Biomembr 1988;20:291–311.

113. Ozawa T, Tanaka M, Sugiyama S, et al. Multiple mitochondrial DNA deletions exist in cardiomyocytes of patients with hypertrophic or dilated cardiomyopathy. Biochem Biophys Res Commun 1990;170:830–6.

114. Channer KD, Channer JL, Campbell MJ, et al. Cardiomyopathy in Kearns-Sayre syndrome. Br Heart J 1988;59:486–90.

115. Poulton J, Deadman ME, Ramacharan S, et al. Germ-line deletions of mtDNA in mitochondrial myopathy. Am J Hum Genet 1991;48:649–53.

116. Moraes CT, DiMauro S, Zeviani M, et al. Mitochondrial DNA deletions in progressive external ophthalmoplegia and Kearns-Sayre syndrome. N Engl J Med 1989;320:1293–9.

117. Moraes CT, Schon EA, DiMauro S, et al. Heteroplasmy of mitochondrial genomes in clonal cultures from patients with Kearns-Sayre syndrome. Biochem Biophys Res Commun 1989;160:765–71.

118. Suomalainen A, Kollmann P, Octave J-N, et al. Quantification of mitochondrial DNA carrying tRNA[8344Lys] point mutation in myoclonus epilepsy and ragged-red fiber disease. Eur J Hum Genet 1993;1:88–95.

119. Tanno Y, Yoneda M, Nonaka I, et al. Quantitation of mitochondrial DNA carrying tRANLys mutation in MERRF patients. Biochem Biophys Res Commun 1991;179:880–5.

120. Shoffner JM, Lott MI, Lezza AM, et al. Myoclonic epilepsy and ragged-red fiber disease (MERRF) is associated with a mitochondrial DNA tRNA(Lys) mutation. Cell 1990;61:931–7.

121. Nakamura M, Nakano S, Goto Y, et al. A novel point mutation in the mitochondrial tRNA[Ser(UCN)] gene detected in a family with MERFF/MELAS overlap syndrome. Biochem Biophys Res Commun 1995;214:86–93.

122. Silvestri G, Moraes CT, Shanske S, et al. A new mtDNA mutation in the tRNA(Lys) gene associated with myoclonic epilepsy and ragged-red fibers (MERRF). Am J Hum Genet 1992;51:1213–7.

123. Fukuhara N. Clinicopathologic features of MERRF. Muscle Nerve 1995;3:590–4.

Arrhythmogenic Forms of Heart Failure in Children

Stuart Berger, MD[a],*, Anne M. Dubin, MD[b]

KEYWORDS

- Arrhythmia • Cardiomyopathy • Heart failure
- Tachycardia-induced cardiomyopathy

Arrhythmia is commonly associated with cardio-myopathy, whether the cardiomyopathy is dilated, hypertrophic, or restrictive in nature. Both atrial and ventricular arrhythmias have been seen with each of these cardiomyopathies. Therefore, it is not uncommon to see a patient with both dilated cardiomyopathy and incessant tachycardia, and it is often difficult to deter-mine whether the tachycardia is primary or secondary. Arrhythmias have been implicated as a causative factor in dilated cardiomyopathy, specifically in arrhythmogenic right ventricular dysplasia, pacing-induced cardiomyopathy, and tachycardia-induced cardiomyopathy.

ARRHYTHMOGENIC RIGHT VENTRICULAR DYSPLASIA

Arrhythmogenic right ventricular dysplasia (ARVD), also known as arrhythmogenic right ventricular cardiomyopathy, is a genetic abnormality charac-terized by ventricular arrhythmias and a thinned, fibrotic right ventricle.[1,2] It is often characterized by fatty infiltration of the right ventricular free wall, and arrhythmia or sudden death. It can be quite difficult to diagnose, and multiple imaging tech-niques have been used to help in this investigation.

Anatomy

The classic findings in ARVD are RV dilatation and myocardial thinning.[2,3] The RV myocardium is re-placed with fibrous and fatty tissue (**Fig. 1**). This is usually seen within the triangle of dysplasia, an

area on the free wall bordered by the apex, inflow tract, and outflow tract.[3] Histologic study of these patients shows an active inflammatory process with mononuclear infiltrates surrounding necrotic myocytes. There is also myocardial atrophy and thinning with fatty replacement. The fibro/fatty replacement can be quite patchy, and is not uniformly distributed throughout the right ventricle.

ARVD can also affect the left ventricle with the characteristic histology seen in the left ventricle. This tends to be seen in older patients, who tend to have worse long-term outcome with a higher incidence of left-sided ventricular arrhythmias and heart failure.[4]

Genetics/Pathophysiology

Approximately 30% of ARVD is familial, and 2 patterns of inheritance have been described: an autosomal dominant and an autosomal recessive form.[5,6]

The autosomal recessive form is commonly called Naxos disease. This is a cardiocutaneous disease with the cardiac features of ARVD along with hyperkeratosis of the palms and soles and wooly hair.[7] This disease develops during adoles-cence; children have no cardiac symptoms, but may have ECG abnormalities. By adolescence there is 100% penetrance with development of RV fatty infiltration, ventricular tachycardia (VT) and ECG abnormalities.[8,9] This disease has been linked to chromosome 17q21, and a 2–base pair deletion in the plakoglobin gene. Plakoglobin is

a Department of Pediatrics, Children's Hospital of Wisconsin, Medical College of Wisconsin, 9000 West Wisconsin Avenue, Milwaukee, WI 53217, USA
b Department of Pediatrics, Lucile Packard Children's Hospital, Stanford University Medical School, 750 Welch Road, Suite 325, Palo Alto, CA 9430, USA
* Corresponding author.
E-mail address: SBerger@chw.org

Heart Failure Clin 6 (2010) 471–481
doi:10.1016/j.hfc.2010.05.006
1551-7136/10/$ – see front matter © 2010 Elsevier Inc. All rights reserved.

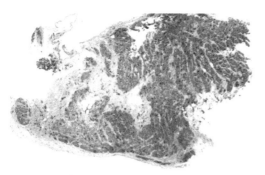

Fig. 1. Fibrofatty replacement of myocardium in patient with ARVD. (*Courtesy of* Jane Crosson, MD, Baltimore, MD.)

critical in maintaining tight cell-cell adhesions that are disrupted in this disease.

The autosomal dominant form of ARVD has been associated with at least 9 different loci in familial studies (ARVD 1-9) (**Table 1**).[10] The first gene mutation identified was within the N-terminal portion of the desmoplakin gene, affecting the plakoglobin-binding domain of desmoplakin.[6] This defect is seen in ARVD8, which is considered the classic ARVD associated with arrhythmia, sudden death, and eventual LV involvement. Desmoplakin is important in maintaining tight cell-cell adhesions. When these junctions are disrupted, cell death and fibrofatty replacement occur.

Plakophilin-2, demsoglein-2, desmocillin-2, and transmembrane potential (TMEM) 43 gene mutations have also been identified with this disease.[11–14] These genes all affect cell adhesion or in the case of TMEM43 can cause dysregulation of adipogenic pathways and may increase fibrofatty replacement of myocardium.

Thus, ARVD appears to be closely linked with the function of desmosomal proteins. The present model for ARVD suggests that impaired desmosome function causes myocyte detachment and cell death when the cell is subjected to mechanical stress. This results in inflammation with ultimate fibrofatty replacement of the damaged myocytes.[15]

Clinical Presentation

Most patients with ARVD are diagnosed secondary to arrhythmia or (missed) sudden death. The disease usually manifests itself anywhere between 10 and 50 years of age with a mean age of diagnosis at 30.[10,16,17] It is extremely uncommon to see this disease in children younger than 10 years and it is not seen in infancy.

Patients usually complain of dizziness, palpitations, or syncope. In one study of 130 patients, palpitations were the most common presenting symptoms noted in 67% of patients, followed by

Table 1
Genetics of ARVD

Genetic Variant	Inheritance	Chromosome	Gene	Comment
ARVD 1	AD	14q24.3		Progressive degeneration of RV myocardium
ARVD 2	AD	1q42-q43	Cardiac ryanodine receptor	Associated with catecholaminergic polymorphic VT
ARVD 3	AD	14q11-q12		
ARVD 4	AD	2q32.1-q32.3		Associated with localized left-ventricular involvement
ARVD 5	AD	3p23	TMEM43	Fully penetrant, sex-influenced high-risk form of ARVD
ARVD 6	AD	10p12-14		Early onset, high penetrance
ARVD 7	AD	10q22		Associated with myofibrillar myopathy
ARVD 8	AD/AR	6p23-24	Desmoplakin	Associated with palmoplantar keratoderma and wooly hair
Naxos	AR	17q21	Plakoglobin	Associated with palmoplantar keratoderma and wooly hair
ARVD	AD	12p11	Plakophilin-2	Intercellular disruption and ARVC

Abbreviations: AD, autosomal dominant; AR, autosomal recessive; ARVD, arrhythmogenic right ventricular dysplasia; RV, right ventricular; VT, ventricular tachycardia.

Data from Calkins H. Arrhythmogenic right ventricular dysplasia/cardiomyopathy. Curr Opin Cardiol 2006;21:55–63.

syncope and atypical chest pain in 32% and 27% respectively.[17] It is extremely rare to see signs of RV failure.

Approximately 50% of patients present with symptomatic ventricular arrhythmias.[17,18] These can range from premature ventricular contraction (PVC) to sustained VT with a left bundle branch block (LBBB) pattern originating from the RV (**Fig. 2**).

Sudden death may be the initial presenting sign of this disease. In an autopsy study of 1930 cases of unexplained sudden cardiac death, 10% were associated with ARVD.[18] Most of these occurred during routine activities with only 3.5% occurring while participating in sports.

Diagnostic Criteria

Making the diagnosis of ARVD can be quite difficult. A definitive diagnosis requires histologic confirmation of transmural fibrofatty replacement of the RV at autopsy or surgery. Biopsy is not

highly sensitive (67%) because of the patchy nature of the disease.[19]

The task force on ARVD from the European Society of Cardiology has proposed a schema of major and minor criteria to diagnose ARVD.[20,21] These criteria are classified into 6 major categories: family history, arrhythmias, conduction abnormalities on ECG (depolarization and repolarization abnormalities), fatty replacement of the RV free wall, and RV dysfunction (**Table 2**). The diagnosis depends on the presence of 2 major criteria, 1 major and 2 minor, or 4 minor criteria.

With the advent of genetic testing, the utility of these criteria have been shown to be limited. Recent study of several families with confirmed ARVD showed that use of the criteria identified 10 of 11 probands with disease and 20 of 24 asymptomatic family members. Just as importantly, by these clinical criteria, 5 family members were identified as affected yet were later found to be negative via gene testing.[13]

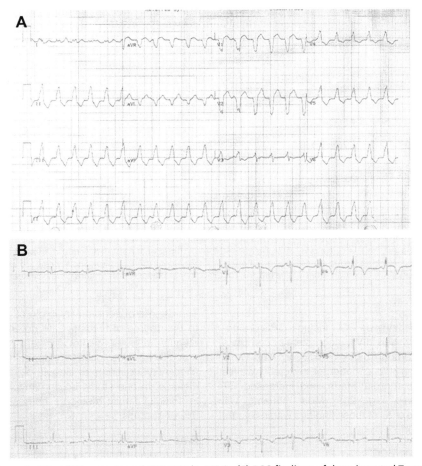

Fig. 2. (*A*) Characteristic LBBB, superior axis VT seen in ARVD, (*B*) ECG findings of deep inverted T waves in V2-V4, and epsilon wave seen in lead V1. (*Courtesy of* Jane Crosson, MD, Baltimore, MD.)

Table 2
ARVD criteria

	Major Criteria	Minor Criteria
Family history	Familial disease confirmed at autopsy or surgery	Family history of premature sudden death (<35) caused by suspected ARVD Family history (clinical diagnosis based on present criteria)
ECG depolarization abnormalities	Epsilon waves or localized prolongation (>110 ms) of the QRS complex in the right precordial leads (V1-V3)	Late potentials seen on signal average ECG
Repolarization abnormalities		Inverted T waves in right precordial leads (V2 and V3) in patients >12 years old and in the absence of right bundle branch block
Tissue characterization of walls	Fibrofatty replacement of myocardium on endomyocardial biopsy	
Global and/or regional dysfunction and structural alterations (detected by echocardiography, angiography, MRI, or radionuclide scintigraphy)	Severe dilation and reduction of RV ejection fraction with no or mild left ventricular impairment Localized right ventricular aneurysms (akinetic or dyskinetic areas with diastolic bulging) Severe segmental dilation of the right ventricle	Mild global right ventricular dilation and/or ejection fraction reduction with normal left ventricle Mild segmental dilation of the right ventricle Regional right ventricular hypokinesia
Arrhythmias		Left bundle branch block type ventricular tachycardia (sustained or nonsustained) documented on ECG, Holter monitoring or during exercise testing Frequent ventricular extrasystoles (more than 1000/24 hours) on Holter monitoring

Abbreviations: ARVD, arrhythmogenic right ventricular dysplasia; RV, right ventricular.
From McKenna WJ, Thiene G, Nava A, et al. Diagnosis of arrhythmogenic right ventricular dysplasia/cardiomyopathy. Task Force of the Working Group Myocardial and Pericardial Disease of the European Society of Cardiology and of the Scientific Council on Cardiomyopathies of the International Society and Federation of Cardiology. Br Heart J 1994;71:215.

ECG

The classic findings on ECG include QRS prolongation, usually seen in V1, incomplete or complete right bundle branch block (RBBB), epsilon wave (usually seen in 30% of patients), inverted T waves in the right precordial leads, and increased QT dispersion (see **Fig. 2**).[22] Most patients will develop some or all of these findings within 6 years of presentation.

Signal average ECG

Most patients who have fulfilled the criteria for ARVD have abnormal signal average ECGs.[23,24]

The degree of abnormality is directly proportional to the degree of fibrosis. Late potentials seem to identify risk of ventricular arrhythmias. This modality has been used in family members of identified ARVD patients to aid with screening for the disease. In one study, late potentials were found in 16% of family members compared with only 3% of controls.[5]

Echo

Echo findings in this disease include RV dilatation and regional wall motion abnormalities.[10] Dyskinesis, akinesis, and diastolic bulging can also be appreciated and this could vary with disease severity.

MRI

MRI is the modality most widely used for the diagnosis of ARVD. Common findings on MRI include myocardial fat, late gadolinium enhancement, and RV wall motion abnormalities (**Fig. 3**).[25] MRI has been found to be very sensitive, with a high negative predictive value; however, at present there is a high rate of false positive examinations, and a great deal of inter-observer variability.[26]

Electrophysiology testing

Electrophysiology (EP) testing (and ablation) may be useful in patients with ARVD. Electroanatomic mapping can show low voltage local electrograms that can identify dysplastic regions.[27] This can help differentiate ARVD from the more benign RV outflow tract (RVOT) VT, which has normal electrograms. Ablation may be useful in lessening arrhythmia burden.

Angiography

Angiography can help further delineate the RV structure and function in patients with suspected ARVD. The classic angiographic findings include transversely arranged hypertrophic trabeculae separated by deep fissure and coarse trabeculae in the apical region. RV volume is also increased.[28]

Biopsy

Biopsy is not usually performed in this disease, as it is neither sensitive nor specific.[29] Sampling error, secondary to the patchy nature of the disease, and because the septum is rarely involved limits its utility. There is also an increased risk of myocardial perforation secondary to the thinning of the RV free wall.

Therapy

The possibility of sudden cardiac death is probably the most serious manifestation of this disease. Several approaches have been suggested in this disease state with regard to the prevention of ventricular arrhythmias and sudden death.

The American College of Cardiology/American Heart Association/European Society of Cardiology (ACC/AHA/ESC) have proposed guidelines for management of patients with ARVD, and in particular have evaluated the role of the implantable cardioverter defibrillator (ICD) in this disease.[30] ICD implantation is considered appropriate in secondary prevention of sudden cardiac death in patients with ARVD. It is also considered appropriate therapy in high-risk patients for primary prevention. Unfortunately, precise indications for primary prevention have not been developed.

There have been several studies that have considered the efficacy of an ICD in this disease.[16,31,32] A multicenter study of 132 patients with a combination of indications including sudden death, syncope, and sustained VT showed that appropriate device discharges occurred in 48% by 39 months with a survival rate of 96%.[31]

Antiarrhythmics have been shown to lessen the ventricular tachycardia burden in patients with ARVD, but, as in most cardiomyopathies, these drugs do not reduce the risk of sudden death.[33] Sotalol has been shown to be the drug of choice in this condition. It has been shown to reduce the incidence of VT on ambulatory monitoring and at EP study. The ACC/AHA/ESC guidelines suggest the use of antiarrhythmics to suppress or lessen VT burden, or in the event that an ICD cannot be implanted.[34]

Radiofrequency ablation has been used to lessen arrhythmia load in patients with VT and ARVD, but is not considered a sole therapy of this disease secondary to the patchy nature of the disease. However in patients with ICDs and frequent shocks, or those in whom an ICD cannot be used, radiofrequency ablation has been shown to decrease the ventricular arrhythmias. Multiple small series have shown that ablation was initially successful in most studies, with a recurrence rate of about 25% to 75% by 3 years after ablation.[35–37] Before widespread use of ICD therapy, surgical disconnection of the RV free wall was

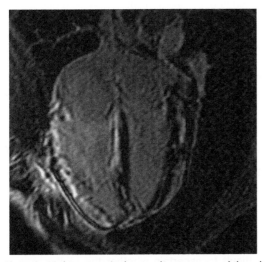

Fig. 3. Right ventricular enlargement, delayed enhancement and fibrosis in anterior wall on MRI of patient with ARVD. (*Courtesy of* Jane Crosson, MD, Baltimore, MD.)

used in patients who were refractory to drug therapy.[38] This decreased sudden death risk by 2 mechanisms: first, the ventricular mass available to fibrillate was diminished, and second, the VT focus was isolated and unable to affect the LV. Unfortunately, RV failure is a known complication of this therapy.

Prognosis

When discussing prognosis there are 2 major patient groups to discuss: those who are asymptomatic and those who have had ventricular tachycardia.

With new advances in genetic testing, it is becoming more common to identify patients with the genetic signature of ARVD, but who are asymptomatic. A study of 37 families of patients with ARVD revealed that approximately 10% of asymptomatic patients (identified secondary to a family member with the disease) will develop echocardiographically diagnosed structural signs of the disease during a follow-up of 8.5 years, whereas 50% will have symptomatic arrhythmias.[10] Thus, these patients warrant close follow-up.

There are conflicting reports with regard to patients with ARVD and VT fare. In a study of 37 families from Italy, only 1 of 49 patients with VT who were treated with antiarrhythmics died during a mean follow-up of 8.5 years, and this was after discontinuation of drug therapy.[10] However, Hulot and colleagues[17] found that 21 of 102 patients with ARVD died of cardiovascular causes in an 8-year follow-up.

At present, there are groups that have been identified as at a high-risk for sudden death, and therapy should be tailored accordingly. These include younger patients, those with recurrent syncope, and those with a history of missed sudden death.[31,39] Several genetic mutations have also been associated with an increased risk of sudden death. These include patients with ARVD2 and ARVD5.[11,40] Patients with Naxos disease are also considered to be higher risk.[9] These higher-risk groups should be restricted from competitive athletics; ICDs are strongly recommended for secondary prevention of sudden death and should be seriously considered for primary prevention.

Dyssynchronous Forms of Cardiomyopathy

Electrical and mechanical dyssynchrony, either secondary to a pacemaker or to abnormal electrical activation of the ventricle, have recently become recognized as potentially important factors in the development of cardiomyopathy.

It is well known that right ventricular pacing can be deleterious to cardiac function. Traditional RV apical pacing can cause disturbed coronary perfusion, alter myocardial work, and ultimately cause systolic and diastolic dysfunction.[41–43] It is also known that 5% to 30% of patients with congenital complete heart block secondary to maternal anti-SSA, SSB antibodies will develop dilated cardiomyopathy.[44,45]

Cardiac reverse remodeling (ie, improvement in ventricular size) has been seen in the pediatric population following resynchronization. Takabayashi and colleagues[46] reported a patient with AV block following congenital heart surgery who developed LV dysfunction 5 years following surgery. Cardiac resynchronization therapy (CRT) was instituted and 1-year follow-up showed a decreased end-diastolic diameter (EDD) and end-systolic diameter (ESD) and improved LV systolic function (LVSF). These findings were confirmed by Moak and colleagues[47] who reported 6 patients with heart block and dilated left ventricles. Each of these patients was also treated with CRT. Echocardiographic findings at a mean follow-up of 13 months demonstrated mechanical remodeling with improved ejection fraction (EF), and decreased LVEDD and LVESD.

Wolff-Parkinson-White Syndrome

There have been several case reports and one recent small series that suggest that patients with Wolff-Parkinson-White syndrome (WPW) and septal pathways may manifest septal dyskinesia and can lead to global LV dysfunction.[48–50] Kwon and colleagues[49] recently published a series of 62 children with WPW who underwent echocardiograms to assess mechanical synchrony. They found that patients with septal pathways have significantly lower EFs (53% vs 61% for right and left lateral pathways) and marked intraventricular dyssynchrony. All patients with dyskinesia had marked improvement in EF and measures of dyssynchrony following radiofrequency ablation.

TACHYCARDIA-INDUCED CARDIOMYOPATHY

Tachycardia-induced cardiomyopathy (TIC) is a relatively uncommon form of dilated cardiomyopathy thought to be secondary to a rapid abnormal heart rate. In circumstances where a nonsinus tachycardia is associated with LV dysfunction/dilated cardiomyopathy, it may be difficult to ascertain whether the tachycardia is the primary event or whether it is secondary to the cardiomyopathy and poor function. If the cardiomyopathy is truly secondary to the tachyarrhythmia, the control of the rhythm and rate has the potential to reverse the ventricular dysfunction, especially if recognized promptly and successfully treated as soon as possible. The definitive diagnosis is often a retrospective diagnosis in that the patient may improve clinically with resolution of ventricular dysfunction over time once the rhythm and rate are controlled.

Pathophysiology

There are several experimental models of TIC that have afforded us an understanding of some of the pathophysiologic mechanisms associated with the biventricular systolic and diastolic dysfunction evident in this condition. The specific etiology for the development of dysfunction, however, is not completely clear.

Spinale and colleagues[51] investigated a model of paced supraventricular tachycardia (SVT) on LV function and myocardial structure in the newborn pig model. They found that SVT was associated with a dilated cardiomyopathy comparable to that found in the adult swine model. The changes in LV function were associated with a decrease in cellular contractile proteins and were comparable to the changes noted in mature animals.

Chrysostomakis and colleagues[52] induced both atrial and ventricular fibrosis in a goat model with rapidly conducting atrial fibrillation. Thus, rapid conduction could equally influence fibrosis development in both atrial and ventricular tissue. This model demonstrated a beneficial effect in atrial remodeling with the use of angiotensin II type 1 receptor blockade.

An experimental canine model of TIC was established by rapid atrial pacing at 350 to 400 beats per minute for 8 weeks in 11 dogs.[53] Ventricular dilatation and systolic dysfunction occurred after 1 week of rapid atrial pacing with concomitant structural damage to myofibrils, mitochondria, and the sarcoplasmic reticulum with intercalated disc discontinuity. Levels of connexion[15] decreased significantly and gap junction remodeling occurred. This suggested that TIC may be multifactorial.

Potassium and calcium channel activity have also been implicated in other models of TIC. Akar and colleagues[54] found that there was significant down-regulation of K currents, probably secondary to post-transcriptional modifications, whereas Lavergne and colleagues[55] found abnormalities in calcium channel activity and sarcoplasmic reticulum transport. The severity of calcium cycling abnormality

correlated with the degree of LV dysfunction, suggesting that a decreased calcium availability to myocytes resulted in a subsequent reduction in contractility.

Other abnormalities have been found in models of TIC including at diminished Na-K-ATPase activity and diminution in myocardial levels of ATP, procreatine, and creatine suggesting depleted high-energy myocardial stores.[56] Such changes have also been well documented in ischemic myocardial injury.[57] Where myocardial ischemia fits in the scheme of TIC is unclear and which is the cause versus the effect is also unknown.

Decreased beta-receptor responsiveness and down-regulation of beta-1 receptor density has also been described in animal models.[58] Oxidative stress injury of the myocardium may also result in the accumulation of peroxynitrite and subsequent modification of myofibrillar proteins and energetics. The concomitant imbalance of pro-oxidant and antioxidant pathways may be associated with cardiac dysfunction.[59]

Histologic abnormalities that have been described in TIC include myocyte hyperplasia, myocyte lengthening, myocardial fibrosis, impaired coronary reserve, and apoptosis.[60]

It has been hypothesized that there may be a genetic basis for TIC. There is an association between the ACE gene (D) and DD (deletion) phenotype, which result in elevated angiotensin-converting enzyme and TIC.[61]

Hemodynamic Abnormalities

The hemodynamic abnormalities encountered in TIC are typical of the findings noted in dilated cardiomyopathy. Low cardiac output, elevation of left and right heart-filling pressures, elevation in pulmonary artery pressure, and elevated systemic vascular resistance all can be seen in this disease. As in all etiologies of heart failure, there is an associated neurohumoral activation that includes an elevation in plasma atrial and brain natriuretic peptide levels and epinephrine and norepinephrine levels, as well as renin and aldosterone activity.

Types of Primary Arrhythmia Associated with Cardiomyopathy

Both atrial and ventricular tachycardias have been associated with dilated cardiomyopathy/ ventricular dysfunction. Probably the most common chronic tachycardia associated with TIC is ectopic atrial tachycardia (Fig. 4). This is probably because patients can remain hemodynamically compensated for longer periods of

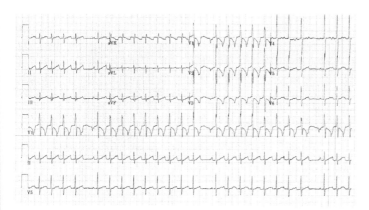

Fig. 4. A 10-year-old who presented with ectopic atrial tachycardia and an ejection fraction of 15%. Radiofrequency ablation resulted in elimination of tachycardia and complete resolution of systolic dysfunction in 2 months.

time in this rhythm. However, other atrial arrhythmias including atrial flutter, atrial fibrillation, and reentrant rhythms including atrialventricular reentrant and atrioventricular nodal reentrant tachycardia (AVNRT) rhythm can be associated with TIC. Additionally, sustained ventricular tachycardia can also result in LV dysfunction. **Box 1** summarizes the common causes of TIC.

Box 1
Dysrhythmias that have been associated with dilated cardiomyopathy

Supraventricular

Junctional ectopic tachycardia, postoperative

Junctional ectopic tachycardia, congenital

Ectopic atrial tachycardia

Atrial flutter

Atrial fibrillation

Atrioventricular re-entry tachycardia

Atrioventricular tachycardia

Permanent junctional reciprocating tachycardia (PJRT)

Ventricular

Right ventricular outflow tract origin

Left ventricular origin

Bundle branch reentry origin

Premature ventricular contractions

Other associated causes

Thyrotoxicosis

Pacemaker mediated tachycardia

Pacemaker associated cardiomyopathy

WPW

Clinical Manifestations

Patients with TIC present with the clinical signs and symptoms seen with heart failure of any etiology. These symptoms may be age specific. In small children, presenting symptoms may include poor feeding and weight gain, easy fatigability, and shortness of breath. In the older child and adolescent, exercise intolerance, chest pain, anorexia, or abdominal pain may be seen. Interestingly, palpitations are only occasionally reported. The physical examination may also be relatively nonspecific and may include signs of both right- and left-sided heart failure such as edema, poor perfusion tachycardia, a gallop rhythm, murmurs of AV valve insufficiency, pulmonary congestion, jugular venous distension, and hepatomegaly. It has been reported that TIC should be considered if the degree of tachycardia is out of proportion to the degree of heart failure or if the heart rate is relatively fixed. A 12-lead ECG should be obtained in all cases of newonset heart failure to specifically rule out a TIC. Echocardiography can help determine the degree of systolic and diastolic dysfunction and AV valve regurgitation. Additional studies would also include a chest radiograph to assess the degree of cardiomegaly and pulmonary congestion, and routine blood analysis including serum brain natriuretic peptide (BNP), electrolytes, blood urea nitrogen (BUN), creatinine, complete blood count, and liver function studies.

Therapy

In addition to the general therapies for heart failure (diuretics, ACE inhibitors, beta blockers), the patient with TIC requires a prompt return to sinus rhythm. This may be achieved by antiarrhythmics, cardioversion, or catheter ablation, depending on the rhythm and severity of disease. After successful conversion to sinus rhythm, improvement in ventricular function, if it occurs, tends to occur over a period of several weeks. In the interim, ongoing medical therapy for heart failure is typically used.

Prognosis

Prognosis of patients with TIC varies with age, the degree of ventricular dysfunction, and the degree and chronicity of the tachycardia. Neonates and infants and those in whom the tachyarrhythmia are diagnosed early tend to have a more rapid and more complete recovery. Often the definitive diagnosis can be made only retrospectively, with recovery after control of the rate and rhythm. In some patients in whom the rate and rhythm abnormalities are long-standing or unremitting, improvement in ventricular function may not occur, requiring chronic heart failure therapy including antiarrhythmic medications, ventricular assist devices, and ultimately cardiac transplantation.

SUMMARY

There are various underlying causes of TIC and it is critical that it be considered in any patient who presents with a newly diagnosed dilated cardiomyopathy. Unlike most other forms of cardiomyopathy, TIC should be considered a treatable form of cardiomyopathy and it is imperative that the diagnosis be fully considered. A 12-lead ECG should be obtained in all patients with a dilated cardiomyopathy. Prompt diagnosis and therapy of this relatively uncommon cause of heart failure is critical and has the potential to completely reverse the ventricular dysfunction that may be present in this abnormality.

REFERENCES

1. Gemayel C, Pelliccia A, Thompson PD. Arrhythmogenic right ventricular cardiomyopathy. J Am Coll Cardiol 2001;38:1773.
2. Sen-Chowdhry S, Lowe MD, Sporton SC, et al. Arrhythmogenic right ventricular cardiomyopathy: clinical presentation, diagnosis, and management. Am J Med 2004;117:685.
3. Marcus FI, Fontaine GH, Guiraudon G, et al. Right ventricular dysplasia: a report of 24 adult cases. Circulation 1982;65:384.
4. Corrado D, Basso C, Thiene G, et al. Spectrum of clinicopathologic manifestations of arrhythmogenic right ventricular cardiomyopathy/dysplasia: a multicenter study. J Am Coll Cardiol 1997;30:1512.
5. Hermida JS, Minassian A, Jarry G, et al. Familial incidence of late ventricular potentials and electrocardiographic abnormalities in arrhythmogenic right ventricular dysplasia. Am J Cardiol 1997;79:1375.
6. Rampazzo A, Nava A, Malacrida S, et al. Mutation in human desmoplakin domain binding to plakoglobin causes a dominant form of arrhythmogenic right ventricular cardiomyopathy. Am J Hum Genet 2002;71:1200.
7. Protonotarios N, Tsatsopoulou A, Patsourakos P, et al. Cardiac abnormalities in familial palmoplantar keratosis. Br Heart J 1986;56:321.
8. Kaplan SR, Gard JJ, Protonotarios N, et al. Remodeling of myocyte gap junctions in arrhythmogenic right ventricular cardiomyopathy due to a deletion in plakoglobin (Naxos disease). Heart Rhythm 2004;1:3.
9. Protonotarios N, Tsatsopoulou A, Anastasakis A, et al. Genotype-phenotype assessment in autosomal recessive arrhythmogenic right ventricular cardiomyopathy (Naxos disease) caused by a deletion in plakoglobin. J Am Coll Cardiol 2001;38:1477.
10. Nava A, Bauce B, Basso C, et al. Clinical profile and long-term follow-up of 37 families with arrhythmogenic right ventricular cardiomyopathy. J Am Coll Cardiol 2000;36:2226.
11. Merner ND, Hodgkinson KA, Haywood AF, et al. Arrhythmogenic right ventricular cardiomyopathy type 5 is a fully penetrant, lethal arrhythmic disorder caused by a missense mutation in the TMEM43 gene. Am J Hum Genet 2008;82:809.
12. Pilichou K, Nava A, Basso C, et al. Mutations in desmoglein-2 gene are associated with arrhythmogenic right ventricular cardiomyopathy. Circulation 2006;113:1171.
13. Syrris P, Ward D, Asimaki A, et al. Clinical expression of plakophilin-2 mutations in familial arrhythmogenic right ventricular cardiomyopathy. Circulation 2006; 113:356.
14. Syrris P, Ward D, Evans A, et al. Arrhythmogenic right ventricular dysplasia/cardiomyopathy associated with mutations in the desmosomal gene desmocollin-2. Am J Hum Genet 2006;79:978.
15. Sen-Chowdhry S, Prasad SK, McKenna WJ. Arrhythmogenic right ventricular cardiomyopathy with fibrofatty atrophy, myocardial oedema, and aneurysmal dilation. Heart 2005;91:784.
16. Dalal D, Nasir K, Bomma C, et al. Arrhythmogenic right ventricular dysplasia: a United States experience. Circulation 2005;112:3823.
17. Hulot JS, Jouven X, Empana JP, et al. Natural history and risk stratification of arrhythmogenic right ventricular dysplasia/cardiomyopathy. Circulation 2004; 110:1879.
18. Tabib A, Loire R, Chalabreysse L, et al. Circumstances of death and gross and microscopic observations in a series of 200 cases of sudden death associated with arrhythmogenic right ventricular cardiomyopathy and/or dysplasia. Circulation 2003;108:3000.

19. Angelini A, Basso C, Nava A, et al. Endomyocardial biopsy in arrhythmogenic right ventricular cardiomyopathy. Am Heart J 1996;132:203.

20. Hamid MS, Norman M, Quraishi A, et al. Prospective evaluation of relatives for familial arrhythmogenic right ventricular cardiomyopathy/dysplasia reveals a need to broaden diagnostic criteria. J Am Coll Cardiol 2002;40:1445.

21. McKenna WJ, Thiene G, Nava A, et al. Diagnosis of arrhythmogenic right ventricular dysplasia/cardiomyopathy. Task Force of the Working Group Myocardial and Pericardial Disease of the European Society of Cardiology and of the Scientific Council on Cardiomyopathies of the International Society and Federation of Cardiology. Br Heart J 1994;71:215.

22. Jaoude SA, Leclercq JF, Coumel P. Progressive ECG changes in arrhythmogenic right ventricular disease. Evidence for an evolving disease. Eur Heart J 1996;17:1717.

23. Leclercq JF, Coumel P. Late potentials in arrhythmogenic right ventricular dysplasia. Prevalence, diagnostic and prognostic values. Eur Heart J 1993; 14(Suppl E):80.

24. Turrini P, Angelini A, Thiene G, et al. Late potentials and ventricular arrhythmias in arrhythmogenic right ventricular cardiomyopathy. Am J Cardiol 1999;83:1214.

25. Bluemke DA, Krupinski EA, Ovitt T, et al. MR imaging of arrhythmogenic right ventricular cardiomyopathy: morphologic findings and interobserver reliability. Cardiology 2003;99:153.

26. Tandri H, Castillo E, Ferrari VA, et al. Magnetic resonance imaging of arrhythmogenic right ventricular dysplasia: sensitivity, specificity, and observer variability of fat detection versus functional analysis of the right ventricle. J Am Coll Cardiol 2006;48:2277.

27. Boulos M, Lashevsky I, Reisner S, et al. Electroanatomic mapping of arrhythmogenic right ventricular dysplasia. J Am Coll Cardiol 2001;38:2020.

28. Daliento L, Rizzoli G, Thiene G, et al. Diagnostic accuracy of right ventriculography in arrhythmogenic right ventricular cardiomyopathy. Am J Cardiol 1990; 66:741.

29. Basso C, Ronco F, Marcus F, et al. Quantitative assessment of endomyocardial biopsy in arrhythmogenic right ventricular cardiomyopathy/dysplasia: an in vitro validation of diagnostic criteria. Eur Heart J 2008;29:2760.

30. Zipes DP, Camm AJ, Borggrefe M, et al. ACC/AHA/ESC 2006 guidelines for management of patients with ventricular arrhythmias and the prevention of sudden cardiac death: a report of the American College of Cardiology/American Heart Association Task Force and the European Society of Cardiology Committee for Practice Guidelines (Writing Committee to Develop Guidelines for Management of Patients With Ventricular Arrhythmias and the Prevention of Sudden Cardiac Death). J Am Coll Cardiol 2006;48:e247.

31. Corrado D, Leoni L, Link MS, et al. Implantable cardioverter-defibrillator therapy for prevention of sudden death in patients with arrhythmogenic right ventricular cardiomyopathy/dysplasia. Circulation 2003;108:3084.

32. Wichter T, Paul M, Wollmann C, et al. Implantable cardioverter/defibrillator therapy in arrhythmogenic right ventricular cardiomyopathy: single-center experience of long-term follow-up and complications in 60 patients. Circulation 2004;109:1503.

33. Wichter T, Borggrefe M, Haverkamp W, et al. Efficacy of antiarrhythmic drugs in patients with arrhythmogenic right ventricular disease. Results in patients with inducible and noninducible ventricular tachycardia. Circulation 1992;86:29.

34. Zipes DP, Camm AJ, Borggrefe M, et al. ACC/AHA/ESC 2006 guidelines for management of patients with ventricular arrhythmias and the prevention of sudden cardiac death—executive summary: a report of the American College of Cardiology/American Heart Association Task Force and the European Society of Cardiology Committee for Practice Guidelines (Writing Committee to Develop Guidelines for Management of Patients with Ventricular Arrhythmias and the Prevention of Sudden Cardiac Death) Developed in collaboration with the European Heart Rhythm Association and the Heart Rhythm Society. Eur Heart J 2006;27:2099.

35. Dalal D, Jain R, Tandri H, et al. Long-term efficacy of catheter ablation of ventricular tachycardia in patients with arrhythmogenic right ventricular dysplasia/cardiomyopathy. J Am Coll Cardiol 2007; 50:432.

36. Marchlinski FE, Zado E, Dixit S, et al. Electroanatomic substrate and outcome of catheter ablative therapy for ventricular tachycardia in setting of right ventricular cardiomyopathy. Circulation 2004;110:2293.

37. Verma A, Kilicaslan F, Schweikert RA, et al. Short- and long-term success of substrate-based mapping and ablation of ventricular tachycardia in arrhythmogenic right ventricular dysplasia. Circulation 2005; 111:3209.

38. Damiano RJ Jr, Asano T, Smith PK, et al. Functional consequences of the right ventricular isolation procedure. J Thorac Cardiovasc Surg 1990;100:569.

39. Turrini P, Corrado D, Basso C, et al. Noninvasive risk stratification in arrhythmogenic right ventricular cardiomyopathy. Ann Noninvasive Electrocardiol 2003;8:161.

40. Bauce B, Nava A, Rampazzo A, et al. Familial effort polymorphic ventricular arrhythmias in arrhythmogenic right ventricular cardiomyopathy map to chromosome 1q42-43. Am J Cardiol 2000;85:573.

41. Karpawich PP, Justice CD, Cavitt DL, et al. Developmental sequelae of fixed-rate ventricular pacing in the immature canine heart: an electrophysiologic, hemodynamic, and histopathologic evaluation. Am Heart J 1990;119:1077.

42. Karpawich PP, Rabah R, Haas JE. Altered cardiac histology following apical right ventricular pacing in patients with congenital atrioventricular block. Pacing Clin Electrophysiol 1999;22:1372.

43. Prinzen FW, Augustijn CH, Arts T, et al. Redistribution of myocardial fiber strain and blood flow by asynchronous activation. Am J Physiol 1990;259:H300.

44. Kim JJ, Friedman RA, Eidem BW, et al. Ventricular function and long-term pacing in children with congenital complete atrioventricular block. J Cardiovasc Electrophysiol 2007;18:373.

45. Villain E, Coastedoat-Chalumeau N, Marijon E, et al. Presentation and prognosis of complete atrioventricular block in childhood, according to maternal antibody status. J Am Coll Cardiol 2006;48:1682.

46. Takabayashi S, Shimpo H, Mitani Y, et al. Pediatric cardiac remodeling after cardiac resynchronization therapy. Pediatr Cardiol 2006;27:485.

47. Moak JP, Hasbani K, Ramwell C, et al. Dilated cardiomyopathy following right ventricular pacing for AV block in young patients: resolution after upgrading to biventricular pacing systems. J Cardiovasc Electrophysiol 2006;17:1068.

48. Emmel M, Balaji S, Sreeram N. Ventricular preexcitation associated with dilated cardiomyopathy: a causal relationship? Cardiol Young 2004;14:594.

49. Kwon BS, Bae EJ, Kim GB, et al. Septal dyskinesia and global left ventricular dysfunction in pediatric Wolff-Parkinson-White syndrome with septal accessory pathway. J Cardiovasc Electrophysiol 2010; 21(3):290–5.

50. Mulpuru SK, Vasavada BC, Hejmadi PS, et al. Unique wall motion abnormalities on stress echocardiogram associated with Wolff-Parkinson-White pattern electrocardiogram: a case report. Int J Cardiol 2007;119:e68.

51. Spinale FG, Fulbright BM, Mukherjee R, et al. Relation between ventricular and myocyte function with tachycardia-induced cardiomyopathy. Circ Res 1992;71:174.

52. Chrysostomakis SI, Karalis IK, Simantirakis EN, et al. Angiotensin II type 1 receptor inhibition is associated with reduced tachyarrhythmia-induced ventricular interstitial fibrosis in a goat atrial fibrillation model. Cardiovasc Drugs Ther 2007;21:357.

53. Zhong JQ, Zhang W, Gao H, et al. Changes in connexin 43, metalloproteinase and tissue inhibitor of metalloproteinase during tachycardia-induced cardiomyopathy in dogs. Eur J Heart Fail 2007; 9:23.

54. Akar FG, Tomaselli GF. Conduction abnormalities in nonischemic dilated cardiomyopathy: basic mechanisms and arrhythmic consequences. Trends Cardiovasc Med 2005;15:259.

55. Lavergne T, Sebag C, Ollitrault H, et al. [Arrhythmic cardiomyopathy]. Arch Mal Coeur Vaiss 2001;94(2): 45 [in French].

56. Schotten U, Greiser M, Benke D, et al. Atrial fibrillation-induced atrial contractile dysfunction: a tachycardiomyopathy of a different sort. Cardiovasc Res 2002;53:192.

57. Shinbane JS, Wood MA, Jensen DN, et al. Tachycardia-induced cardiomyopathy: a review of animal models and clinical studies. J Am Coll Cardiol 1997;29:709.

58. Spinale FG, Tempel GE, Mukherjee R, et al. Cellular and molecular alterations in the beta adrenergic system with cardiomyopathy induced by tachycardia. Cardiovasc Res 1994;28:1243.

59. Masullo P, Venditti P, Agnisola C, et al. Role of nitric oxide in the reperfusion induced injury in hyperthyroid rat hearts. Free Radic Res 2000;32:411.

60. Spinale FG, Hendrick DA, Crawford FA, et al. Chronic supraventricular tachycardia causes ventricular dysfunction and subendocardial injury in swine. Am J Physiol 1990;259:H218.

61. Moe GW, Stopps TP, Angus C, et al. Alterations in serum sodium in relation to atrial natriuretic factor and other neuroendocrine variables in experimental pacing-induced heart failure. J Am Coll Cardiol 1989;13:173.

Myocarditis in Children

Uwe Kühl, MD, PhD*, Heinz-Peter Schultheiss, MD

KEYWORDS

- Lymphocytic myocarditis • Viral myocarditis
- Inflammatory cardiomyopathy • Heart failure
- Myocardial cell loss • Coxsackie-adenoviral receptor

In the absence of structural heart diseases lymphocytic myocarditis accounts for around 10% of recent onset cardiomyopathy in adults and this figure may be higher in children. Viruses are the main causes in developed countries; other infectious agents predominate as the cause of myocarditis in rural countries. Early fulminant disease is associated with high mortality despite in-time intensive care. In recent years, improvement in early intensive care including mechanical support with biventricular assist devices has improved the prognosis of children of all age groups and often allows complete recovery from fulminant disease or bridging to transplantation. Patients who survive the critical phase have a fairly good prognosis and survival from myocarditis in children and adults is similar at around 80%. In the remaining patients, progressive chronic heart failure and unpredictable sudden cardiac death remain a serious concern. In contrast to fulminant disease, nonfulminant myocarditis is more likely to result in a progressive course with death or transplantation being required.

The kind and extent of acute and chronic myocardial compromise depends on the nature of the offending infectious agent, the affected cardiac structures, and myocardial lesions caused by cytolytic viruses, or by the innate and adaptive antiinfectious immune responses.[1] Myocardial cell loss is caused by different pathogenic mechanisms including cytokine production contributing to disease severity, viral persistence, which may interfere with the integrity of myocardial matrix, viral invasion of vascular endothelium causing vascular spasms with reperfusion injury, or heart-reactive autoimmune responses.

Irreversible injury is associated with compensatory myocyte hypertrophy, interstitial fibrosis, scarring, and chamber dilatation. In time, administration of symptomatic heart failure therapy may delay onset or progression of severe heart failure but often cannot prevent development of end-stage dilated cardiomyopathy (DCM) in those patients. However, spontaneous recovery is frequently seen in patients with acute or subacute heart failure caused by myocarditis. This indicates that severe hemodynamic compromise at first presentation is not necessarily caused by irreversible cardiac injury. This justifies more invasive diagnostic procedures such as biopsy to establish a specific diagnosis, which is the only basis for any specific therapy option.

This article focuses on the current information on epidemiology, cause, diagnosis, and treatment of childhood myocarditis. Current differential diagnostics that have consistently improved over the years and thus provided the basis for first successful treatment studies in children and well-characterized subgroups of adults are discussed, bearing in mind that the causes leading to acute or chronic myocardial damage in viral and immune myocarditis resulting in heart failure, arrhythmias, and developing cardiomyopathy are not yet exactly defined for all of the infectious pathogens and immune processes discussed.

Department of Cardiology and Pneumology, University Medicine Berlin, Campus Benjamin-Franklin, Medical Clinic II, Hindenburgdamm 30, Berlin 1210, Germany
* Corresponding author.
E-mail address: uwe.kuehl@charite.de

Heart Failure Clin 6 (2010) 483–496
doi:10.1016/j.hfc.2010.05.009

DEFINITION AND HISTOLOGIC FEATURES OF MYOCARDITIS AND INFLAMMATORY CARDIOMYOPATHY

Histologically, active myocarditis is characterized by an initial focal mononuclear cellular infiltrate with myocytolysis and/or degeneration of adjacent myocytes (**Fig. 1**).[2] In addition to lymphocytes, the inflammatory infiltrate may also include mixed types of inflammatory cells consisting of lymphocytes, leukocytes, monocytes, and macrophages. Approximately 10% to 12% of adult patients with cardiomyopathy of recent onset who undergo early endomyocardial biopsy (EMB) have this condition but higher numbers have been reported for children.[3] In rare cases, mutinucleated giant cells or eosinophils dominate the active inflammatory process although these rare conditions are frequently less detected than in adults (see **Fig. 1**).[4–7]

The term chronic active myocarditis histologically describes a persistent active myocarditis more than 3 months after onset of acute symptoms or detected in follow-up biopsies.[3,7,8] Myocyte degeneration, reactive fibrosis, and focal scars, which refer to areas of fibrotic replacement of single or few damaged myocytes are already present in addition to atrophic and/or hypertrophic cardiomyocytes indicating ongoing myocardial burden. In borderline myocarditis, inflammatory cells but no active myocyte necrosis is found.[2]

In a clinical setting classified as chronic myocarditis with respect to the onset of the disease or chronic inflammatory cardiomyopathy, the more diffuse inflammatory infiltrates are less prominent and without frank myocyte necroses. In the histologic sections these low lymphocyte numbers are frequently overlooked. Newer histologic criteria rely on inflammatory cell-specific antigens directed against distinct cellular surface antigens such as anti-CD3, anti-CD4, anti-CD8, anti-CD68/Mac-1, and cellular adhesion molecules such as antihuman leukocyte antigen, anti-CD54/ICAM-1, or anti-CD106/VCAM-1 (see **Fig. 1**). The procedural low sensitivity of the conventionally stained myocardial tissue sections is significantly improved by such immunhohistological staining techniques, which allow detection, characterization, and quantification of low-grade inflammatory cell subsets and inflammation-associated proteins such as vascular CAMs.[9,10]

PATHOPHYSIOLOGY

Viral infections of the heart develop within pathologically distinct phases with most information on this issue derived from enteroviral and adenoviral infections of the heart (**Fig. 2**).[1,11] Both viruses enter the heart as a secondary target organ and infect cardiomyocytes after binding to the coxsackie-adenoviral receptor (CAR).[12,13] The co-localization of CAR with the coreceptors for adenovirus internalization $av\beta3$ and $av\beta5$ at the myocyte surface suggests that this gap junctional protein is an important molecular determinant for the cardiotropism of both viruses in viral heart disease.[14] Erythroviruses and human herpesvirus 6 genomes, on the other hand, infect vascular endothelial cells and/or other cardiac cells including myocytes (HHV-6).[15–17] These different infection sites in cardiac tissue, in addition to different virus variants and virus loads, may explain the heterogenicity of viral heart disease with respect to expression of its phenotype, clinical presentation, and prognosis.

In enterovirus infections the virus RNA is predominantly located in areas showing an inflammatory cell infiltrate and myofiber necrosis. Such findings suggest that during the early disease direct lytic infection of myocytes by virus is responsible for myocarditis in these cases, rather than an autoimmune process.[18] The innate and adaptive antiviral immune responses initiate a further step in the development of viral heart disease.[1,11] Virus-infected cardiac cells are destroyed by immune-effector cells at the expense of further loss of infected myocytes.[19] The ensuing myocardial damage depends on the scale of the cellular virus infection and increases with growing virus dispersion, which, in addition to the early virus-mediated injury, contributes to later tissue remodeling and possible progression of the disease.[10,20] Virus clearance from infected cardiomyocytes therefore takes place at the expense of a partial destruction of myocardial tissue that is not capable of regeneration. This may account for a clinical picture that is consistent with DCM.

The presentation of viral antigens that evoke an antiviral immune response that aims at viral elimination is not necessarily detrimental to the heart. However, this immune response is a double-edged sword. Molecular mimicry and perhaps genetically predisposing conditions can secondarily target cryptic myocardial antigens. In the case of postviral autoimmunity, this immune response can continue despite elimination of the viral genome. On the other hand, chronic viral persistence maintains the anticardiac immune response. Activated B lymphocytes produce antibodies that can cross-react with myocardial antigens and may also contribute to impairment of cardiac contractility. Numerous autoantibodies have been identified in patients with DCM, targeting the ADP/ATP carrier, the $\beta1$ adrenoreceptor,

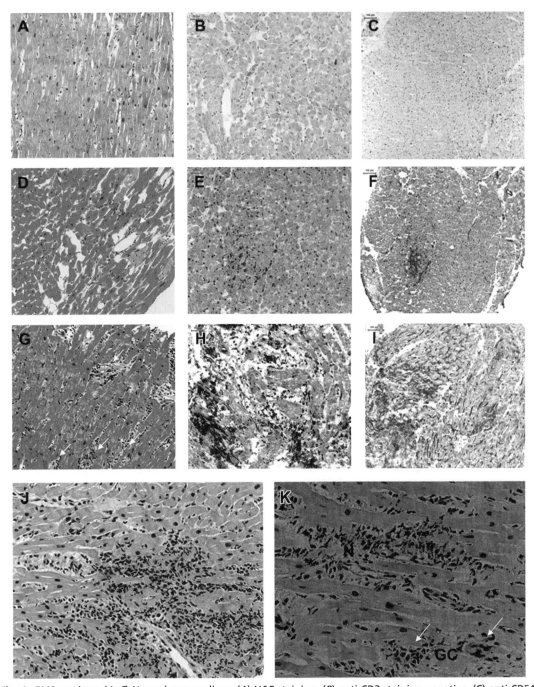

Fig. 1. EMB sections. (*A–C*) Normal myocardium. (*A*) H&E staining, (*B*) anti-CD3 staining negative, (C) anti-CD54/ICAM-1staining with minimal endothelial ICAM-expression in noninflamed myocardium. (*D–F*) Focal lymphocytic borderline myocarditis. (*D*) H&E staining, (*E*) single focus of anti-CD3–positive lymphocytes, (*F*) focally enhanced anti-CD54/ICAM-1 expression nearby the cellular infiltrate. (*G–I*) Mild focal lymphocytic myocarditis with myocyte necroses. (*G*) H&E staining, (*H*) multiple anti-CD3–positive infiltrates, (*I*) enhanced anti-CD54/ICAM-1 expression. (*J*) Lymphocytic myocarditis, (*K*) giant cell myocarditis.

and further mitochondrial and contractile proteins. The pathogenic relevance of autoantibodies may have been questioned in the past as epiphenomena of the immune response, but recent experiments have proved the pathogenic principle of stimulating antibodies directed against the second extracellular β1-receptor loop, because sera transferred from immunized rats induces

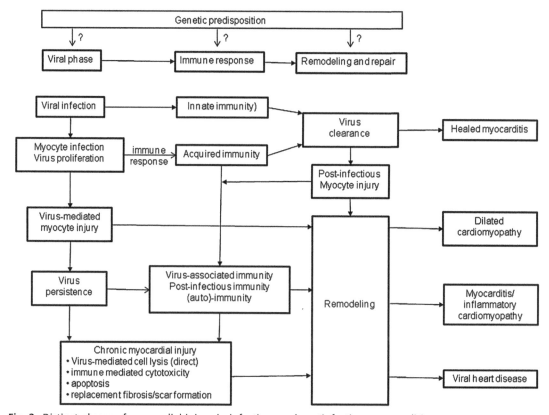

Fig. 2. Distinct phases of myocardial injury in infectious and postinfectious myocarditis.

DCM in healthy littermates. Furthermore, positive results from immunoadsorption studies indicate a causative role for autoantibodies in DCM.

In addition, cardiodepressive cytokines induced by the immune system can directly impair cardiac contractility. Cytokines promote an imbalance between metalloproteinases (MMP) and their tissue inhibitors (TIMP), contributing to remodeling. Preliminary results indicate a relationship between MMP/TIMP expression patterns and left ventricular function. Cytokines may also induce cell adhesion molecules (CAMs) on the endothelium, which mediate transendothelial migration of immunocompetent cells into the myocardium. CAM interactions are also involved in the continuous loss of cardiomyocytes, mediated specifically by cytotoxic T lymphocytes.

INCIDENCE OF MYOCARDITIS

Many cases of myocarditis remain unrecognized because of their often subclinical presentation and misinterpretation of unspecific symptoms and therefore, the true incidence of myocarditis is unknown. Because EMB is infrequently used in routine clinical practice, unambiguous histologic confirmation of myocarditis within a patient's

lifetime is rare even in those with a typical history and clinical presentation. In the past, most information has been obtained from postmortem studies and biopsy-based data have only recently been reported.

Estimates of myocarditis from autopsy reports range from 0.12% to 12%, and 9.6% of myocarditis was documented in adult patients with unexplained heart failure.[21–24] A review of the results of all autopsies (n = 1516) of children aged 0 to 18 years of age in a single pediatric center over a 10-year period demonstrated that histologically proven myocarditis was present in 28 cases (1.8%, age range 10 days to 16 years, median age 10 months), of which 16 (57%) presented as sudden death.[25] More than half of all cases with myocarditis are reported in infants less than 1 year of age, accounting for 2% of infant deaths referred for autopsy, compared with around 5% of childhood deaths over the age of 5 years. In almost 40% of cases there were no macroscopic cardiac abnormalities, the diagnosis being entirely dependent on routine histologic examination of the heart.

In a population-based cohort of children less than 16 years of age reported from 2 regions of the United States, New England, and the central southwest, myocarditis was also the most frequent cause in children with known causes of DCM (46%), followed by neuromuscular diseases (26%).[26] DCM accounts for around 50% of cardiomyopathies in those less than 18 years of ages with myocarditis being among the most common known causes.[26–32] In this age group myocarditis has been diagnosed in around 10% of all registered cardiomyopathies and 18% of cases of pediatric DCM.[31] These figures based on pure clinical diagnosis are underestimated. Probable or confirmed diagnosis based on histologic criteria elicited a higher incidence of myocarditis especially in children less than 10 years of age, with highest detection rates within the first year of life.[29,33] In children who underwent EMB within 4 to 6 weeks after onset of acute DCM, 40% of patients were histologically positive.[3,25]

CAUSE OF MYOCARDITIS

Causes include viruses, protozoa, bacteria, fungi, toxins, drugs, and myocardial involvement caused by systemic autoimmune diseases but often the underlying cause cannot be identified (**Table 1**). In developed countries, viral infections cause most cases of myocarditis. Apart from enteroviruses, which traditionally have been considered the most common agent in myocarditis and DCM, distinct genotypes of erythroviruses, human herpesvirus type 6, adenoviruses, human immunodeficiency virus, cytomegalovirus, herpes simplex type 2 virus, hepatitis C virus, and others have

Table 1
Virus-associated heart disease. Infectious pathogens in acquired viral myocarditis/inflammatory cardiomyopathy and postinfectious of heart failure

Virus	Virus	Cardiotropic Subtypes/Variants	Treatment (Heart Failure Therapy Plus)
RNA viruses	Picornavirus		
	Coxsackie A+B	CVB 1–6, A2, 5	Interferon-β
	Echovirus	Echo 30	
	Poliovirus		
	Hepatitis virus	C	Interferon-α
	Orthomyxoviren		
	Influenza	A, B, C	
	Paramyxoviren		
	RSV		
	Mumps		
	Togaviruses		
	Rubella		
	Flaviviruses		
	Dengue fever		
	Yellow fever		
DNA viruses	Adenovirus	A 1, 2 ,3 and 5	
	Erythrovirus	1 (B19V), 2	
	Herpesvirus		
	Human herpes virus 6	A, B	Val-/ganciclovir
	Cytomegalovirus		
	Epstein-Barr virus		
	Varicella-zoster virus		
	Retrovirus		
	HIV		
Postinfectious cardiomyopathy	Autoimmune myocarditis and DCMi		Immunosuppression (cortisone, azathioprine, cyclosporine)
	DCM		Symptomatic (angiotensin-converting enzyme inhibitors, β-blockers, diuretics)

been identified with varying degrees of frequency.[27,34–46]

Because EMB has been infrequently used in children, a lot of information has to be extrapolated from adults. If biopsy studies were done, virus was detected with similar, sometimes higher frequencies.[27,34–36,47–50] In one study virus was detected in 9 (36%) of the 25 cases in whom virological analyses were performed. The histologic features were all similar, with an interstitial inflammatory cell infiltrate, predominantly lymphocytic, with focal myocyte necrosis and interstitial edema.[33] Recent reports indicate that adenoviruses may be more frequent than enteroviruses.[34,36]

Although numerous bacterial and other infectious and noninfectious causes such as fungi, protozoa, parasites, or toxins, immune-mediated diseases, and physical conditions cause myocarditis, these causes are far less common than virus-induced myocarditis (**Table 2**).[51] As a result of effective eradication of the protozoa, acute Chagas myocarditis has declined in Brazil in recent years. Lyme disease caused by *Burrelia burgdorferi* can result in acute and chronic myocarditis in around 16% with nearly half of the children (n = 207) presenting with advanced atrioventricular heart block.[52] Progression to DCM is rare. Drugs can induce myocardial inflammation by either direct toxic effects on heart tissue or by inducing hypersensitivity reactions, which is often associated with an eosinophilic myocarditis (see **Table 2**).[53] Eosinophils are also observed in myocardial inflammatory processes that are associated with Churg-Strauss or hypereosinophilic syndromes, vaccination for several diseases, or caused by helminthic and parasitic infections (see **Table 2**).

EPIDEMIOLOGY

Myocarditis varies as a function of circulating virus populations and may correlate with virus outbreaks.[43,54–61] In children and adults, individual and outbreak-associated cases of myocarditis are frequently recognized in a seasonal distribution depending on the viral species.

The prevalence of virus-associated acute myocarditis is highest during the neonatal period and in infants infected during the first year of life.[36,57,62,63] The cause of sudden infant death syndrome (SIDS) is an unresolved problem of high relevance and several studies have indicated a role of myocarditis and viral infections.[64] In 62 SIDS victims studied, enteroviruses were detected in 14 (22.5%), adenoviruses in 2 (3.2%), Epstein-Barr viruses in 3 (4.8%), and parvovirus B19 in 7 (11.2%). Control group samples (n = 7) were completely virus negative.[65] A male preponderance

---

Table 2
Nonviral causes of myocarditis

Bacteria	Drugs
Chlamydia (C pneumonia/psittacosis), Haemophilus influenzae, Legionella pneumophilia, Brucella clostridium, Francisella tularensis, Neisseria meningitis, Mycobacterium tuberculosis, Salmonella, Staphylococcus, Streptococcus A, S pneumonia, tularemia, tetanus, syphilis, Vibrio cholerae	Aminophyllin, amphetamine, anthracyclin, catecholamines, chloramphenicol, cocaine, cyclophosphamide, doxorubicin, 5-fluoruracil, mesylate, methylsergit, phenytoin, trastuzumab, zidovudine
Spirocheta	**Hypersensitivity reactions (drugs)**
Borrelia recurrentis, Leptospira, Treponema pallidum	Azitromycin, benzodiazepines, clozapine, cephalosporins, dapsone, dobutamin, lithium, diuretics, thiazide, methyldopa, mexiletine, streptomycin, sulfonamides, nonsteroidal antiinflammatory drugs, tetanus toxoid, tetracycline, tricyclic antidepressives
Reckettsia	
Coxiella burnettii, R rickettsii/prowazekii	
Fungi	**Hypersensitivity reactions (venoms)**
Actinomyces, Aspergillus, Candida, Cryptokokkus, Histoplasma nocardia	Bee, wasp, black widow spider, scorpion, snakes
Protozoa	**Autoimmune diseases**
Entamoeba histolytica, Leishmania, Plasmodium falciparum, trypanosoma cruzi, trypanosoma brucei, toxoplasma gondii	Dematomyositis, inflammatory bowel disease, rheumatoid arthritis, Sjögren syndrome, systemic lupus erythematodes, Wegner granulomatosis, giant cell myocarditis
Helmintic	**Systemic diseases**
Ascaris, Echinococcus granulosus, Schistosoma, Trichinella spiralis, Wuchereria bancrofti	Churg-Strauss syndrome, collagen diseases, sarcoidosis, Kawasaki disease, scleroderma

has been noted with coxsackievirus B infections of the heart; differences between the sexes are unknown for other virus infections.[66]

HISTORY AND CLINICAL PRESENTATION

Clinical presentation ranges from mild flu-like symptoms with no hemodynamic consequences to congestive heart failure, ventricular dysfunction, arrhythmias, and sudden cardiac death. Newborns and infants are often more severely affected and in contrast to older children, they are more likely to have circulatory shock and present as acute DCM.[3] A viral prodrome may precede the onset of myocarditis by several days to a few weeks. Newborns, infants, toddlers, and preschool children may have a history of respiratory or gastrointestinal infection, present with anorexia, abdominal pain, poor appetite, vomiting or lethargy, seizure, sinus tachycardia out of proportion to fever, or syncope.[67,68] Often patients are diagnosed as having gastroenteritis, pneumonia, asthma, or bronchiolitis, which are common diagnoses in children. At an older age, children may complain of chest pain, shortness of breath, exercise intolerance, myalgias, arthralgias, fatigue, or palpitations.[69] Acute myocarditis may mimic typical angina, be associated with electrocardiographic changes such as ST-segment increase and abnormally increased creatine kinase or troponin I. If the prevailing symptoms develop with a variable delay after a viral illness, they are often not recognized as symptoms of an underlying infectious heart disease.[28,32]

DIAGNOSIS

The initial diagnosis of myocarditis is highly dependent on clinical suspicion because diagnosis based on EMB is not performed routinely. In the past, myocarditis has more often been a clinically derived diagnosis of exclusion, than a specifically proven diagnosis. Because of the enormous spectrum of presentations of pediatric myocarditis, which may range from asymptomatic presentation to manifest heart failure or sudden cardiac death, the diagnosis may easily be missed and the true underlying disease may only be obvious in cases in which fulminant disease and histologic confirmation are present.[28]

Information from pediatric and adult disease have confirmed that information from noninvasive clinical procedures or imaging data alone is insufficient to establish an unambiguous diagnosis and myocardial history cannot reliably be predicted from history and clinical presentation.[3,10,70,71]

NONINVASIVE SCREENING

The electrocardiogram may reveal several abnormalities raging from unspecific T-wave changes, ST-segment increase or decrease, pathologic Q waves, and nearly any kind of arrhythmia. The electrocardiogram may resemble changes seen in acute myocardial infarction or pericarditis but its sensitivity for myocarditis is less than 50%.[72] Pericardial effusion, pulmonary venous congestion, interstitial infiltrates, and pleural effusions may be recognized on chest radiographs but lack of detection does not exclude acute or chronic myocardial inflammation. Abnormal laboratory markers are not necessarily present. If detected they are increased during the early phase of the disease and at this time point, they confirm an infectious disease rather than myocardial involvement. Increased serum markers of inflammation can therefore not be used to diagnose myocarditis. Creatine kinase level (muscle and brain type) may be increased and an increased troponin level has been reported to have a specificity of 83% and a sensitivity of 71% in childhood myocarditis.[73,74] Mild myocardial injury, indirectly documented by often low increase of cardiac biomarkers, is attributed to the persistence of cytolytic virus and the antiviral immune response, and may rapidly decline without adverse prognostic myocardial damage after effective virus clearance. In such cases, increased cardiac biomarkers indicate myocardial involvement but not persistent myocardial inflammation.

IMAGING TECHNIQUES

In the past decade, a major shift in the diagnostic evaluation of myocarditis away from EMB and histologic confirmation toward noninvasive diagnosis and prognostication of acute myocarditis. Imaging techniques such as echocardiography are useful as an initial diagnostic evaluation in children to detect the presence and severity of regional or global ventricular dysfunction that often but not regularly accompanies acute myocardial inflammation. Parameters of ventricular remodeling including chamber dilation and regional hypertrophy, and regional wall motion abnormalities are often seen with this condition, but these changes may be indistinguishable from that of myocardial ischemia or infarction at the outset. The absence of matching regional coronary disease in older patients, and evidence of rapid recovery of ventricular dysfunction during follow-up are general clues to the diagnosis of myocarditis.

Echo may also distinguish fulminant from nonful-minant forms of myocarditis, with the former showing less diastolic dimensional increase, but increased septal thickness, and the latter showing much greater degree of ventricular dilatation. Echocardiographic features are not specific for myocarditis and major diagnostic and prognostic contributions are needed to evaluate the severity of myocardial involvement and rule out other causes of heart failure.[75]

Cardiac magnetic resonance (CMR) imaging is attractive for the detection of myocarditis because of its ability to characterize tissue according to water content and changes in contrast kinetics. Inflammation-associated changes in membrane permeability, tissue edema, and ultimately tissue fibrosis directly affect the T_2 relaxation parameters of the tissues, which are dependent on water content.[76] Extracellular contrast agents such as gadolinium diethylenetriamine pentaacetic acid distribute and clear differently in inflamed or scarred tissue compared with normal tissue, leading to changes in T1 relaxation and thus contrast changes or delayed enhancement on T1-weighted images.[77] CMR also allows visualiza-tion of the myocardium, and is thus well suited to detect the local patchy nature of the myocarditic lesions. It has been recommended because some of the magnetic resonance imaging (MRI) characteristics seen in pediatric patients with acute myocarditis may serve as predictors of outcome.[78]

This holds true for cases in which the sponta-neous natural course of the disease can be awaited after symptomatic stabilization of the patient but may raise considerable problems as soon as decisions for specific management and treatment are concerned. At the early stage (<4 weeks), areas of inflammatory cell infiltrates and myofiber necrosis are predominantly located around small foci of viral RNA and thus are too small to be detected by MRI with an actual resolu-tion of structures greater than 4 mm. At later stages (>8–10 weeks), myocardial inflammation may have resolved leaving MRI-detectable tissue alterations; the substrate that would be targeted by immunosuppression is no longer present.[79] Persistence of viruses and low-grade inflammation at the cellular level cannot be distinguished by any imaging procedure from postinfectious or postin-flammatory myocardial damage.

Indications for antiviral or antiinflammatory treatment and delay of permanent treatments such as a pacemaker, an implantable cardioverter-defibrillator (ICD), or a heart trans-plant demand an exact diagnosis that can only be provided by EMB.

BIOPSY-BASED MANAGEMENT

The gold standard of diagnosing acute and chronic myocarditis and the possible underlying causes is the histologic, immunohistological, and polymerase chain reaction–based analysis of endomyocardial biopsies if its time-dependent and methological limi-tations are kept in mind.[1,10,80–82] Despite such limi-tations, the EMB technique is highly sensitive in children with myocardial disorders and a major diag-nostic tool for invasive but safe detection of myocar-dial disease.[10,25,36,81,83–87] In experienced hands EMB can be performed with very low morbidity in children of all age groups and adults.[88–93]

TREATMENT
Treatment of Myocarditis and Postinfectious Inflammation

Myocardial inflammatory processes or autoimmu-nity may survive myocardial virus elimination and warrant immunosuppressive treatment to prevent later immune-mediated myocardial injury.[94–96] Frequently administered antiinflammatory drugs are immunoglobulins, corticosteroids, azathio-prine, and cyclosporine, which are administered in addition to regular heart failure medication.

The role of immunosuppressive therapy is not clearly established in the pediatric age group because of the limited number of studies and the lack of respective controls. Initial data from chil-dren presenting with presumed acute myocarditis treated with intravenous immunoglobulin (IVIG) suggested that use of high-dose IVIG for treatment of acute myocarditis is associated with improved recovery of left ventricular function and with a tendency toward better survival during the first year after presentation.[97] Later investigations and randomized studies revealed that the treatment with IVIG was not effective.[98] Freedom from death or transplantation was 81% at 1 year, and 74% at 5 years, with no difference between the modes of treatments. The median time to recovery of func-tion was also comparable between the groups. Thus, treatment with IVIG seemed to confer no advantage to steroid therapy alone.[99]

Only few data on immunosuppression in chil-dren with myocarditis are available.[80,100] One early report has indicated that immunosuppres-sion with cortisone, azathioprine, or closporine improves the outcome in acute pediatric disease.[101] In another cohort of 68 children with severe DCM (aged 10 months to 15 years), 43 presented with active myocarditis diagnosed by EMB.[102] Eight months of immunosuppressive therapy with azathioprine or cyclosporine associ-ated with prednisone improved the prognosis in

23 of 29 children (79%) with active myocarditis and severe ventricular dysfunction, but only 5 out of 21 children (24%) submitted to conventional therapy alone or conventional therapy plus prednisone improved. Of the children who received prednisolone, 10% died of cardiogenic shock during treatment.

In adults, a clinical benefit of immunosuppression demands exclusion of virus from treated patients.[94,103] Whether undiagnosed viral infection applies for the unfavorable outcome of some of the treated children is unknown. A recent report in children has questioned this observation obtained from adult patients.[27] Active myocarditis was diagnosed in 10 of 30 patients (9 months to 12 years of age) who presented with left ventricular ejection fraction of 22.8 $\pm$ 4.1%. Viral genomes were present in 50% of the patients with myocarditis. Because immunosuppression resulted in a significant increase in left ventricular ejection fraction from 25.2 $\pm$ 2.8% to 45.7 $\pm$ 8.6% (vs 20.0 $\pm$ 4.0% to 22.0 $\pm$ 9.0% in historical controls, $P<.01$) regardless of the presence of viral genomes, the authors concluded that virus-positive patients with acute myocarditis respond as well as virus-negative individuals.

Such a recommendation taken from data of a small cohort of virus-positive patients is of limited value for general treatment decisions. It is known that different viruses and even different virus subtypes respond in a distinct and unpredictable way to treatment. Furthermore, virus load and the type of the infected cells, both of which influence the course of the disease and drug response, have to be taken into consideration. Immunosuppression should be avoided in virus-positive patients because most of the available data from adult cohorts and animal studies predict adverse outcomes.[103–105]

Antiviral Treatment Strategies

Because of a lack of specific symptoms pointing at heart involvement, the early phase of a viral disease preceding heart-cell infection is generally missed in most patients. Elimination of viral translation, transcription, and proliferation with the use of any antiviral medication that targets viral attachment to host-cell receptors, virus entry, or virus uncoating, such as Pleconaril, WIN 54954, or CAR-Fc antibodies, are of limited use in patients with virus-associated heart disease because symptomatic patients generally present when organ infection is already established.[106,107] The current challenge of any antiviral therapy in patients with cardiac viral infections is the establishment of treatment strategies that prevent further virus spreading and to achieve in-time virus clearance before chronically infected heart tissue has been damaged irreversibly.

Interferons serve as a natural defense against many viral infections. Their innate production is associated with clinical recovery from viral infection and subsequent sequelae; exogenous administration is protective. Type I interferons therefore constitute a promising choice for treatment. Respective data from interferon treatment in children are not available. Adult patients with chronic enteroviral and adenoviral cardiomyopathy get considerable clinical and hemodynamic benefit from antiviral therapy. IFN-β 1a therapy effectively clears enterovirus and adenovirus, which constitute the 2 most frequent viruses associated with childhood myocarditis, in all treated patients.[108] Complete elimination of viral genome was proved by biopsy, and virus eradication was paralleled by a significant improvement in left ventricular function, decrease in ventricular size, amelioration of heart failure symptoms, and a significant decrease of infiltrating inflammatory cells; no patient deteriorated. Other viruses respond less well with respect to virus clearance although such patients may improve clinically following normalization of endothelial dysfunction despite incomplete virus clearance.[109] Clearance of those viruses may need other antiviral treatment regimens (see **Table 1**), but effective treatment conditions for viruses other than enterovirus and adenovirus have not yet been tested.

Despite promising results from several uncontrolled pediatric studies using immunosuppressive and/or immunomodulating therapy with intravenous γ-globulin, the translation of these results into a recommended routine therapy for pediatric myocarditis has been complicated by the high rate of spontaneous improvement of myocarditis with supportive care and the lack of demonstrable benefit for such therapies in blinded, randomized, placebo-controlled trials in adult myocarditis.[78] In acute disease it is actually difficult to decide whether immunosuppression or the spontaneous course has been responsible for reported improved outcome.[22,110]

PROGNOSIS

In children, myocarditis often presents with acute heart failure and prognosis and subsequent need for treatment are considerably influenced by the kind of underlying inflammatory process or the age of the child. Fulminant lymphocytic myocarditis with severe hemodynamic compromise has a high early mortality of more than 40% in adults and more than 75% in children especially during the neonatal period and the first years of life.[101,111] In addition to an age less than 1 year, abrupt onset of heart failure and lack of spontaneous ventricular improvement in the short-term is associated with high mortality.[26,98,101,112] Extracorporeal membrane oxygenation is a valuable tool to rescue children with severe cardiorespiratory compromise related to myocarditis.[113–115] Female gender, arrhythmia on extracorporeal membrane oxygenation, and the need for dialysis during extracorporeal membrane oxygenation were associated with increased mortality.[114]

Management is first of all supportive and is not aimed at the causative agent. Rapid aggressive support of cardiac function including inotropic therapy, mechanical circulatory support, and arrhythmia management may be a life-saving measure by bridging the interval for return to improved or native ventricular function or providing a bridge to transplantation.[116] In patients with myocarditis, therapy for arrhythmias is supportive, because even severe arrhythmias may resolve completely after the acute phase of the disease. Because spontaneous resolution of severe myocardial inflammation can last several weeks, implantation of a pacemaker or ICD sometimes cannot be avoided.

In patients who survive the initial critical phase, the long-term outcome seems favorable and better than that for patients presenting with more insidious chronic disease.[46,111,113] Histologic evidence of myocarditis as the cause of pediatric DCM has been considered to be a positive prognostic indicator for recovery, and single-center studies have reported a 50% to 80% chance for resolution of DCM from myocarditis within 2 years after presentation.[98,113] Although hemodynamic improvement often occurs within the first months of presentation, spontaneous improvement may be delayed up to 2 years. However, progression to severe heart failure with the need for transplantation may develop with a considerable delay after onset or initial clinical improvement of the disease.[26]

The histologic diagnosis of noninflammatory DCM, which may constitute a postinflammatory state, is associated with poorer outcome.[70,117] Furthermore, compared with cardiomyopathies and congenital heart diseases, the incidence of acute rejection seems to be highest in pediatric patients with myocarditis, resulting in a poor outcome for this population.[118] Heart transplantation in older children, which has a limited 15-year survival of 50%, should therefore be considered only when all available diagnostic tools have been applied and maximal supportive therapy does not lead to improvement.[113,119–121]

SUMMARY

DCM is the most common form of cardiomyopathy and reason for cardiac transplantation in adults and children. The spectrum of disease etiologies in childhood is different from that reported in adults, because myocarditis, a potentially life-threatening disease, is the most common cause of pure DCM. Deaths continue to occur years after presentation and the continuing mortality risk contradicts the reported high recovery rate for this condition. Such data from chronic disease and the high early mortality in acute myocarditis presenting as acute DCM especially in the youngest patients indicates a strong need for an early and exact diagnosis to identify the respective cohort of patients. An unambiguous diagnosis, infectious and/or inflammatory, is mandatory to initiate any specific treatment in addition to symptomatic therapy, and to avoid unnecessary interventions and improve prognosis in many patients with acute and chronic disease.

REFERENCES

1. Liu PP, Schultheiss HP. Myocarditis. In: Libby P, Bonow RO, Mann DL, editors. Baunwald's heart disease a textbook of cardiovascular medicine. 8th edition. Philadelphia: WB Saunders; 2008. p. 1775–92.

2. Aretz HT, Billingham ME, Edwards WD, et al. Myocarditis. A histopathologic definition and classification. Am J Cardiovasc Pathol 1987;1:3–14.

3. Kleinert S, Weintraub RG, Wilkinson JL, et al. Myocarditis in children with dilated cardiomyopathy: incidence and outcome after dual therapy immunosuppression. J Heart Lung Transplant 1997;16:1248–54.

4. Laufs H, Nigrovic PA, Schneider LC, et al. Giant cell myocarditis in a 12-year-old girl with common variable immunodeficiency. Mayo Clin Proc 2002; 77:92–6.

5. Lind-Ayres MR, Abramowsky C, Mahle WT. Pediatric giant cell myocarditis and orbital myositis. Pediatr Cardiol 2009;30:510–2.

6. Cooper LT. Giant cell myocarditis in children. Prog Pediatr Cardiol 2007;24:47–9.

7. Kodama M, Oda H, Okabe M, et al. Early and long-term mortality of the clinical subtypes of myocarditis. Jpn Circ J 2001;65:961–4.

8. Gagliardi MG, Bevilacqua M, Squitieri C, et al. Dilated cardiomyopathy caused by acute myocarditis in pediatric patients: evolution of myocardial damage in a group of potential heart transplant candidates. J Heart Lung Transplant 1993;12:S224–9.

9. Kühl U, Noutsias M, Seeberg B, et al. Immunohistological evidence for a chronic intramyocardial

inflammatory process in dilated cardiomyopathy. Heart 1996;75:295–300.

10. Kuhl U, Schultheiss HP. Viral myocarditis: diagnosis, aetiology and management. Drugs 2009; 69:1287–302.

11. Mason JW. Myocarditis and dilated cardiomyopathy: an inflammatory link. Cardiovasc Res 2003; 60:5–10.

12. Bergelson JM, Cunningham JA, Droguett G, et al. Isolation of a common receptor for Coxsackie B viruses and adenoviruses 2 and 5. Science 1997; 275:1320–3.

13. Bergelson JM. Receptors mediating adenovirus attachment and internalization. Biochem Pharmacol 1999;57:975–9.

14. Noutsias M, Fechner H, de Jonge H, et al. Human coxsackie-adenovirus receptor is colocalized with integrins alpha(v)beta(3) and alpha(v)beta(5) on the cardiomyocyte sarcolemma and upregulated in dilated cardiomyopathy: implications for cardiotropic viral infections. Circulation 2001;104:275–80.

15. Bultmann BD, Klingel K, Sotlar K, et al. Fatal parvovirus B19-associated myocarditis clinically mimicking ischemic heart disease: an endothelial cell-mediated disease. Hum Pathol 2003;34:92–5.

16. Bock CT, Klingel K, Aberle S, et al. Human Parvovirus B19: a new emerging pathogen of inflammatory cardiomyopathy. J Vet Med B Infect Dis Vet Public Health 2005;52:340–3.

17. Klingel K, Sauter M, Bock CT, et al. Molecular pathology of inflammatory cardiomyopathy. Med Microbiol Immunol (Berl) 2004;193:101–7.

18. Hilton DA, Variend S, Pringle JH. Demonstration of Coxsackie virus RNA in formalin-fixed tissue sections from childhood myocarditis cases by in situ hybridization and the polymerase chain reaction. J Pathol 1993;170:45–51.

19. Liu PP, Opavsky MA. Viral myocarditis: receptors that bridge the cardiovascular with the immune system? Circ Res 2000;86:253–4.

20. Levi D, Alejos J. Diagnosis and treatment of pediatric viral myocarditis. Curr Opin Cardiol 2001;16: 77–83.

21. Gravanis MB, Sternby NH. Incidence of myocarditis. A 10-year autopsy study from Malmo, Sweden. Arch Pathol Lab Med 1991;115:390–2.

22. Mason JW. Immunopathogenesis and treatment of myocarditis: the United States Myocarditis Treatment Trial. J Card Fail 1996;2:S173–7.

23. Doolan A, Langlois N, Semsarian C. Causes of sudden cardiac death in young Australians. Med J Aust 2004;180:110–2.

24. Kyto V, Saraste A, Voipio-Pulkki LM, et al. Incidence of fatal myocarditis: a population-based study in Finland. Am J Epidemiol 2007;165:570–4.

25. Webber SA, Boyle GJ, Jaffe R, et al. Role of right ventricular endomyocardial biopsy in infants and children with suspected or possible myocarditis. Br Heart J 1994;72:360–3.

26. Towbin JA, Lowe AM, Colan SD, et al. Incidence, causes, and outcomes of dilated cardiomyopathy in children. JAMA 2006;296:1867–76.

27. Camargo PR, Okay TS, Yamamoto L, et al. Myocarditis in children and detection of viruses in myocardial tissue: implications for immunosuppressive therapy. Int J Cardiol 2009. [Epub ahead of print].

28. Durani Y, Egan M, Baffa J, et al. Pediatric myocarditis: presenting clinical characteristics. Am J Emerg Med 2009;27:942–7.

29. Nugent AW, Daubeney PE, Chondros P, et al. The epidemiology of childhood cardiomyopathy in Australia. N Engl J Med 2003;348:1639–46.

30. Wilkinson JD, Sleeper LA, Alvarez JA, et al. The pediatric cardiomyopathy registry: 1995–2007. Prog Pediatr Cardiol 2008;25:31–6.

31. Cox GF, Sleeper LA, Lowe AM, et al. Factors associated with establishing a causal diagnosis for children with cardiomyopathy. Pediatrics 2006;118: 1519–31.

32. Lipshultz SE, Sleeper LA, Towbin JA, et al. The incidence of pediatric cardiomyopathy in two regions of the United States. N Engl J Med 2003;348: 1647–55.

33. Weber MA, Ashworth MT, Risdon RA, et al. Clinicopathological features of paediatric deaths due to myocarditis: an autopsy series. Arch Dis Child 2008;93:594–8.

34. Calabrese F, Rigo E, Milanesi O, et al. Molecular diagnosis of myocarditis and dilated cardiomyopathy in children: clinicopathologic features and prognostic implications. Diagn Mol Pathol 2002;11:212–21.

35. Bowles NE, Kearney DL, Ni J, et al. The detection of viral genomes by polymerase chain reaction in the myocardium of pediatric patients with advanced HIV disease. J Am Coll Cardiol 1999;34:857–65.

36. Bowles NE, Ni J, Kearney DL, et al. Detection of viruses in myocardial tissues by polymerase chain reaction. Evidence of adenovirus as a common cause of myocarditis in children and adults. J Am Coll Cardiol 2003;42:466–72.

37. Carturan E, Milanesi O, Kato Y, et al. Viral detection and tumor necrosis factor alpha profile in tracheal aspirates from children with suspicion of myocarditis. Diagn Mol Pathol 2008;17:21–7.

38. Comar M, D'Agaro P, Campello C, et al. Human herpes virus 6 in archival cardiac tissues from children with idiopathic dilated cardiomyopathy or congenital heart disease. J Clin Pathol 2009;62:80–3.

39. Dettmeyer R, Baasner A, Schlamann M, et al. Coxsackie B3 myocarditis in 4 cases of suspected sudden infant death syndrome: diagnosis by immunohistochemical and molecular-pathologic investigations. Pathol Res Pract 2002;198:689–96.

40. Gouton M, Di Filippo S, Sassolas F, et al. [Acute infectious myocarditis in children. Apropos of 2 series from Lyon]. Arch Mal Coeur Vaiss 1995;88:753–9 [in French].

41. Martin AB, Webber S, Fricker FJ, et al. Acute myocarditis. Rapid diagnosis by PCR in children. Circulation 1994;90:330–9.

42. Munro K, Croxson MC, Thomas S, et al. Three cases of myocarditis in childhood associated with human parvovirus (B19 virus). Pediatr Cardiol 2003;24:473–5.

43. Savon C, Acosta B, Valdes O, et al. A myocarditis outbreak with fatal cases associated with adenovirus subgenera C among children from Havana City in 2005. J Clin Virol 2008;43:152–7.

44. Schowengerdt KO, Ni J, Denfield SW, et al. Association of parvovirus B19 genome in children with myocarditis and cardiac allograft rejection: diagnosis using the polymerase chain reaction. Circulation 1997;96:3549–54.

45. Talsma MD, Kroos MA, Visser G, et al. A rare presentation of childhood pompe disease: cardiac involvement provoked by Epstein-Barr virus infection. Pediatrics 2002;109:e65.

46. Vare D, Vare B, Dauphin C, et al. [Acute myocarditis in children. Study of 11 clinical cases]. Arch Mal Coeur Vaiss 2000;93:571–9 [in French].

47. Baboonian C, Treasure T. Meta-analysis of the association of enteroviruses with human heart disease. Heart 1997;78:539–43.

48. Batmaz G, Villain E, Bonnet D, et al. [Therapy and prognosis of infectious complete atrioventricular block in children]. Arch Mal Coeur Vaiss 2000;93:553–7 [in French].

49. Dancea AB. Myocarditis in infants and children: a review for the paediatrician. Paediatr Child Health 2001;6:543–5.

50. Khaleduzzaman M, Francis J, Corbin ME, et al. Infection of cardiomyocytes and induction of left ventricle dysfunction by neurovirulent polytropic murine retrovirus. J Virol 2007;81:12307–15.

51. Guarner J, Paddock CD, Shieh WJ, et al. Histopathologic and immunohistochemical features of fatal influenza virus infection in children during the 2003–2004 season. Clin Infect Dis 2006;43:132–40.

52. Costello JM, Alexander ME, Greco KM, et al. Lyme carditis in children: presentation, predictive factors, and clinical course. Pediatrics 2009;123:e835–41.

53. Taliercio CP, Olney BA, Lie JT. Myocarditis related to drug hypersensitivity. Mayo Clin Proc 1985;60:463–8.

54. Press S, Lipkind RS. Acute myocarditis in infants. Initial presentation. Clin Pediatr (Phila) 1990;29:73–6.

55. Amvrosieva TV, Paklonskaya NV, Biazruchka AA, et al. Enteroviral infection outbreak in the Republic of Belarus: principal characteristics and phylogenetic analysis of etiological agents. Cent Eur J Public Health 2006;14:67–73.

56. Mounts AW, Amr S, Jamshidi R, et al. A cluster of fulminant myocarditis cases in children, Baltimore, Maryland, 1997. Pediatr Cardiol 2001;22:34–9.

57. Schoub BD, Johnson S, McAnerney JM, et al. Epidemic Coxsackie B virus infection in Johannesburg, South Africa. J Hyg (Lond) 1985;95:447–55.

58. Valdes O, Acosta B, Pinon A, et al. First report on fatal myocarditis associated with adenovirus infection in Cuba. J Med Virol 2008;80:1756–61.

59. Wang DM, Zhao GC, Zhuang SM, et al. An epidemic of encephalitis and meningoencephalitis in children caused by echovirus type 30 in Shanghai. Chin Med J (Engl) 1993;106:767–9.

60. Yodfat Y, Nishmi M. Clinical virology in family practice: epidemiological and clinical observations of an outbreak of Coxsackievirus B type 1 infection in a kibbutz. J Fam Pract 1977;5:201–7.

61. Zurynski YA, Lester-Smith D, Festa MS, et al. Enhanced surveillance for serious complications of influenza in children: role of the Australian Paediatric Surveillance Unit. Commun Dis Intell 2008;32:71–6.

62. Adekanmbi AF, Ogunlesi TA, Olowu AO, et al. Current trends in the prevalence and aetiology of childhood congestive cardiac failure in Sagamu. J Trop Pediatr 2007;53:103–6.

63. Chehab G, Shalak W, Gerbaka B, et al. [Inflammatory heart diseases in childhood: Lebanese epidemiological survey]. J Med Liban 2006;54:124–31 [in French].

64. Rajs J, Hammarquist F. Sudden infant death in Stockholm. A forensic pathology study covering ten years. Acta Paediatr Scand 1988;77:812–20.

65. Dettmeyer R, Baasner A, Schlamann M, et al. Role of virus-induced myocardial affections in sudden infant death syndrome: a prospective postmortem study. Pediatr Res 2004;55:947–52.

66. Woodruff JF. Viral myocarditis. A review. Am J Pathol 1980;101:425–84.

67. Chang YJ, Chao HC, Hsia SH, et al. Myocarditis presenting as gastritis in children. Pediatr Emerg Care 2006;22:439–40.

68. Chavda KK, Dhuper S, Madhok A, et al. Seizures secondary to a high-grade atrioventricular block as a presentation of acute myocarditis. Pediatr Emerg Care 2004;20:387–90.

69. da Silva MA, da Silva RP, de Morais SC, et al. [Clinical aspects and development of dilated cardiomyopathy in infants and children]. Arq Bras Cardiol 1991;56:213–8 [in Portuguese].

70. Nugent AW, Davis AM, Kleinert S, et al. Clinical, electrocardiographic, and histologic correlations in children with dilated cardiomyopathy. J Heart Lung Transplant 2001;20:1152–7.

71. Mangnani JW, Dec GW. Myocarditis: current trends in diagnosis and treatment. Circulation 2006;113: 876–90.

72. Morgera T, Di Lenarda A, Dreas L, et al. Electrocardiography of myocarditis revisited: clinical and prognostic significance of electrocardiographic changes. Am Heart J 1992;124: 455–67.

73. Smith SC, Ladenson JH, Mason JW, et al. Elevations of cardiac troponin I associated with myocarditis. Experimental and clinical correlates. Circulation 1997;95:163–8.

74. Soongswang J, Durongpisitkul K, Nana A, et al. Cardiac troponin T: a marker in the diagnosis of acute myocarditis in children. Pediatr Cardiol 2005;26:45–9.

75. Pinamonti B, Alberti E, Cigalotto A, et al. Echocardiographic findings in myocarditis. Am J Cardiol 1988;62:285–91.

76. Abdel-Aty H, Boye P, Zagrosek A, et al. Diagnostic performance of cardiovascular magnetic resonance in patients with suspected acute myocarditis: comparison of different approaches. J Am Coll Cardiol 2005;45:1815–22.

77. Friedrich MG, Sechtem U, Schulz-Menger J, et al. Cardiovascular magnetic resonance in myocarditis: a JACC White Paper. J Am Coll Cardiol 2009;53:1475–87.

78. Vashist S, Singh GK. Acute myocarditis in children: current concepts and management. Curr Treat Options Cardiovasc Med 2009;11:383–91.

79. Gutberlet M, Spors B, Thoma T, et al. Suspected chronic myocarditis at cardiac MR: diagnostic accuracy and association with immunohistologically detected inflammation and viral persistence. Radiology 2008;246:401–9.

80. Balaji S, Wiles HB, Sens MA, et al. Immunosuppressive treatment for myocarditis and borderline myocarditis in children with ventricular ectopic rhythm. Br Heart J 1994;72:354–9.

81. Baughman KL. Diagnosis of myocarditis: death of Dallas criteria. Circulation 2006;113:593–5.

82. Schultheiss HP, Kuehl U. Cardiovascular viral infections. In: Lennette EH, editor. Lennette's laboratory diagnosis of viral infections. 4th edition. New York (NY): Informa Healthcare; 2010. p. 304–18, Chapter 18.

83. Celiker A, Ozkutlu S, Ozer S, et al. Endomyocardial biopsy in children. Usefulness in various myocardial disorders. Jpn Heart J 1991;32:227–37.

84. Chandra RS. The role of endomyocardial biopsy in the diagnosis of cardiac disorders in infants and children. Am J Cardiovasc Pathol 1987;1: 157–72.

85. Gagliardi MG, Bevilacqua M, Parisi F, et al. [Endomyocardial biopsy in childhood]. G Ital Cardiol 1992;22:963–8 [in Italian].

86. Narula N, Narula J, Dec GW. Endomyocardial biopsy for non-transplant-related disorders. Am J Clin Pathol 2005;123(Suppl):S106–18.

87. Schmaltz AA, Apitz J, Hort W. Endomyocardial biopsy in infants and children: technique; indications and results. Eur J Pediatr 1982;138:211–5.

88. Cowley CG, Lozier JS, Orsmond GS, et al. Safety of endomyocardial biopsy in children. Cardiol Young 2003;13:404–7.

89. Pass RH, Trivedi KR, Hsu DT. A new technique for endomyocardial biopsy in infants and small children. Catheter Cardiovasc Interv 2000;50: 441–4.

90. Schmaltz AA, Apitz J, Hort W, et al. [Endomyocardial biopsy in childhood–experiences in 60 pediatric patients]. Z Kardiol 1987;76:563–9 [in German].

91. Yoshizato T, Edwards WD, Alboliras ET, et al. Safety and utility of endomyocardial biopsy in infants, children and adolescents: a review of 66 procedures in 53 patients. J Am Coll Cardiol 1990;15: 436–42.

92. Parisi F. Why do we not perform routine endomyocardial biopsies in childhood cardiomyopathy? J Heart Lung Transplant 2009;28(12):1249–51.

93. Holzmann M, Nicko A, Kühl U, et al. Complication rate of right ventricular endomyocardial biopsy via the femoral approach. A retrospective and prospective study analyzing 3048 diagnostic procedures over an 11-year period. Circulation 2008;118:1722–8.

94. Frustaci A, Russo MA, Chimenti C. Randomized study on the efficacy of immunosuppressive therapy in patients with virus-negative inflammatory cardiomyopathy: the TIMIC study. Eur Heart J 2009;30:1995–2002.

95. Kühl U, Strauer BE, Schultheiss HP. Methylprednisolone in chronic myocarditis. Postgrad Med J 1994; 70:S35–42.

96. Wojnicz R, Nowalany-Kozielska E, Wojciechowska C, et al. Randomized, placebo-controlled study for immunosuppressive treatment of inflammatory dilated cardiomyopathy: two-year follow-up results. Circulation 2001;104:39–45.

97. Drucker NA, Colan SD, Lewis AB, et al. Gamma-globulin treatment of acute myocarditis in the pediatric population. Circulation 1994;89:252–7.

98. English RF, Janosky JE, Ettedgui JA, et al. Outcomes for children with acute myocarditis. Cardiol Young 2004;14:488–93.

99. Klugman D, Berger JT, Sable CA, et al. Pediatric patients hospitalized with myocarditis: a multi-institutional analysis. Pediatr Cardiol 2009;31(2): 222–8.

100. Chan KY, Iwahara M, Benson LN, et al. Immunosuppressive therapy in the management of acute myocarditis in children: a clinical trial. J Am Coll Cardiol 1991;17:458–60.

101. Nunes T, Vaz T, Monterroso J, et al. [Myocarditis in early childhood. Two years' experience at the pediatric cardiology unit at the S. Joao Hospital]. Rev Port Cardiol 1991;10:511–6 [in Portuguese].

102. Camargo PR, Snitcowsky R, da Luz PL, et al. Favorable effects of immunosuppressive therapy in children with dilated cardiomyopathy and active myocarditis. Pediatr Cardiol 1995;16:61–8.

103. Frustaci A, Chimenti C, Calabrese F, et al. Immunosuppressive therapy for active lymphocytic myocarditis: virological and immunologic profile of responders versus nonresponders. Circulation 2003;107:857–63.

104. Khatib R, Reyes MP, Smith F, et al. Enhancement of coxsackievirus B4 virulence by indomethacin. J Lab Clin Med 1990;116:116–20.

105. Costanzo-Nordin MR, Reap EA, O'Connell JB, et al. A nonsteroid anti-inflammatory drug exacerbates Coxsackie B3 murine myocarditis. J Am Coll Cardiol 1985;6:1078–82.

106. Abzug MJ. Presentation, diagnosis, and management of enterovirus infections in neonates. Paediatr Drugs 2004;6:1–10.

107. Liu Z, Yuan J, Yanagawa B, et al. Coxsackievirus-induced myocarditis: new trends in treatment. Expert Rev Anti Infect Ther 2005;3:641–50.

108. Kühl U, Pauschinger M, Schwimmbeck PL, et al. Interferon-beta treatment eliminates cardiotropic viruses and improves left ventricular function in patients with myocardial persistence of viral genomes and left ventricular dysfunction. Circulation 2003;107:2793–8.

109. Schmidt-Lucke C, Spillmann F, Bock T, et al. Interferon-beta modulates endothelial damage in patients with cardiac persistence of human parvovirus b19 infection. J Infect Dis 2009;201(6):936–45.

110. Stanton C, Mookadam F, Cha S, et al. Greater symptom duration predicts response to immunomodulatory therapy in dilated cardiomyopathy. Int J Cardiol 2008;128:38–41.

111. McCarthy RE 3rd, Boehmer JP, Hruban RH, et al. Long-term outcome of fulminant myocarditis as compared with acute (nonfulminant) myocarditis. N Engl J Med 2000;342:690–5.

112. Torres F, Anguita M, Tejero I, et al. [Acute myocarditis with severe cardiac dysfunction in the pediatric population. The evolution and differential characteristics with respect to adult myocarditis]. Rev Esp Cardiol 1995;48:660–5 [in Spanish].

113. Lee KJ, McCrindle BW, Bohn DJ, et al. Clinical outcomes of acute myocarditis in childhood. Heart 1999;82:226–33.

114. Rajagopal SK, Almond CS, Laussen PC, et al. Extracorporeal membrane oxygenation for the support of infants, children, and young adults with acute myocarditis: a review of the Extracorporeal Life Support Organization registry. Crit Care Med 2009;38(2):382–7.

115. Duncan BW, Bohn DJ, Atz AM, et al. Mechanical circulatory support for the treatment of children with acute fulminant myocarditis. J Thorac Cardiovasc Surg 2001;122:440–8.

116. Stiller B, Weng Y, Hubler M, et al. Pneumatic pulsatile ventricular assist devices in children under 1 year of age. Eur J Cardiothorac Surg 2005;28:234–9.

117. Matitiau A, Perez-Atayde A, Sanders SP, et al. Infantile dilated cardiomyopathy. Relation of outcome to left ventricular mechanics, hemodynamics, and histology at the time of presentation. Circulation 1994;90:1310–8.

118. Parisi F, Carotti A, Esu F, et al. Intermediate and long-term results after pediatric heart transplantation: incidence and role of pretransplant diagnosis. Transpl Int 1998;11(Suppl 1):S493–8.

119. Amabile N, Fraisse A, Bouvenot J, et al. Outcome of acute fulminant myocarditis in children. Heart 2006;92:1269–73.

120. Bohn D, Benson L. Diagnosis and management of pediatric myocarditis. Paediatr Drugs 2002;4:171–81.

121. Kirk R, Naftel D, Hoffman TM, et al. Outcome of pediatric patients with dilated cardiomyopathy listed for transplant: a multi-institutional study. J Heart Lung Transplant 2009;28(12):1322–8.

Pathophysiology and Management of Heart Failure in Repaired Congenital Heart Disease

Paul F. Kantor, MB, BCh, DCH, FRCPC*,
Andrew N. Redington, MD, FRCP

KEYWORDS

- Heart failure • Congenital heart disease • Fontan
- Remodeling • Right ventricle

Transient myocardial dysfunction during the early postoperative course is a common sequela of open heart surgery in children, which for the vast majority seems to resolve completely. However, whether related to this perioperative insult or a more chronic effect of the disease, its treatment, or residual abnormalities, established heart failure in children with congenital heart disease may occur at any time in their postoperative course. This article details the current knowledge of congenital disease-related heart failure (CDHF), alluding to common themes in the pathophysiology of systemic ventricular dysfunction, which inform the clinician regarding treatment. These aspects are examined in the context of specific lesions, and treatment options are discussed.

PERSISTENT VENTRICULAR DYSFUNCTION FOLLOWING SURGICAL REPAIR

In the contemporary era, advances in perfusion, anesthesia, and early postoperative supportive care/drug therapy have resulted in a "new normal," in which relatively few patients manifest overt ventricular dysfunction after the first 72 postsurgical hours. However, certain high-risk lesions persist in manifesting late ventricular dysfunction, even when the primary correction is expertly done. These include

- Hypoplastic left heart syndrome during its staged repair.
- The Fontan repair for single-ventricle physiology of various sorts.
- Congenitally corrected transposition of the great arteries requiring surgical intervention.

In many respects, the substrate for late ventricular failure is evident in early childhood and is amplified over years and decades because of one or more persistent hemodynamic problems. Operative repair is frequently imperfect, but how often this actually results in symptoms that could reasonably be described as heart failure can be questioned. In a meta-analysis, Verheugt and colleagues[1] reviewed the published literature from 1980 to 2007, identifying 35 case series describing the course of 7984 patients with postoperative congenital heart disease. Although survival was generally good, they were also able to identify the prevalence of New York Heart Association (NYHA) I status for the major common diagnoses (**Fig. 1**). Overall, 93% of patients from follow-up studies commencing in the pediatric age range survived, and of these, around 80% were in NYHA I class. However, only 50% of cases with a systemic right ventricle (RV) were symptom-free at a mean age of 20 to 25 years. The importance of the solitary or

University of Toronto, Division of Cardiology, Hospital for Sick Children, 555 University Avenue, Toronto, ON M5G 1X8, Canada
* Corresponding author.
E-mail address: Paul.Kantor@sickkids.ca

Heart Failure Clin 6 (2010) 497–506
doi:10.1016/j.hfc.2010.06.002

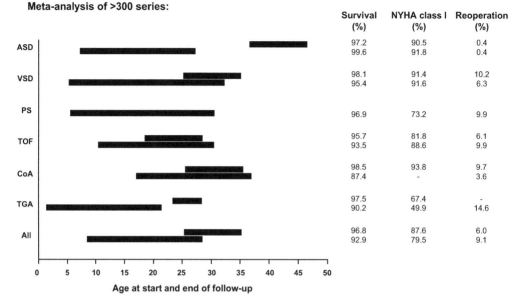

Fig. 1. Meta-analysis of the prognosis of congenital heart disease, including 35 series incorporating 7984 patients followed between 1980 and 2007. Horizontal bars represent studies clustered according to follow-up duration and age (either pediatric or adult range), arranged according to the major diagnostic groups. Percentage survival, NYHA I symptomatic class, and reoperation status at last follow-up are represented in the right hand columns for each diagnostic group and age stratum. (*From* Verheugt CL, Uiterwaal CS, Grobbee DE, et al. Long-term prognosis of congenital heart defects: a systematic review. Int J Cardiol 2008;131(1):25–32 [Review]; with permission.)

systemic RV as the substrate for failure is further supported by work from Norozi and colleagues[2] in a single-center series, in which more than 20% of patients with a single ventricle or a systemic RV (as well as with tetralogy of Fallot) had both a reduction in aerobic capacity and elevated B-type natriuretic peptide (BNP) levels by age 20 years. These specific situations are examined in more detail.

THE SINGLE VENTRICLE: HEART FAILURE DURING INTERSTAGE PALLIATION
Scope of the Problem

Many of the conditions that fall under the umbrella of functionally single ventricle present in the neonatal period, with some form of heart failure. Those with anatomy that limits systemic blood flow in utero (eg, double inlet left ventricle [LV] with discordant ventriculo-arterial connections, hypoplastic left heart syndrome [HLHS]) are (1) predisposed to aortic arch anomalies that render their systemic circulation duct-dependent, and (2) at risk of rapid development of preoperative heart failure symptoms because of an increasing pulmonary-to-systemic flow ratio

(Qp/Qs), as the pulmonary vascular resistance falls. The key to successful treatment lies in timely surgical palliation, but preoperative management should be directed at maintenance of ductal patency, where appropriate, and manipulation of Qp/Qs. Nowadays this is achieved primarily by modification of systemic vascular resistance (SVR).

Neither strategy is effective if there is limitation of blood flow elsewhere in the circulation. For HLHS in particular, an appropriate interatrial communication is required to avoid pulmonary venous hypertension and its secondary effects on pulmonary blood flow and oxygenation. The success of fetal screening programs has made presentation with cardiovascular collapse a rare event in many units, and consequently, overt early ventricular myocardial failure has become similarly uncommon. As a result, even in the HLHS population, there is remarkably little data pointing to a correlation between preoperative ventricular performance and postoperative outcomes. However, in one study, a poor RV ejection fraction (RVEF), though not associated with early survival, was predictive of poorer late outcomes.[3] The authors' data from a cohort of patients managed in Toronto between 1998 and 2007 suggested an adverse impact of reduced preoperative RVEF on both early and late survival after first-stage Norwood procedure.

Phenotype of the Failing Single Ventricle Palliation

It is beyond the scope of this article to discuss in detail the early postoperative management of the neonate after palliation (most often some form of Norwood palliation). The general principles of preoperative management apply equally, and perhaps more importantly, postoperatively. Residual obstruction to systemic blood flow is poorly tolerated, and in the early postoperative period, manipulation of SVR with intravenous vasodilators has become part of routine care.

Despite this, myocardial dysfunction and associated systemic atrioventricular (AV) valve regurgitation are not infrequent, particularly in HLHS but also in other forms of functionally single ventricle. For some, intrinsic abnormalities of the atrioventricular valve drive a spiral of worsening regurgitation and ventricular dysfunction. These patients may benefit from direct surgical intervention on the valve.[4] For others, the primary abnormality appears to be within the myocardium. While a clear-cut abnormality can sometimes be defined (eg, coronary ischemia in HLHS associated with mitral stenosis and aortic atresia, or LV noncompaction in the setting of pulmonary atresia with intact ventricular septum), most often this appears to reflect the outcome of "multiple hits" conspiring to cause adverse remodeling and potentially

inexorable decline (**Fig. 2**). Unfortunately, the treatment options for this latter group are limited, but are discussed as follows.

Treatment Options for Heart Failure Before Fontan Completion

The prophylactic use of angiotensin-converting enzyme (ACE) inhibitors has become ubiquitous in the postoperative management of the functionally single ventricle, despite there being little data to support their use in this way. Indeed, a recent study completed by the National Institutes of Health-supported Pediatric Heart Network showed no benefit in terms of symptoms or weight gain of ACE inhibition as interstage therapy before the bidirectional Glenn procedure (D Hsu, personal communication, 2009). Proponents of this therapy identify the benefits of afterload reduction in the early postoperative period, and it has become commonplace to wean patients after stage 1 palliation from intravenous vasodilators to oral therapy in the immediate postoperative period. While intuitively attractive, superficially, this logic does not sustain close scrutiny; although many patients also receive intravenous inotropic agents, one would not consider replacing such therapy with an oral inotrope during weaning. Also, little is known of the effects of a chronically reduced afterload. In disease states (eg, vitamin B deficiency, arteriovenous malformations), a chronically reduced afterload can itself lead to high-output failure, with ventricular dilation, atrioventricular valve regurgitation, and ultimately, systolic dysfunction. At the very least, some caution

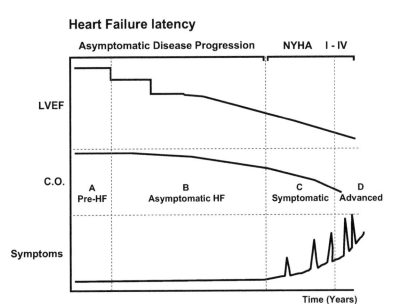

Fig. 2. Schematic depiction of the latency of clinical symptoms and functional deterioration in heart failure. The phase of deteriorating function and diminishing cardiac output greatly exceeds the duration of overt symptoms. In congenital heart disease, much of stage A and B occurs in early childhood, with overt symptoms more frequently developing in later adolescence or adult life. CO, cardiac output; HF, heart failure. (*Adapted from* Liu P, personal communication, 2009; with permission. *Courtesy of* Peter Liu, MD, Toronto, Canada.)

should be exercised in the indiscriminate use of these agents in this setting. Similarly, given the wealth of data from adult trials, the use of β-blockers to treat the ventricular dysfunction associated with congenital heart diseases appears intuitive. However, the data available suggest that such therapy may have overtly adverse effects on the systemic RV[5]; these agents, if used, should be used under strict (ideally research-driven) protocols and cannot be recommended for routine or prophylactic therapy.

THE FONTAN CIRCULATION

Introduced in the 1970s[6] as a means of increasing pulmonary blood flow in adults without a distinct RV circulation, this palliation has undergone several iterations, taking a routine place in the staged palliation of children with a single ventricle. Early failure of the Fontan operation and associated takedown have become an uncommon event (<2%) in the current era because of more cautious patient selection, transplantation emerging as a viable option, and, to some extent, improved perioperative techniques. Patients operated on before 1985 predominantly using an atriopulmonary or atrioventricular anastomosis technique had a mortality of 30% at a median of 12 years, with a high degree of risk for reintervention. Most of these deaths occurred in the perioperative phase.[7] In contrast, more recent series suggest survival exceeding 90% at 10 years.[8] While early surgical mortality (now also <2%) has therefore declined dramatically,[9] 10-year mortality has also decreased from around 20% to less than 10%.

Ventricular Morphology

The substrate upon which a Fontan operation is constructed matters, perhaps as much as the construction itself. The prelude to a Fontan operation involves a volume-loaded ventricle and, in some cases, a pressure load as well because of pulmonary arterial (PA) banding in infancy. This is especially true for patients from the previous era who were not subject to staging via an early cavopulmonary shunt and takedown of the initial palliative Blalock-Taussig shunt.[10] As a result, the substrate of the Fontan operation is an imperfect ventricle, often hypertrophied and dilated. The subsequent reduction in inflow after the Fontan operation results in an underfilled and hypertrophied heart. Also, there is good evidence from the Pediatric Heart Network multicentre study[11] that RV morphology of the single ventricle is closely related to late ventricular dysfunction and, predictably, to AV valve failure as well. However, these are not the only mechanisms of

Fontan failure and death. Most series describe a spectrum of overlapping risks for these patients, including arrhythmic events and sudden death, thromboembolism, and heart failure, occurring in about 6% in the historic series.[7] These investigators described independent predictors of heart-failure death as being protein-losing enteropathy (hazard ratio [HR], 7.1; $P = .0043$), single morphologically RV (HR, 10.5; $P = .0429$), and higher right atrial pressure (HR, 1.3 per 1 mm Hg; $P = .0016$).

Traditional Measures of Heart Failure

Are these features then a hallmark of all patients with this circulation, or only those from an earlier era? A recent report from Rotterdam suggests that many patients (32%) do not maintain sinus rhythm and that ventricular ejection fraction at rest is lower than in controls but still in the normal range.[12] Aerobic exercise capacity is well known to be reduced in these patients,[13] with both cardiopulmonary and peripheral muscle factors implicated. Ventricular function is difficult to characterize in this setting. Simple measures, such as ejection fraction, suggest normal range cavity displacement in about three-quarters of patients, with diastolic dysfunction being far more pervasive and detectable in about 70% of patients.[11] Many have stated that the Fontan circulation is preload-limited, and it is clear that the transpulmonary pressure gradient that determines this preload is precarious. With an age-related increment in systemic ventricular diastolic pressure, one can anticipate that diastolic function of the systemic ventricle becomes the weakest link in the chain for Fontan-circulation patients.

The Phenotype of a Failing Fontan

There is unfortunately no simple definition of Fontan failure, and indeed, it and may not overlap completely with obvious ventricular function problems: protein losing enteropathy, plastic bronchitis, intrapulmonary arteriovenous malformations, and atrial arrhythmias are all well described in the presence of normal ventricular function in these patients. Hence, some have argued that ventricular and cavopulmonary failure are separate entities and distinguishable by BNP levels, which remain normal in the latter[14] but are moderately elevated in Fontan patients with ventricular dysfunction.

Treatment of the Failing Fontan

Some of the elements alluded to earlier and others not discussed (persistent shunts, leaks, and venovenous collateral connections) are treatable lesions. AV valve repair and Fontan conversion are well recognized to improve symptoms and reduce the arrhythmia burden, which is one of the major drivers of symptoms. The treatment of protein-losing enteropathy, plastic bronchitis, and AV malformations is less well established, with long-term success proving to be elusive in many. In these situations, cardiac transplantation should be considered. Medical therapy for ventricular failure in the Fontan circulation is often attempted and seldom successful in the authors' experience. Diuretics, including aldosterone antagonists, have a sound theoretical basis and are indicated. ACE inhibitors and β-adrenoceptor blockers have a lesser role and cannot be endorsed at this time. It is possible that vasodilation may worsen symptoms for many patients.

CONGENITALLY CORRECTED TRANSPOSITION AND THE ATRIAL SWITCH OPERATION

Few situations are as enigmatic and vexing from a therapeutic point of view as the RV in the systemic position, either by virtue of nature or surgical design. Congenitally corrected transposition of the great arteries (CCTGA) exists within a range of disorders of AV connections, and it is characterized by discordance of AV connections, with ventriculoarterial discordance. Hence, the circulation is physiologically corrected, but as observed by Van Praagh, little else is correct, and these hearts are at high risk of ventricular failure for many reasons.

Natural History and Surgical Options for CCTGA

The natural history of unoperated CCTGA is unfavorable, reported to be a survival of 72.3% at age 3 years in a recent Eastern European series[15] and 64% at 10 years of follow-up in a institution-based historic cohort reported by Huhta and colleagues.[16]

There are several reasons for symptoms and death in these patients, especially in those with associated lesions. The tricuspid valve subjected to systemic pressures is prone to failure, and tricuspid regurgitation alone can account for much of the excess mortality seen in CCTGA.[17] In addition, the presence of a ventricular septal defect (VSD) and subpulmonary stenosis may also result in oxygen desaturation, and, because the conduction axis passes anteriorly along the free wall of the LV and is elongated and susceptible, complete AV block is reported in about 2% of patients per year, reaching up to 45% in long-term follow-up.[18] For all symptomatic patients, especially those with associated lesions, surgery remains the first and possibly the only meaningful strategy.

Surgical remediation of this disorder is typically undertaken by one of the 2 approaches:

1. Closing the existing VSD and addressing subpulmonary obstruction by placing an LV-to-PA conduit without correcting anatomic relations (a classic or physiologic repair); the tricuspid valve remains in the systemic circulation and may also be repaired or replaced.

2. Restoration of functional connections along morphologic grounds: restoring the LV from a subpulmonary to a subaortic position and re-routing atrial inflow to the appropriate morphologic ventricle; this double switch is typically accomplished by a combination of a Mustard or Senning atrial baffle and an arterial switch or interventricular tunnel connecting the accompanying VSD to the aorta and placing an RV-to-PA conduit (a variant of the Rastelli procedure).

Modifications incorporating volume unloading for the subpulmonary ventricle by a cavopulmonary anastomosis have been advocated.[19] Even the Fontan operation is an available option for surgical palliation. Other considerations include repair or replacement of the tricuspid valve, which is commonly dysplastic and regurgitant, and, most importantly, retraining of the low-pressure subpulmonary LV to regain near-systemic pressure before a switch procedure by serial PA banding in most individuals.

The success of surgery for this condition has been mixed, and although surgical survival is improving in the current era, it is still unclear whether this can be attributed to a particular surgical approach. A Toronto group have argued for the protective effect of a Rastelli-type anatomic repair by modeling data from 124 patients in a meta-analysis.[20] Others, describing single-center data acquired over decades, are able to show an improving survival with time but cannot attribute this clearly to a particular surgical strategy.[21] Regardless of surgical strategy, the tricuspid valve and the systemic RV are probably the underlying reasons for heart failure in surgical survivors.[22]

Phenotype of Heart Failure in CCTGA

Most often, patients are noticed in 1 of the 3 scenarios:

1. No prior surgical intervention, with progressive cyanosis indicating a VSD and subpulmonary stenosis

2. Previous surgical palliation leaving the tricuspid valve in the systemic position, with RV failure

3. Previous surgical palliation with secondary LV dysfunction and frequently combined ventricular dysfunction.

Recently, Szymanski and colleagues[23] attempted to codify the features of systemic RV failure in symptomatic and asymptomatic patients with a systemic RV. These investigators found that 54.2% of their patients had no RV systolic dysfunction, 23.8 % had asymptomatic RV dysfunction, and the remainder had dysfunction and symptoms; conversely, 11.9% of patients had heart failure symptoms with normal (preserved) systolic RV function, frequently in the presence of tricuspid regurgitation. They found that normal BNP levels were a good predictor of normal RV function in all patients. Other investigators reported that amino-terminal proBNP (NT-proBNP) was significantly elevated in all patients with a systemic RV, correlating with magnetic resonance imaging (MRI)-derived RVEF and with tissue Doppler-derived annular velocity, even in asymptomatic patients. MRI assessment of the systemic RV has further revealed a significant prevalence of fibrosis, as indicated by late Gadolinium enhancement (of the right ventricle in several recent studies).

The Treatment of Heart Failure in CCTGA

The best answer to what can be done to manage the failing systemic RV is also likely to address the underlying cause; because there are several surgically remediable issues, this is always a logical first step. Hence, the unoperated patient requires careful assessment to determine the most appropriate repair strategy. In those who have undergone a classic/physiologic repair, tricuspid valve regurgitation may respond to PA banding, with the attendant shift in the septal position and volume unloading of the morphologic RV that results. Similarly, tricuspid valve repair may be attempted. There is good experiential evidence that PA banding may be a preemptive therapy to systemic RV deterioration in young patients and that it may constitute a destination therapy in older patients, reducing symptoms substantially.[24] However, later data from a Birmingham group portray a pessimistic view of staged LV retraining toward completion of an arterial switch, with 45% of patients subjected to complete morphologic LV retraining developing moderate-to-severe LV dysfunction and/or requiring cardiac transplantation.[25] Medical therapy on failure of the systemic RV has so far proven unpersuasive. There are few reports of β-blocker therapy having any beneficial effect in these patients; however, one small series in adults, most of whom had undergone an atrial repair for simple TGA,[26] demonstrated a short-term benefit for the use of carvedilol, with reverse remodeling of RV volume and improvement in RVEF and LVEF while aerobic capacity remained unaltered. No controlled trials are available to assess this strategy. Similarly, the value of inhibiting the pathway of angiotensin production or cardiac binding has proven to be questionable at best. Several small studies of ACE inhibitors (see Winter and colleagues,[27] for a review of this topic), including one well-conducted placebo-controlled trial of losartan,[28] have failed to show any benefit to function of the systemic RV. The authors' current practice is to use diuretics and aldosterone (as a means to preempt cardiac fibrosis), with no routine indication for β-adrenoceptor blockers or ACE antagonists.

NOVEL APPROACHES TO HEART FAILURE IN CONGENITAL HEART DISEASE

If the foregoing portrays the limitations of conventional wisdom in dealing with heart failure following congenital heart disease repair, perhaps alternative approaches are required.

Resynchronization Therapy

In 1992, Gibson and colleagues[29] reported that a reduction in the AV coupling interval by AV sequential pacing in patients with dilated cardiomyopathy had marked effects on cardiac index and exercise tolerance. Few could have predicted the ramifications of this finding. Later, it became clear that septal pacing and, eventually, 4-chamber pacing had similar effects; shortly thereafter, Blanc and colleagues[30] offered the first analysis of the effects of multisite pacing on ventricular performance. Over the subsequent decade, the concepts of electrical and mechanical ventricular dyssynchrony have been refined, and biventricular pacing has become a proven therapy for heart failure, primarily of nonischemic cause, in adult patients.

What of the congenital heart disease population? Bundle branch block is present in most patients who have had a ventriculotomy, and hence, one would expect that clear signal of mechanical dyssynchrony could also easily be demonstrated. Vogel and colleagues[31] showed greater QRS duration and dispersion as well as systolic and diastolic velocity reversal in the RV free wall of patients with repaired Fallot tetralogy (TOF). Others have further explored this phenomenon and have implicated biventricular dyssynchrony as being present and possibly important in patients with repaired TOF.[32,33] Although sudden death appears to be associated with QRS duration,[34] a clear and progressive link between interventricular mechanoelectrical dyssynchrony and an eventual decline in systemic ventricular function is yet to be demonstrated. However, encouraging results have been noted from the use of resynchronization therapy in a wide variety of children with congenital heart disease and prolonged QRS duration with ventricular dysfunction.[35] Recently, a small but carefully executed study measured the effects of resynchronization on young patients with systemic RV (surgically or congenitally corrected), heart failure, and QRS duration of 160 ± 30 millisecond.[36] The investigators reported that after 19.4 ± 8.1 months of cardiac resynchronization therapy (CRT), mean QRS duration decreased from 160 ± 31 to 120 ± 28 millisecond ($P = .03$); intraventricular delay, from 104 ± 27 to 14 ± 15 millisecond ($P = .01$); and NYHA functional class, from 3.0 to 1.57 ($P = .01$) with peak oxygen consumption increasing from 13.8 ± 2.5 to 22.8 ± 6.7 mL/kg/min ($P = .03$). While systematic studies identifying patients with congenital heart disease and heart failure who should receive CRT are still awaited, current intuitive guidelines suggest that the presence of RV or LV dysfunction with a prolonged QRS duration would be grounds for a trial of multisite pacing. Unfortunately, the technical challenges in patients with atrial baffles, multiple prior surgeries, and abnormal native conduction pathways are still formidable.

Diastolic Heart Failure

While the understanding of systolic dysfunction in postoperative congenital heart disease is maturing, the understanding of diastolic dysfunction (as a driver of symptoms and a cause of heart failure) is very much in its infancy. Nonetheless, there is good evidence that diastolic dysfunction is an important element of the circulatory disturbance characteristic of the exemplars discussed earlier. Some have long recognized that abnormal diastolic function is the most obvious myocardial functional abnormality detectable during staged palliation of functionally single ventricles. The acute preload reduction associated with conversion from parallel systemic and pulmonary circulations to the series bidirectional Glenn or Fontan circulation is associated with major changes in ventricular geometry and diastolic function, originally demonstrated in patients transitioning directly to a Fontan circulation.[37,38] This abrupt reduction in preload and therefore ventricular end-diastolic volume, in the setting of maintained systolic shortening and unchanged ventricular

mass, was associated with an acute increase in ventricular wall thickness. The same phenomenon is seen in those transitioning to a bidirectional Glenn procedure as part of 3-stage palliation.[39] The end-effect is profound ventricular incoordination leading to early relaxation abnormalities, with prolongation of the time constant of relaxation and the isovolumic relaxation period and reduced early rapid filling. The functional importance of these abnormalities was not examined in the early studies, but recently it has been shown that patients with greater degrees of diastolic function have more postoperative complications and longer postoperative stay.[40,41] Furthermore, these relaxation abnormalities persist in long-term follow-up, and there is emerging evidence that a gradual reduction in ventricular compliance also occurs at the same time.[11,42] The functional consequences of this shift are not yet well defined; however, reduced early rapid filling with insidious reduction in late diastolic filling because of increasing ventricular stiffness could be a cause of reduced cardiac output and declining circulatory performance in this tenuous circulation and, ultimately, of Fontan failure. This area deserves more research.

A wholly different form of diastolic dysfunction has been described in patients with surgically corrected TGA. The poor stroke volume responses to exercise and during provocative testing in these patients was often attributed to poor systemic RV function in earlier studies.[43] However, in a later study using conductance catheter assessment of ventricular responses to dobutamine stress in patients after the Mustard and Senning procedures, there seemed to be appropriate systolic (load-independent indices, ventriculo-vascular coupling) and some diastolic (time constant of relaxation, end-diastolic pressure-volume relationships) responses.[44] Despite these myocardial responses, the RV filling rate was unchanged, and consequently, the tachycardia (and reduced diastolic filling time) related to increasing doses of dobutamine was associated with a progressive decrease in stroke volume. This phenomenon is almost certainly a reflection of abnormal atrioventricular coupling resulting from the abnormal capacitance and reduced contractile function of the restrictive atrial pathways after such operations. These findings have subsequently been reproduced by others[45]; they provide for a better understanding of pathophysiology and the well-known lack of response to ACE inhibitors and angiotensin-receptor blockers, as discussed earlier, and they further endorse the fact that intuitive assumptions are often proven to be incorrect in congenital heart disease. Detailed study of

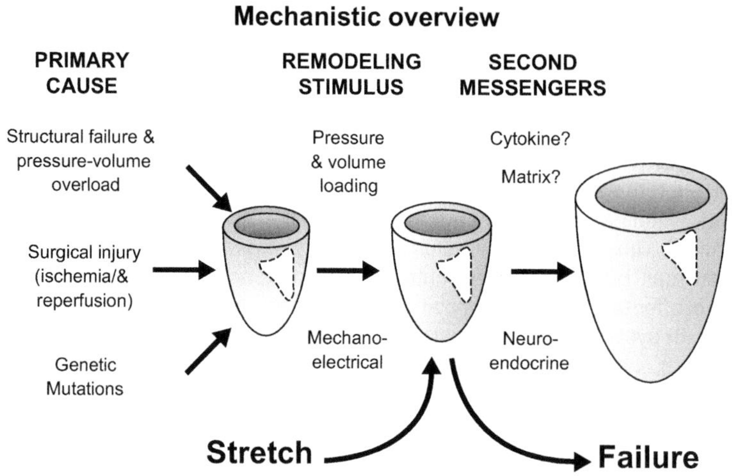

Mechanistic overview

| PRIMARY CAUSE | REMODELING STIMULUS | SECOND MESSENGERS |

Structural failure & pressure-volume overload

Surgical injury (ischemia/& reperfusion)

Genetic Mutations

Pressure & volume loading

Mechano-electrical

Cytokine?

Matrix?

Neuro-endocrine

Stretch ⟶ **Failure**

Fig. 3. Mechanistic hypothesis of the pathogenesis of heart failure in congenital heart disease. The primary mechanisms are those of structural failure resulting in hemodynamic (pressure and volume) stress, exacerbated by ischemia, and reperfusion injury. Genetic modifiers of the response are probably also important in explaining individual variation. The common pathway of structural remodeling is promoted by pressure and volume loading and by dyssynchronous mechano-electrical coupling. Lastly, second messengers of classic heart failure progression become evident; neuroendocrine activation is definitively evident, but the specific role of cytokines and matrix remodeling factors is poorly defined. (*Adapted from* Liu P, personal communication, 2009; with permission. *Courtesy of* Peter Liu, MD, Toronto, Canada.)

individual lesions and corrective procedures applied to them are likely to help develop rational and successful treatments for the heart failure that is associated with them.

SUMMARY

The overall picture that emerges regarding heart failure following congenital heart disease is that it may take years or decades to develop. As a working construct, the authors have proposed that 3 elements are necessary, as illustrated in **Fig. 3**.

1. An underlying primary cause: in most cases the lesion is the end result of an attempted palliation, leaving a residual abnormality of function; coexisiting factors, such as recurrent ischemia, and disease modifiers of a genomic nature may also play a role in determining the severity of the primary underlying cause.
2. A remodeling stimulus: typically, during the latent phase of the disease, there is a requirement for long-lasting hemodynamic remodeling to be operating in the form of a volume load (such as a regurgitant tricuspid valve) or a persistent pressure load (unrelieved LV outflow obstruction); more recognition is now given to the probable importance of mechanical and electrical dyssynchrony as a mechanism of progressive remodeling in these patients.

3. A second messenger: operating as a signaling mechanism by one of several pathways, including neurohormonal activation, matrix remodeling, or inflammatory or apoptosis-provoking stimuli; these messengers become more evident in the symptomatic phase of the disease.

Based on the above construct, it is possible to rationalize and identify the timing and role of specific therapies for each given situation.

REFERENCES

1. Verheugt CL, Uiterwaal CS, Grobbee DE, et al. Long-term prognosis of congenital heart defects: a systematic review. Int J Cardiol 2008;131(1): 25–32 [Review].
2. Norozi K, Wessel A, Alpers V, et al. Incidence and risk distribution of heart failure in adolescents and adults with congenital heart disease after cardiac surgery. Am J Cardiol 2006;97(8):1238–43 [Research Support, Non-U.S. Gov't].
3. Altmann K, Printz BF, Solowiejczky DE, et al. Two-dimensional echocardiographic assessment of right ventricular function as a predictor of outcome in hypoplastic left heart syndrome. Am J Cardiol 2000;86(9):964–8.
4. Kanter KR, Forbess JM, Fyfe DA, et al. De Vega tricuspid annuloplasty for systemic tricuspid regurgitation in children with univentricular physiology. J Heart Valve Dis 2004;13(1):86–90.

5. Shaddy RE, Boucek MM, Hsu DT, et al. Carvedilol for children and adolescents with heart failure: a randomized controlled trial. [see comment]. JAMA 2007;298(10):1171–9 [Multicenter Study Randomized Controlled Trial Research Support, Non-U.S. Gov't].

6. Fontan F, Baudet E. Surgical repair of tricuspid atresia. Thorax 1971;26(3):240–8.

7. Khairy P, Fernandes SM, Mayer JE Jr, et al. Long-term survival, modes of death, and predictors of mortality in patients with Fontan surgery. [see comment]. Circulation 2008;117(1):85–92 [Research Support, Non-U.S. Gov't].

8. Kim SJ, Kim WH, Lim HG, et al. Outcome of 200 patients after an extracardiac Fontan procedure. J Thorac Cardiovasc Surg 2008;136(1):108–16 [Evaluation Studies].

9. Freedom RM, Yoo SJ, Mikailian H, et al. In: Freedom RM, Yoo SJ, Mikailian H, et al, editors. The natural and modified history of congenital heart disease. Elmsford (NY): Blackwell Publishing; 2004. p. 457–9.

10. Gewillig M. The Fontan circulation. Heart 2005;91(6): 839–46 [Review].

11. Anderson PA, Sleeper LA, Mahony L, et al. Contemporary outcomes after the Fontan procedure: a Pediatric Heart Network multicenter study. [see comment]. J Am Coll Cardiol 2008;52(2):85–98 [Multicenter Study Research Support, N.I.H., Extramural].

12. Robbers-Visser D, Kapusta L, van Osch-Gevers L, et al. Clinical outcome 5 to 18 years after the Fontan operation performed on children younger than 5 years. J Thorac Cardiovasc Surg 2009;138(1):89–95.

13. Brassard P, Bedard E, Jobin J, et al. Exercise capacity and impact of exercise training in patients after a Fontan procedure: a review. Can J Cardiol 2006;22(6):489–95 [Research Support, Non-U.S. Gov't Review].

14. Law YM, Ettedgui J, Beerman L, et al. Comparison of plasma B-type natriuretic peptide levels in single ventricle patients with systemic ventricle heart failure versus isolated cavopulmonary failure. Am J Cardiol 2006;98(4):520–4 [Comparative Study].

15. Samanek M, Voriskova M. Congenital heart disease among 815,569 children born between 1980 and 1990 and their 15-year survival: a prospective Bohemia survival study. Pediatr Cardiol 1999;20(6): 411–7 [Research Support, Non-U.S. Gov't].

16. Huhta JC, Danielson GK, Ritter DG, et al. Survival in atrioventricular discordance. Pediatr Cardiol 1985; 6(2):57–60 [Research Support, U.S. Gov't, P.H.S.].

17. Prieto LR, Hordof AJ, Secic M, et al. Progressive tricuspid valve disease in patients with congenitally corrected transposition of the great arteries. Circulation 1998;98(10):997–1005.

18. Fyler DC. Nadas' pediatric cardiology. St Louis (MO): Mosby: Mosby Year-Book; 1992. 701–8.

19. Mavroudis C, Backer CL. Physiologic versus anatomic repair of congenitally corrected transposition of the great arteries. Semin Thorac Cardiovasc Surg Pediatr Card Surg Annu 2003;6:16–26 [Comparative Study Review].

20. Alghamdi AA, McCrindle BW, Van Arsdell GS. Physiologic versus anatomic repair of congenitally corrected transposition of the great arteries: meta-analysis of individual patient data. Ann Thorac Surg 2006;81(4):1529–35 [Comparative Study Meta-Analysis].

21. Horer J, Schreiber C, Krane S, et al. Outcome after surgical repair/palliation of congenitally corrected transposition of the great arteries. Thorac Cardiovasc Surg 2008;56(7):391–7 [Comparative Study].

22. Rutledge JM, Nihill MR, Fraser CD, et al. Outcome of 121 patients with congenitally corrected transposition of the great arteries. Pediatr Cardiol 2002; 23(2):137–45.

23. Szymanski P, Klisiewicz A, Lubiszewska B, et al. Application of classic heart failure definitions of asymptomatic and symptomatic ventricular dysfunction and heart failure symptoms with preserved ejection fraction to patients with systemic right ventricles. Am J Cardiol 2009;104(3):414–8.

24. Winlaw DS, McGuirk SP, Balmer C, et al. Intention-to-treat analysis of pulmonary artery banding in conditions with a morphological right ventricle in the systemic circulation with a view to anatomic biventricular repair. Circulation 2005;111(4):405–11 [Evaluation Studies].

25. Quinn DW, McGuirk SP, Metha C, et al. The morphologic left ventricle that requires training by means of pulmonary artery banding before the double-switch procedure for congenitally corrected transposition of the great arteries is at risk of late dysfunction. J Thorac Cardiovasc Surg 2008;135(5):1137–44 [Comparative Study].

26. Giardini A, Napoleone CP, Specchia S, et al. Conversion of atriopulmonary Fontan to extracardiac total cavopulmonary connection improves cardiopulmonary function. Int J Cardiol 2006;113(3):341–4.

27. Winter MM, Bouma BJ, Groenink M, et al. Latest insights in therapeutic options for systemic right ventricular failure: a comparison with left ventricular failure. Heart 2009;95(12):960–3 [Comparative Study Research Support, Non-U.S. Gov't Review].

28. Dore A, Houde C, Chan KL, et al. Angiotensin receptor blockade and exercise capacity in adults with systemic right ventricles: a multicenter, randomized, placebo-controlled clinical trial. Circulation 2005;112(16):2411–6 [Multicenter Study Randomized Controlled Trial Research Support, Non-U.S. Gov't].

29. Brecker SJ, Xiao HB, Sparrow J, et al. Effects of dual-chamber pacing with short atrioventricular delay in dilated cardiomyopathy. [see comment]

[erratum appears in Lancet 1992 Dec 12;340 (8833):1482]. Lancet 1992;340(8831):1308—12 [Research Support, Non-U.S. Gov't].

30. Blanc JJ, Etienne Y, Gilard M, et al. Evaluation of different ventricular pacing sites in patients with severe heart failure: results of an acute hemodynamic study. Circulation 1997;96(10):3273—7 [Clinical Trial Comparative Study].

31. Vogel M, Sponring J, Cullen S, et al. Regional wall motion and abnormalities of electrical depolarization and repolarization in patients after surgical repair of tetralogy of Fallot. Circulation 2001;103(12): 1669—73 [Clinical Trial Controlled Clinical Trial Research Support, Non-U.S. Gov't].

32. D'Andrea A, Caso P, Sarubbi B, et al. Right ventricular myocardial activation delay in adult patients with right bundle branch block late after repair of Tetralogy of Fallot. [see comment]. Eur J Echocardiogr 2004;5(2):123—31 [Comparative Study Evaluation Studies Research Support, Non-U.S. Gov't].

33. Uebing A, Gibson DG, Babu-Narayan SV, et al. Right ventricular mechanics and QRS duration in patients with repaired tetralogy of Fallot: implications of infundibular disease. [see comment]. Circulation 2007; 116(14):1532—9 [Research Support, Non-U.S. Gov't].

34. Gatzoulis MA, Till JA, Somerville J, et al. Mechanoelectrical interaction in tetralogy of Fallot. QRS prolongation relates to right ventricular size and predicts malignant ventricular arrhythmias and sudden death. Circulation 1995;92(2):231—7 [see comment].

35. Dubin AM, Janousek J, Rhee E, et al. Resynchronization therapy in pediatric and congenital heart disease patients: an international multicenter study. J Am Coll Cardiol 2005;46(12):2277—83 [Evaluation Studies Multicenter Study Research Support, Non-U.S. Gov't].

36. Jauvert G, Rousseau-Paziaud J, Villain E, et al. Effects of cardiac resynchronization therapy on echocardiographic indices, functional capacity, and clinical outcomes of patients with a systemic right ventricle. Europace 2009;11(2):184—90.

37. Penny DJ, Rigby ML, Redington AN. Abnormal patterns of intraventricular flow and diastolic filling after the Fontan operation: evidence for incoordinate ventricular wall motion. Br Heart J 1991;66(5):375—8 [Research Support, Non-U.S. Gov't].

38. Penny DJ, Redington AN. Angiographic demonstration of incoordinate motion of the ventricular wall after the Fontan operation. Br Heart J 1991;66(6): 456—9 [Research Support, Non-U.S. Gov't].

39. Fogel MA, Gupta KB, Weinberg PM, et al. Regional wall motion and strain analysis across stages of Fontan reconstruction by magnetic resonance tagging. Am J Physiol 1995;269(3 Pt 2):H1132—52 [Research Support, Non-U.S. Gov't Research Support, U.S. Gov't, P.H.S.].

40. Border WL, Syed AU, Michelfelder EC, et al. Impaired systemic ventricular relaxation affects postoperative short-term outcome in Fontan patients. J Thorac Cardiovasc Surg 2003;126(6): 1760—4.

41. Garofalo CA, Cabreriza SE, Quinn TA, et al. Ventricular diastolic stiffness predicts perioperative morbidity and duration of pleural effusions after the Fontan operation. Circulation 2006;114(1 Suppl): I56—61 [Research Support, N.I.H., Extramural].

42. Cheung YF, Penny DJ, Redington AN. Serial assessment of left ventricular diastolic function after Fontan procedure. Heart 2000;83(4):420—4.

43. Tulevski II, van der Wall EE, Groenink M, et al. Usefulness of magnetic resonance imaging dobutamine stress in asymptomatic and minimally symptomatic patients with decreased cardiac reserve from congenital heart disease (complete and corrected transposition of the great arteries and subpulmonic obstruction). Am J Cardiol 2002;89(9): 1077—81 [Clinical Trial Controlled Clinical Trial Research Support, Non-U.S. Gov't].

44. Fratz S, Hager A, Busch R, et al. Patients after atrial switch operation for transposition of the great arteries can not increase stroke volume under dobutamine stress as opposed to patients with congenitally corrected transposition. Circ J 2008; 72(7):1130—5 [Comparative Study].

45. Vogt M, Kuhn A, Wiese J, et al. Reduced contractile reserve of the systemic right ventricle under Dobutamine stress is associated with increased brain natriuretic peptide levels in patients with complete transposition after atrial repair. Eur J Echocardiogr 2009;10(5):691—4.

Genetics of Heart Failure and Sudden Death

Matteo Vatta, PhD[a,b],*, Michael J. Ackerman, MD, PhD[c,d,e]

KEYWORDS

• Heart failure • Coronary artery disease • Sudden death

Sudden cardiac death (SCD) is a major cause of mortality in western populations, accounting for about 350,000 deaths in the United States alone each year.[1] Most SCDs originate from arrhythmic events in subjects with acute coronary artery disease (CAD) and ischemia, followed by primary cardiomyopathies of viral, idiopathic, sporadic, or familial genetic etiology.[1–4] In cases where a negative autopsy is ascertained, primary arrhythmogenic disorders such as long QT syndrome (LQTS) and Brugada syndrome (BrS) may be to blame. Until recently, these cardiac channelopathies were thought to stem from mutations in the *KCNQ1*, *KCNH2*, *SCN5A*, *KCNE,1* and *KCNE2* genes encoding for the alpha and beta subunits of cardiac potassium and sodium channels that govern the cardiac action potential.[1]

Among decedents with an unremarkable autopsy, however, one cannot exclude the occurrence of a subclinical myocardial remodeling unnoticed by the morphologic and histologic analysis. The genetic and molecular studies investigating the underlying causes of primary cardiomyopathies demonstrated the incidence of cytoskeletal proteins defects that, in the long term, lead the myocardium to an uncompensated state characterized by structural, morphologic, hemodynamic, and electrical changes.

This cardiac remodeling predisposes the subjects to a higher susceptibility for electrical defects including ventricular arrhythmias with high morbidity and mortality that can even precede the expression of an overt cardiomyopathy.

In the past, the development of cardiac arrhythmias often was believed to stem from the extracellular matrix (ECM) remodeling and the increased collagen deposition in the interstitial space left empty by the myocyte cell loss.[5] The ECM remodeling, however, does not always explain the baseline electrocardiogram (ECG) alterations observed even in asymptomatic subjects with familial or sporadic cardiomyopathy. This phenomenon led the authors to investigate alternative mechanisms leading to arrhythmogenesis in such cardiomyopathic individuals. In particular, in the last few years, basic science investigations discovered that cytoskeletal proteins such as dystrophin (DMD), alpha-actinin-2 (ACTN2), telethonin (TCAP), alpha-1-syntrophin (SNTA1), and caveolin-3 (CAV3), previously identified to be mutated in subjects with cardiomyopathies and muscular dystrophy with cardiac involvement,

---

[a] Department of Pediatrics (Cardiology), Texas Children's Hospital, Baylor College of Medicine, Houston, TX, USA
[b] Department of Molecular Physiology and Biophysics, Texas Children's Hospital, Baylor College of Medicine, Houston, TX, USA
[c] Division of Cardiovascular Diseases, Department of Medicine, Windland Smith Rice Sudden Death Genomics Laboratory, Guggenheim 501, Mayo Clinic, Rochester, MN 55905, USA
[d] Division of Pediatric Cardiology, Department of Pediatrics, Windland Smith Rice Sudden Death Genomics Laboratory, Guggenheim 501, Mayo Clinic, Rochester, MN 55905, USA
[e] Department of Molecular Pharmacology and Experimental Therapeutics, Windland Smith Rice Sudden Death Genomics Laboratory, Mayo Clinic, Rochester, MN, USA
* Corresponding author. Phoebe Willingham Muzzy, Molecular Cardiology Research Laboratory, Texas Children's Hospital, Baylor College of Medicine, 1102 Bates Street F.C. 430.04, Houston, TX 77030.
E-mail address: mvatta@bcm.edu

Heart Failure Clin 6 (2010) 507–514
doi:10.1016/j.hfc.2010.05.008

associate and modulate the function of ion channels such as $Na_v1.5$, $Ca_v1.2$, and $K_v11.1$, and $K_v7.1$ (**Table 1**).[6–10] These ion channels are the major determinants of phases 0, 2, and 3 of the cardiac action potential, respectively.[6–10]

Recent studies demonstrated that mutations in the aforementioned cytoskeletal protein-encoding genes are able to alter ion channel function and mimic the alterations caused by primary mutations in ion channel-encoding genes (phenocopy).[11–14] This brief synopsis will examine these new lines of investigation that further illuminate the relationship between the cytoskeleton and ion channels, thus representing a novel level of complexity in the finely tuned cardiac electric homeostasis, and holding new possible approaches to the genetic and molecular research and their application to patient management.

ELECTROCARDIOGRAPHIC ALTERATIONS IN HEART FAILURE

Heart failure (HF) is among the major determinants of morbidity and mortality in western populations, and it causes more than 5 million cases and 800,000 hospitalizations in the United States per year. HF is characterized by reduced cardiac output due to either systolic or diastolic dysfunction, and it often is associated with the development of rhythm disturbances such as ventricular tachycardia (VT) and ventricular fibrillation (VF), both frequent causes of SCD.[15]

In fact, patients with HF caused by ischemic cardiomyopathy or dilated cardiomyopathy (DCM), present with specific ECG alterations, including QT interval prolongation, QT dispersion, ST segment elevation, and T wave alternans (especially during exercise), as well as conduction defects such as right or left bundle branch block (RBBB or LBBB) and AV block. Diffuse myocardial damage caused by cardiomyopathy can present with LBBB, while RBBB with right axis deviation and P wave alteration can suggest right ventricular hypertrophy secondary to pulmonary hypertension.[15] Interestingly, the previously mentioned HF-associated ECG alterations are also evident among the primary arrhythmogenic syndromes such as LQTS, BrS, or CPVT, diseases that are not normally associated with obvious morphologic and structural changes, such as myocardial remodeling.[15]

PRIMARY CARDIOMYOPATHIES

Cardiomyopathies are diseases of the myocardium associated with ventricular dysfunction. The HF caused by the progression of the cardiomyopathy is a significant and increasing health care and social issue that has not been adequately supported by resources for basic, translational, and clinical research, given the diffusion and proportion of this problem. Therefore, despite the technological and scientific advance, the therapies currently available to the HF patient mostly focus on the management of the symptoms rather than on the prevention and decrease of the disease progression.[2] The classification of the cardiomyopathies has usually followed morphologic and functional criteria that subdivided them into four major categories: dilated cardiomyopathy (DCM), hypertrophic cardiomyopathy (HCM), arrhythmogenic right ventricular cardiomyopathy (ARVC), and restrictive cardiomyopathy (RCM).[2–4]

Over the past two decades, cardiomyopathy investigations have generated new evidence about the impact of the genetic factors into the development and progression of the clinical picture in HF patients. In particular, the investigation of familial forms of cardiomyopathies allowed the authors to recognize the inheritability of these diseases and the importance of genetic factors that precipitate a large percentage of cardiomyopathies. Genetic cardiomyopathies can be inherited as autosomal-dominant, autosomal-recessive, X-linked, matrilineal, or mitochondrial traits. In addition to the familial forms, there are also sporadic forms stemming from de novo mutations.[2–4]

For many years, the molecular genetic analysis has focused mostly on the monogenic inherited cardiomyopathies, which are those diseases caused generally by mutations in a single gene. These studies allowed the identification of a large number of genes and a plethora of associated mutations. Most of these mutations are private, thus identified in a single index case, if the case is sporadic, or present in the proband and the affected family members of a single pedigree with familial cardiomyopathy (see **Table 1**).[2–4]

Although most mutations have been identified in genes encoding for cytoskeletal proteins, gene alterations involving the SCN5A gene, which encodes for the alpha subunit of the cardiac sodium channel Nav1.5, have been found recently in patients with either a sporadic or familial phenotype of DCM and abnormal conduction.[16,17] Recent studies showed that SCN5A mutations can be observed in 2.6% of the analyzed subjects.[18] However, the detailed mechanism leading SCN5A mutations to the development of the cardiac remodeling and hemodynamic dysfunction characterizing a DCM heart remains unknown.

The authors' recent studies on primary arrhythmogenic syndromes demonstrated that cytoskeletal proteins of the cardiomyocyte are not only able to physically interact with, but also modulate

Table 1
Genes identified in long QT syndrome subjects

Genotype	Gene	Definition	Locus	Protein	Current	Probable Cytoskeletal Partner
LQT1	KCNQ1	KQT-like voltage-gated potassium channel 1	11p15.5	$K_v7.1$	I_{Ks}	AKAP9; CDKN1C
LQT2	KCNH2	Potassium channel, voltage-gated, H2	7q36.1	$K_v11.1$	I_{Kr}	AKAP9; CDKN1C
LQT3	SCN5A	Alpha polypeptide of voltage-gated sodium channel type V	3p21	$Na_v1.5$	I_{Na}	CAV3, SNTA1, ANK2, ANK3, GJA5, GPD1L, TCAP
LQT4	ANK2	Ankyrin-B	4q25–q27	Ankyrin-B	I_{Na}	OBSCN
LQT5	KCNE1	Voltage-gated potassium channel, Isk-related subfamily, member 1	21q22.1–q22.2	Isk/β1	I_{Ks}/I_{Kr}	TCAP
LQT6	KCNE2	Voltage-gated potassium channel, Isk-related subfamily, member 2	21q21.1	MiRP1/β2	I_{Kr}/I_{Ks}	ANK2, AKAP9
LQT7	KCNJ2	Potassium inwardly-rectifying channel, subfamily J, member 2	17q23.1–q24.2	Kir2.1		AKAP5, ANK2
LQT8	CACNA1C	Calcium channel, L type, alpha 1 polypeptide isoform	12p13.3	$Ca_v1.2$	$I_{Ca,L}$	ACTN2, DMD
LQT9	CAV3	Caveolin-3	3p25	Caveolin-3	I_{Na}	DMD, SGCA, SGCB, SGCG, SGCD, SGCE, NOS3
LQT10	SCN4B	Sodium channel, voltage-gated, type IV beta subunit	11q23.3	SCN4B	I_{Na}	ANK2, CAV3
LQT11	AKAP9	A-kinase anchor protein-9	7q21–q22	AKAP9		N/A
LQT12	SNTA1	Alpha-1 syntrophin	20q11.2	SNTA1	I_{Na}	DMD, DTNA, SGCA, NOS1

Abbreviations: AKAP9, A-kinase anchor protein 9; ACTN2, alpha-actinin-2; AKAP5, A-kinase anchor protein 5; ANK2, ankyrin-B; ANK3, ankyrin-G; CDKN1C, cyclin-dependent kinase inhibitor 1C; CAV3, caveolin-3; DMD, dystrophin; DTNA, alpha-dystrobrevin; GJA5, Gap junction alpha-5 protein [Connexin-40]; GPD1L, glycerol-3-phosphate dehydrogenase 1-like; NOS1, nitric oxide brain; NOS3, nitric oxide endothelial; OBSCN, obscurin; SGCA, alpha-sarcoglycan; SGCB, beta-sarcoglycan; SGCD, delta-sarcoglycan; SGCE, epsilon-sarcoglycan; SGCG, gamma-sarcoglycan; SNTA1, alpha-1-syntrophin; TCAP, telethonin.

the kinetic of ion channels such as Nav1.5. In addition, other research groups have identified additional cytoskeletal proteins that associate and regulate the function of various ion channels, thus playing a major role as Channel Interacting Proteins (ChIPs).

PRIMARY ARRHYTHMOGENIC SYNDROMES

CADs cause about 80% of all SCD. However, primary arrhythmogenic syndromes, which account for 5% of all SCD, represent a common identifiable cause of autopsy-negative SCD following a molecular autopsy.[19] If no structural myocardial alterations are observed during the autopsy, the most probable causes of SCD are believed to be LQTS, ventricular pre-excitation (Wolff-Parkinson-White syndrome), idiopathic ventricular fibrillation, catecholaminergic polymorphic ventricular tachycardia (CPVT), and BrS, which is characterized by the ST segment elevation in the right precordial leads and an RBBB-like pattern.[1–4] In addition, a proportion of sudden infant death syndrome (SIDS) may be secondary to cardiac causes. Although noncardiac causes, such as asphyxia and brain hypoperfusion, gastrointestinal diseases (GI), metabolic disorders, traumatic accidents, brain malformations, or physical abuse have been implicated in SIDS,[20] a cardiac hypothesis for SIDS speculating that developmental abnormalities in the cardiac sympathetic innervations could predispose infants to lethal arrhythmias was put forward in 1976.[21]

Twenty years later, this hypothesis was supported in a study where the group led by Peter Schwartz[22] reported the analysis of the electrocardiogram (ECG) of 34,442 infants. In this report, the authors observed that in 24 of 34 cases of SIDS, the QTc was prolonged compared with the control infants or with neonates deceased for other causes. Among those 24 cases, 12 neonates (50%) presented with a QTc exceeding the 97.5th percentile value (440 ms) for 3- to 4-day-old infants, thus leading the authors to hypothesize that a prolonged QT interval in the first week of life may be associated with increased risk for SIDS.[22]

Recently, the role of ion channel function alterations (channelopathies) has gained considerable attention as a possible cause of SIDS.[23–26] Recognizing that channelopathic SIDS may account for approximately 10% of SIDS, presentation during infancy may represent an early and more malignant presentation of the aforementioned arrhythmogenic syndromes, of which, the best characterized and studied is surely the LQTS.

THE LQTS

LQTS is characterized by the alteration of the cardiac repolarization, which can be of genetic, sporadic or familial, or acquired origin.[27] LQTS presents with a prolongation of the QTc (>480 ms as the 50th percentile in the authors' LQTS clinic), relative bradycardia, T wave abnormalities, VT, and torsades de pointes.[27] In a significant number of cases, recurrent syncope and epilepsy episodes may represent the first symptom manifestation in LQTS subjects. These symptoms should suggest a more attentive analysis of the ECG, which remains a key diagnostic test in the evaluation of LQTS. Unfortunately, there are many cases in which SCD is the first manifestation, although in some individuals, their family history would have been suggestive of a familial SCD-predisposing disease process.[27]

The familial forms of LQTS generally are transmitted in an autosomal-dominant (vast majority) or recessive (seldom) fashion, while the acquired or secondary form may originate from adverse effects of pharmacologic therapy such as with antibiotics (ie, erythromycin), antihistamines, antidepressants, antifungals, and antiarrhythmic drugs such as quinidine.[27] In addition, metabolic disorders such as diabetes and hypokalemia may delay cardiac repolarization and prolong the QT interval.[27] Finally, syndromic disorders involving syndactyly, the fascioscapulohumeral dystrophy, and Timothy syndrome also have been associated with LQTS.[28,29]

GENETICS OF LQTS

Since 1995, genetic research has made significant progress in the understanding of the genetic basis of LQTS and some phenotypic differences in the various forms of the disease. The autosomal-dominant form of LQTS, historically called Romano-Ward syndrome (RWS), is characterized by the inheritance of the disease-causing gene in 50% of the offspring of an affected individual. The clinical presentation of RWS subjects includes the prolonged QTc, syncope, epilepsy, and SCD.[1,27] Subjects with the relatively rare autosomal-recessive form, also called Jervell and Lange-Nielsen syndrome (JLNS), present with similar symptoms as RWS plus severe sensorineural hearing loss.[1,27] In addition, JLNS individuals are characterized by a more pronounced QTc prolongation, and a more malignant disease progression than RWS patients.[1,27] More recently, however, the group of Dr Silvia G. Piori identified heterozygous mutations in JLNS subjects, thus shaking the concept of a mere autosomal-recessive trait for JLNS.[1,27]

Although the first LQTS-associated locus was reported in 1991, the three major LQTS-susceptibility genes emerged in 1995 and 1996 (see **Table 1**).[30–32] Although there are now approximately 12 LQTS susceptibility genes, mutations in these three canonical genes: *KCNQ1* (LQT1), *KCNH2* (LQT2), and *SCN5A* (LQT3) account for approximately 75% of all LQTS and over 95% of genetically identifiable LQTS.[26] *KCNQ1* encodes for the alpha subunit of the slow rectifier voltage-gated potassium channel (I_{Ks}) and is the most commonly mutated gene in LQTS subjects.[26] *KCNQ1* is expressed in many human tissues, including the heart, inner ear, kidney, lungs, gastric mucosa, placenta, and pancreas, although it is not expressed in skeletal muscle or the liver.[1,27] In addition, *KCNQ1* also was shown to be expressed in the mammalian brain and mice carrying either the p.A341E mutation (p.A341E in humans) or the p.T311I mutation (p.T312I in humans) displaying a complex phenotype, which included prolonged QT interval, bradyarrhythmias, and VF associated with the occurrence of convulsive seizures or frequent partial seizures evolving into electroclinical nonconvulsive status epilepticus.[33] The protein encoded by *KCNQ1* is the alpha subunit ($K_v7.1$), which assembles with the *KCNE1*-encoded beta subunit (minK/Isk) to recapitulate I_{Ks}.[1,27]

So far, the *SCN5A*-encoded $Na_v1.5$, one of approximately 12 different I_{Na} alpha subunits, is the principal cardiac isoform and the only cardiac sodium channel mutated in LQTS (LQT3).[1,27] *SCN5A* is highly expressed in the myocardium and in the brain, although at lower extent, but not in skeletal muscle, liver, or uterus.[1,27] The protein sequence of for the longest $Na_v1.5$ alternatively spliced isoform consists of 2016 amino acids and a putative structure including four transmembrane domains (DI-DIV), each of them containing six transmembrane segments (S1-S6) similar to the potassium channel structure.[1,27] Despite the identification of the aforementioned genes, many LQTS subjects and families have not been associated with those loci, suggesting a high genetic heterogeneity in LQTS.[1,27]

CHIPS AND ARRHYTHMOGENESIS

The discovery of LQTS-causing mutations in the α and β subunits generating the I_{Na}, I_{Ks}, and I_{Kr} currents established LQTS as a channelopathy caused by primary mutations in genes encoding for ion channels subunits. However, the recent discovery of LQTS-causing mutations in the cytoskeletal protein ankyrin-B (*ANK2*), mapping to 4q25-27 (LQT4), revealed a novel arrhythmogenic mechanism leading to abnormal $Na_v1.5$ metabolism.[34–36]

Mutations in *ANK2* that are causing LQTS lead to alteration of sarcolemmal trafficking and $Na_v1.5$ turnover on the cardiomyocyte surface.[34–36] This mechanism diverges from that of primary mutations in potassium channels, which cause a loss of channel function, or in *SCN5A* lead to gain-of-function in which $Na_v1.5$ usually has normal ion permeability with altered channel inactivation kinetics.[27]

In the last few years, the investigation of the ion channel regulation led to the discovery of proteins that associate with and modulate various ion channel subunits. Enzymatic modulation of ion channels kinetics may occur as post-translational modifications such as phosphorylation by protein kinases A and C (PKA and PKC), which add an inorganic phosphate residue to key amino acids such as Serines and Threonines on the ion channel protein to regulate its function.[37] In addition, calcium homeostasis plays a role in ion channels' function, and the increased intracellular Ca^{2+} level initiates the activation of calmodulin (CaM), which can bind to ion channels such as $Na_v1.5$ and modify their channel kinetics.[37]

The evidences accumulated so far linking ion channels and structural proteins indicate that ion channels are forming intricate macromolecular complexes with cytoskeletal proteins acting as channel adaptors. Among those adaptors or ChIPs are important proteins such as dystrophin, syntrophin, yotiao, alpha-actinin, telethonin, and caveolin-3 that bind and modulate ion channels such as $Na_v1.5$, $Ca_v1.2$, $K_v7.1$, and $K_v1.5$.[6–14,25,38]

These aforementioned proteins represented possible targets for the pathogenesis of LQTS or other forms of primary arrhythmogenesis, and this hypothesis recently was demonstrated in a collaborative effort between the authors' two groups with the identification of mutations in *CAV3* and *SNTA1* in subjects with LQTS or SIDS and causing either a prolonged late sodium current or impairing the steady-state activation/inactivation kinetics with subsequent more robust and persistent sodium influx.[12–14,25]

These alterations caused a prolongation of the cardiac action potential secondary to accentuation in the late sodium current consistent with the known pathogenic mechanism for LQT3-associated mutations in the cardiac sodium channel's alpha subunit.[12–14,25]

THERAPEUTIC IMPLICATIONS IN HF AND ARRHYTHMIAS

These novel determinants of electrical and mechanical functions in the myocardium have improved the understanding of the molecular mechanisms of cardiac functions, but they represent a serious challenge for the current therapeutic intervention, thus far often focused on inhibiting the ion channel function without considering what happens to the underlying cytoskeletal structures and during regulatory processes such as phosphorylation and nitrosylation.

Patients with symptomatic HF and arrhythmias often are treated with beta-blockers, which have been demonstrated to be also effective in decreasing the occurrence of torsades de pointes in LQTS subjects with $K_v7.1$ or $K_v11.1$ mutations.[1] In some individuals with LQT3-associated sodium channel mutations, beta-blocker therapy may not be sufficiently protective, while a sodium channel blocker mexiletine could shorten the QTc, thereby decreasing the potential for torsades de pointes.[39–41] However, neither beta-blockers nor late sodium current blockers eliminate entirely the risk for a LQTS-triggered cardiac event. For channelopathies like LQTS, if pharmacologic therapy is not deemed sufficiently protective or if unacceptable adverse effects are encountered, denervation therapy or device therapy can be considered.

For the cardiomyopathies, if conventional therapies are insufficient, heart transplantation remains an option. As a bridge to heart transplantation, or in selected cases as destination therapy, subjects with intractable or refractory HF may be supported by the implantation of a left ventricular assist device (LVAD), which may facilitate reverse remodeling in adults and children.[42–44]

Despite the technological and intellectual advances in the field of genetic heart disease, there is ample need for addition to the currently available therapies for HF and arrhythmias. Whether the insights into cardiomyopathic/channelopathic perturbations in ChIPs will foster novel therapies remains to be determined. It is possible that abnormalities in these ChIPs not only can lead to structural and mechanical impairment, but may also impair ion channel function, thus at least partially explaining the frequent alterations on the baseline ECG, often observed in patients with heart failure. They therefore represent novel therapeutic targets (**Fig. 1**).

It is clear that in the future, knowing the underlying genetic defect and its functional implications may help to not only understand the clinical presentation, but also to tailor more effective anti-arrhythmic and HF therapies. For example, patients with CAV3 or SNTA1 mutations causing prolonged late sodium current may benefit from drugs targeting this specific defect. Recent animal studies with the antiarrhythmic drug ranolazine [(±)-1-piperazineacetamide, *N*-(2,6-dimethylphenyl)-4-[2-hydroxy-3-(2-methoxyphenoxy)propyl]-], which targets the late sodium current, have demonstrated improvement in the cardiac dysfunction caused by the proischemic metabolite Palmitoyl-L-carnitine (PC).[40] In another model of cardiac ischemia, use of the 4-dihydro-N-([2S])-3-([2-hydroxy-3-methylphenyl]thio)-2-methylpropyl-2H-(3R)-1,5-benzoxathiepin-3-amine (2d) (F 15,741) was cardioprotective.[41]

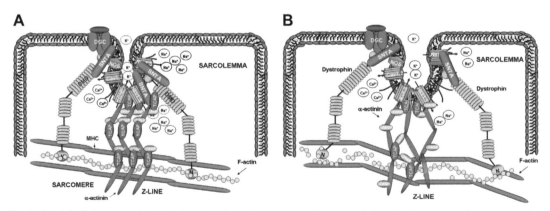

Fig. 1. Model of the secondary ion channel alteration upon cardiac remodeling. In the myocardium, proper ion channel function depends on the maintenance of normal cytoskeletal structure and ion homeostasis. In the cardiomyocyte with intact cytoskeleton, ion channel function is normal. (*A*) In the myocardial cell of a remodeled heart, ion channels may be altered irrespective of the hemodynamic compensatory ability. (*B*) Among subjects with compensated heart failure, ion channel dysregulation may not precipitate any symptoms, although its presence may be electrocardiographically evident. Among individuals with uncompensated hemodynamic function, however, arrhythmias and conduction defects could stem from the secondary insults to the ion channels of the heart.

SUMMARY

Since the sentinel discovery of LQTS as a channel-opathy in 1995, many significant strides have been made related to exposing the pathogenic mechanisms underlying SCD. However, elucidating the most influential genetic and environmental determinants that underlie the variable penetrance and expressivity of the primary syndrome-associated mutation remains a daunting task.

The use of the most advanced genomics and proteomics techniques may provide a new framework to better understand whether genetic variants, gene dosage, gene expression and post-translational modifications such as phosphorylation, methylation, acetylation, glycosylation and nitrosylation, play a significant role in the detailed mechanisms that regulate the ion channel function in the intact as well as in the remodeled myocardium. Such an understanding may enhance the ability to design novel and more efficient therapeutic interventions to alleviate symptoms, halt disease progression, and possibly even prevent the development of disease altogether for this collection of sudden death predisposing cardiomyopathies and channelopathies.

REFERENCES

1. Priori SG, Barhanin J, Hauer RN, et al. Genetic and molecular basis of cardiac arrhythmias; impact on clinical management. Study group on molecular basis of arrhythmias of the Working Group on Arrhythmias of the European Society of Cardiology. Eur Heart J 1999;20(3):174–95.

2. Sinagra G, Di Lenarda A, Moretti M, et al. The challenge of cardiomyopathies in 2007. J Cardiovasc Med (Hagerstown) 2008;9(6):545–54.

3. Elliott P, Andersson B, Arbustini E, et al. Classification of the cardiomyopathies: a position statement from the European Society Of Cardiology Working Group on Myocardial and Pericardial Diseases. Eur Heart J 2008;29(2):270–6.

4. Maron BJ, Towbin JA, Thiene G, et al. Contemporary definitions and classification of the cardiomyopathies: an American Heart Association Scientific Statement from the Council on Clinical Cardiology, Heart Failure and Transplantation Committee; Quality of Care and Outcomes Research and Functional Genomics and Translational Biology Interdisciplinary Working Groups; and Council on Epidemiology and Prevention. Circulation 2006; 113(14):1807–16.

5. Rohr S. Myofibroblasts in diseased hearts: new players in cardiac arrhythmias? Heart Rhythm 2009;6:848–56.

6. Sadeghi A, Doyle AD, Johnson BD. Regulation of the cardiac L-type Ca2+ channel by the actin-binding proteins alpha-actinin and dystrophin. Am J Physiol Cell Physiol 2002;282(6):C1502–11.

7. Lu L, Zhang Q, Timofeyev V, et al. Molecular coupling of a Ca2+-activated K+ channel to L-type Ca2+ channels via alpha-actinin2. Circ Res 2007;100(1):112–20.

8. Barbuti A, Gravante B, Riolfo M, et al. Localization of pacemaker channels in lipid rafts regulates channel kinetics. Circ Res 2004;94:1325–31.

9. Gavillet B, Rougier JS, Domenighetti AA, et al. Cardiac sodium channel Nav1.5 is regulated by a multiprotein complex composed of syntrophins and dystrophin. Circ Res 2006;99(4):407–14.

10. Furukawa T, Ono Y, Tsuchiya H, et al. Specific interaction of the potassium channel beta-subunit minK with the sarcomeric protein T-cap suggests a T-tubule-myofibril linking system. J Mol Biol 2001; 313(4):775–84.

11. Mazzone A, Strege PR, Tester DJ, et al. A mutation in telethonin alters Nav1.5 function. J Biol Chem 2008; 283(24):16537–44.

12. Ueda K, Valdivia C, Medeiros-Domingo A, et al. Syntrophin mutation associated with long QT syndrome through activation of the nNOS-SCN5A macromolecular complex. Proc Natl Acad Sci U S A 2008; 105:9355–60.

13. Wu G, Ai T, Kim JJ, et al. Alpha-1-syntrophin mutation and the long QT syndrome: a disease of sodium channel disruption. Circ Arrhythm Electrophysiol 2008;1:193–201.

14. Vatta M, Ackerman MJ, Ye B, et al. Mutant caveolin-3 induces persistent late sodium current and is associated with long QT syndrome. Circulation 2006; 114(20):2104–12.

15. Hombach V. Electrocardiogram of the failing heart. Card Electrophysiol Rev 2002;6(3):209–14.

16. McNair WP, Ku L, Taylor MR, et al. Familial Cardiomyopathy Registry Research Group. SCN5A mutation associated with dilated cardiomyopathy, conduction disorder, and arrhythmia. Circulation 2004;110(15): 2163–7.

17. Olson TM, Michels VV, Ballew JD, et al. Sodium channel mutations and susceptibility to heart failure and atrial fibrillation. JAMA 2005;293(4):447–54.

18. Hershberger RE, Parks SB, Kushner JD, et al. Coding sequence mutations identified in MYH7, TNNT2, SCN5A, CSRP3, LBD3, and TCAP from 313 patients with familial or idiopathic dilated cardiomyopathy. Clin Transl Sci 2008;1(1):21–6.

19. Tester DJ, Ackerman MJ. Postmortem long QT syndrome genetic testing for sudden unexplained death in the young. J Am Coll Cardiol 2007;49: 240–6.

20. Kinney HC, Thach BT. The sudden infant death syndrome. N Engl J Med 2009;361(8):795–805.

21. Schwartz PJ. Cardiac sympathetic innervation and the sudden infant death syndrome. A possible pathogenetic link. Am J Med 1976;60:167–72.

22. Schwartz PJ, Stramba-Badiale M, Segantini A, et al. Prolongation of the QT interval and the sudden infant death syndrome. N Engl J Med 1998;338:1709–14.

23. Ackerman MJ, Siu BL, Sturner WQ, et al. Postmortem molecular analysis of SCN5A defects in sudden infant death syndrome. JAMA 2001;286(18):2264–9.

24. Wang DW, Desai RR, Crotti L, et al. Cardiac sodium channel dysfunction in sudden infant death syndrome. Circulation 2007;115(3):368–76.

25. Cronk LB, Ye B, Kaku T, et al. Novel mechanism for sudden infant death syndrome: persistent late sodium current secondary to mutations in caveolin-3. Heart Rhythm 2007;4(2):161–6.

26. Ackerman MJ. State of postmortem genetic testing known as the cardiac channel molecular autopsy in the forensic evaluation of unexplained sudden cardiac death in the young. Pacing Clin Electrophysiol 2009;32(Suppl 2):S86–9.

27. Vatta M, Li H, Towbin JA. Molecular biology of arrhythmic syndromes. Curr Opin Cardiol 2000; 15(1):12–22.

28. Trevisan CP, Pastorello E, Armani M, et al. Facioscapulohumeral muscular dystrophy and occurrence of heart arrhythmia. Eur Neurol 2006;56(1):1–5.

29. Splawski I, Timothy KW, Sharpe LM, et al. Ca(V)1.2 calcium channel dysfunction causes a multisystem disorder including arrhythmia and autism. Cell 2004;119(1):19–31.

30. Curran ME, Splawski I, Timothy KW, et al. A molecular basis for cardiac arrhythmia: HERG mutations cause long QT syndrome. Cell 1995; 80(5):795–803.

31. Wang Q, Shen J, Splawski I, et al. SCN5A mutations associated with an inherited cardiac arrhythmia, long QT syndrome. Cell 1995;80(5):805–11.

32. Wang Q, Curran ME, Splawski I, et al. Positional cloning of a novel potassium channel gene: KVLQT1 mutations cause cardiac arrhythmias. Nat Genet 1996;12(1):17–23.

33. Goldman AM, Glasscock E, Yoo J, et al. Arrhythmia in Heart and brain: KCNQ1 mutations link epilepsy and sudden unexplained death. Sci Transl Med 2009;1:1–9.

34. Schott JJ, Charpentier F, Peltier S, et al. Mapping of a gene for long QT syndrome to chromosome 4q25–27. Am J Hum Genet 1995;57:1114–22.

35. Mohler PJ, Schott JJ, Gramolini AO, et al. Ankyrin-B mutation causes type 4 long-QT cardiac arrhythmia and sudden cardiac death. Nature 2003; 421(6923):634–9.

36. Mohler PJ, Splawski I, Napolitano C, et al. A cardiac arrhythmia syndrome caused by loss of ankyrin-B function. Proc Natl Acad Sci U S A 2004;101: 9137–42.

37. Abriel H. Roles and regulation of the cardiac sodium channel Na(v)1.5: recent insights from experimental studies. Cardiovasc Res 2007;76(3):381–9.

38. Vatta M, Faulkner G. Cytoskeletal basis of ion channel function in cardiac muscle. Future Cardiol 2006;2(4):467–76.

39. Schwartz PJ, Priori SG, Locati EH, et al. Long QT syndrome patients with mutations of the SCN5A and HERG genes have differential responses to Na+ channel blockade and to increases in heart rate. Implications for gene-specific therapy. Circulation 1995;92:3381–6.

40. Wu Y, Song Y, Belardinelli L, et al. The late Na+ current (INa) inhibitor ranolazine attenuates effects of palmitoyl-L-carnitine to increase late INa and cause ventricular diastolic dysfunction. J Pharmacol Exp Ther 2009;330(2):550–7.

41. Le Grand B, Pignier C, Létienne R, et al. Na+ currents in cardioprotection: better to be late. J Med Chem 2009;52(14):4149–60.

42. Vatta M, Stetson SJ, Perez-Verdia A, et al. Molecular remodeling of dystrophin in patients with end-stage cardiomyopathies and reversal in patients treated with assistance-device therapy. Lancet 2002;359: 936–41.

43. Vatta M, Stetson SJ, Jimenez S, et al. Molecular normalization of dystrophin in the failing left and right ventricle of patients treated with either pulsatile or continuous flow type ventricular assist devices. J Am Coll Cardiol 2004;43(5):811–7.

44. Mohapatra B, Vick GW 3rd, Fraser CD Jr, et al. Short-term mechanical unloading and reverse remodeling of failing hearts in children. J Heart Lung Transplant 2010;29(1):98–104.

Outpatient Management of Pediatric Heart Failure

Matthew J. O'Connor, MD[a,b,*], David N. Rosenthal, MD[c,d],
Robert E. Shaddy, MD[a,b]

KEYWORDS

- Heart failure • Children • Pediatric • Therapy
- Management • Outpatient

Pediatric heart failure (HF) is an important clinical syndrome that is responsible for morbidity and mortality disproportionate to its frequency in children. In children, HF is a clinical syndrome rather than a specific diagnosis. It encompasses a variety of causes, each having different mechanisms leading to the final common pathway of ventricular dysfunction.[1] The treatment of HF in adults has advanced greatly in the past 3 decades, driven by an impressive accumulation of evidence obtained through large, randomized, placebo-controlled trials with well-defined end points such as all-cause and cardiovascular-related mortality. However, in comparison with this substantial literature, there is less evidence regarding the effect of various therapies on the course of pediatric HF; therefore, with few exceptions, the outpatient management of pediatric HF is largely guided by accumulated clinical experience, expert consensus, small case series, and extrapolation from adult trials. Although pediatric-specific guidelines have been published,[1] practice variation between practitioners and centers is not uncommon.[2] This article reviews outpatient management of the child with HF, paying particular attention to general concepts of patient management and a review of the major pharmacologic therapies applied to children with HF.

DIVERSE CAUSES OF PEDIATRIC HF

The treatment of pediatric HF is aided by an understanding of the underlying mechanism for cardiac dysfunction, the determination of which can be a challenge given the extensive list of potential causes that must be considered by the practitioner. To add to the complexity of diagnosis and management, a single patient with HF may have several contributory mechanisms; for example, consider the patient with left ventricular dysfunction from dilated cardiomyopathy (DCM) and mitral regurgitation who develops right-sided HF from increased pulmonary capillary wedge pressure. When considering the causes of pediatric HF, it is useful to characterize the underlying anatomic substrate. For example, systolic HF in the patient with a biventricular circulation may be approached differently from HF symptoms in a patient with hypoplastic left heart syndrome palliated with a Fontan circulation, whose systemic ventricle is a right ventricle. Similarly, a patient with diastolic dysfunction secondary to cardiomyopathy with restrictive features may be treated in a different

Disclosures: none.
Financial support: none.
[a] Division of Cardiology, The Children's Hospital of Philadelphia, 34th Street and Civic Center Boulevard, Philadelphia, PA 19104-4399, USA
[b] University of Pennsylvania School of Medicine, Philadelphia, PA, USA
[c] Stanford University, Stanford, CA, USA
[d] Pediatric Cardiology, Pediatric Advanced Cardiac Therapies Program, Lucile Packard Children's Hospital, 750 Welch Road, #325, Stanford, CA 94304, USA
* Corresponding author. Division of Cardiology, The Children's Hospital of Philadelphia, 34th Street and Civic Center Boulevard, Philadelphia, PA 19104-4399.
E-mail address: oconnorm@email.chop.edu

Heart Failure Clin 6 (2010) 515–529
doi:10.1016/j.hfc.2010.05.007
1551-7136/10/$ – see front matter © 2010 Elsevier Inc. All rights reserved.

fashion from a patient with a DCM caused by an underlying mitochondrial defect.

Much of the current literature concerning therapy in adults is focused on patients with left ventricular systolic dysfunction, although there is an emerging and growing focus on diastolic HF (HF with preserved ejection fraction).[3,4] Because of a combination of space constraints and a limited evidence base to guide management, this article addresses only the issue of pediatric HF associated with systemic ventricular systolic dysfunction. The treatment of HF from left-to-right shunt lesions, right-sided HF from pulmonary hypertension, and HF from primary diastolic dysfunction is not considered in this discussion.

CLINICAL ASSESSMENT OF THE HF PATIENT

Among the most fundamental tasks required for treatment of the child with HF is the assessment and characterization of the severity of the illness. The clinical spectrum of pediatric HF ranges from an asymptomatic, well-compensated physiologic state to hemodynamic collapse. In an attempt to standardize the description of these states, a variety of disease severity classification schemes have been proposed; these are summarized in **Box 1**. The Ross and New York Health Association (NYHA) classifications are stratified based on the severity of current symptoms, and these classification schemes are most useful for children with illness of at least moderate severity. However, these scales do not reflect intensity of therapy. To more broadly characterize the spectrum and evolution of pediatric HF, the International Society of Heart and Lung Transplantation (ISHLT) classification was developed in 2004.[1] In this scheme, HF stages are described, ranging from stage A (patients at risk of developing HF, but no recognizable abnormalities clinically or by imaging), to stage D (end-stage disease).

To accurately determine the symptom burden of HF in a pediatric patient, a careful history must be tailored to the age and prior activities of the patient. As children reach a stage of disease at which their functional capacity is restricted, they will often simply self-limit their daily activities. Thus, the question of whether a child is symptomatic requires an understanding of what their expected daily activities might be, rather than simply questioning whether they experience breathlessness, chest pain, or other symptoms. For example, a 9 year old might be reporting no symptoms, but is no longer participating in the weekend soccer league that was previously a major part of his or her activities.

At each outpatient visit, meticulous attention to changes in vital signs and the physical examination is mandatory. Patient weight, if properly and consistently measured, can be an important indicator of fluid balance. Significant increases in weight over brief periods of time may indicate pathologic shifts of intravascular volume into the interstitial space, from left-sided HF (manifesting as pulmonary edema) or right-sided HF (manifesting as ascites), or a combination of the two. Conversely, failure to gain weight at an age-appropriate velocity may indicate a catabolic state imposed by the increased metabolic demands of the HF syndrome, or inadequate caloric intake.

Heart rate is a critically important indicator of patient well-being. Knowledge of the patient's heart rate trends is necessary, because a child with compensated HF may have a degree of baseline tachycardia. Changes in heart rate from this baseline should prompt evaluation for underlying infection, arrhythmia, or worsening of ventricular function. An electrocardiogram (ECG) should be considered at each patient visit, with additional consideration given to periodic ambulatory ECG monitoring for surveillance in patients with known or suspected arrhythmias, or those at significant risk for arrhythmias. Other aspects of the physical examination of the child with HF also play an important role in clinical assessment, including respiratory pattern and effort; presence of a gallop; adequacy of peripheral circulation as judged by skin temperature; capillary refill and quality of peripheral pulses; and intravascular fluid status indicated by hepatomegaly, venous distension, and (occasionally) peripheral edema.

Noninvasive imaging plays a major role in the diagnosis and management of HF in children. Patients undergoing initial evaluation for HF require a complete echocardiogram with two-dimensional imaging and color Doppler to accurately identify structural defects potentially mimicking or contributing to HF symptoms (eg, severe aortic stenosis, congenital mitral valve disease). Echocardiography is a valuable noninvasive tool in the chronic management of HF by virtue of its ability to establish trends in left ventricular ejection fraction, left ventricular chamber dimensions, atrioventricular valve regurgitation, and estimates of right ventricular pressure. There may be an emerging role for cardiac magnetic resonance imaging (MRI) in the evaluation of chronic HF, particularly with respect to assessment of remodeling and myocardial viability;[5–7] however, its use in children may be limited by the need for sedation in many younger patients.

Laboratory evaluation of the outpatient with chronic HF should be individualized. Frequent

---

Box 1
Classification of HF symptoms

Proposed Staging in Children from the International Society for Heart and Lung Transplantation

Stage A HF

- At increased risk of developing HF; without symptoms

Stage B HF

- Abnormal cardiac structure or function; without symptoms

Stage C HF

- Abnormal cardiac structure or function; with past or current symptoms

Stage D HF

- Abnormal cardiac structure or function, warranting (1) continuous intravenous inotropic support; (2) continuous prostaglandin E_1 to maintain patency of ductus arteriosus; (3) mechanical ventilatory or circulatory support; (4) cardiac transplantation; or (5) hospice care

Ross Classification for HF in Children

Class I HF

- Asymptomatic

Class II HF

- Mild tachypnea or diaphoresis with feeding in infants; dyspnea on exertion in older children

Class III HF

- Marked tachypnea or diaphoresis with feeding in infants; prolonged feeding times with growth failure resulting from HF; marked dyspnea on exertion in older children

Class IV HF

- Symptoms such as tachypnea, retractions, grunting, or diaphoresis at rest

NYHA Classification for HF in Adults

Class I HF

- Symptoms of HF are only present at levels of exertion that would limit normal individuals

Class II HF

- Symptoms of HF are present at ordinary levels of exertion

Class III HF

- Symptoms of HF are present at less-than-ordinary levels of exertion

Class IV HF

- Symptoms of HF are present at rest

Data from Rosenthal D, Christant MRK, Edens E, et al. International Society for Heart and Lung Transplantation: practice guidelines for management of heart failure in children. J Heart Lung Transplant 2004;23:1333; and Hunt SA, Abraham WT, Chin MH, et al. ACC/AHA 2005 Guideline update for the diagnosis and management of chronic heart failure in the adult: a report of the American College of Cardiology/American Heart Association Task Force on Practice Guidelines (Writing Committee to Update the 2001 Guidelines for the Evaluation and Management of Heart Failure): developed in collaboration with the American College of Chest Physicians and the International Society for Heart and Lung Transplantation: endorsed by the Heart Rhythm Society. Circulation 2005;112:e154–235.

---

monitoring of serum electrolytes is reasonable during initiation and dose titration of diuretics or angiotensin converting enzyme (ACE) inhibitors, but can be performed less frequently once a stable dose has been achieved. In particular, hyponatremia is a concerning finding that has been associated with short- and long-term increases in mortality in adult patients with acute and chronic HF.[8] Hyponatremia, when encountered in HF, is typically a manifestation of fluid overload rather than sodium depletion. Thus, it is not easily treated. Liver function tests, including albumin, may corroborate end-organ dysfunction and injury and can be surrogates of overall nutritional status. The role of anemia in outcomes of pediatric HF has not been well evaluated; in adults with HF, anemia is an independent risk factor for increased mortality.[9] However, the role correction of anemia plays in the improvement in outcomes of HF remains unclear[10] and is not supported in the routine management of adult HF.[11,12]

Evaluation of B-type natriuretic peptide (BNP) in the management of chronic pediatric HF deserves special mention. BNP, first discovered in brain tissue, is a protein secreted by ventricular myocytes in response to mechanical stress.[13] BNP release promotes natriuresis and, in turn, diuresis. In addition, the renin-angiotensin-aldosterone (RAA) system is inhibited by BNP release. Serum BNP levels are increased in acute and chronic ventricular dysfunction, systolic and diastolic HF, and in asymptomatic as well as symptomatic patients. For these reasons, combined with a widely available commercial assay, measurement of plasma BNP levels has become increasingly common in evaluating the severity, response to treatment, and prognosis of HF in children and adults. Normal values have been established in the pediatric population,[14–17] with little crossover between children with and without cardiovascular disease.[18] However, reference values for BNP vary among assays and laboratory-specific normative data must be taken into account when comparing results obtained from different platforms.

Studies in children have found associations between cardiovascular disease and perturbations in BNP levels. In children with decompensated HF in the intensive care unit (ICU) setting, increased BNP levels predict mortality and need for readmission,[19] and have been shown to predict adverse outcomes in pediatric outpatients with HF.[20] BNP has also been shown to be useful in detecting cardiovascular toxicity following anthracycline exposure,[21] left ventricular dysfunction in hypertrophic cardiomyopathy,[22] screening for rejection following heart transplantation (HT),[23] and assessing response to treatment of pulmonary hypertension.[24] In the outpatient setting in patients with established HF, BNP may be useful as an adjunctive method of assessing HF status or response to changes in therapy, but must be taken into context with clinical observation.

ORGANIZATION AND DELIVERY OF CARE

Children with HF comprise a vulnerable group of patients with severe, chronic disease. A subset of severely ill patients will experience frequent hospitalizations. Most will require frequent medical visits and diagnostic tests. Although there is little literature specific to pediatric subjects, it is the authors' opinion that the management of pediatric HF is optimized by dedicated clinical programs. Ideally, these programs will include a multidisciplinary team that is capable of addressing issues such as maintaining adequate nutritional intake, recognizing and treating depression, advocating with school systems for appropriate support services, and monitoring for medication interactions in a disease state in which polypharmacy is often the norm. In addition, long-term consistency of physicians may aid in the early detection of subtle, but important, changes in clinical status. It is also beneficial to children with HF if the team familiar with the outpatient management is an active participant in decision making during hospitalizations. This care model is also increasingly common in programs treating adults with HF. However, there is controversy in the literature concerning the demonstrable benefits of such programs for adults, and there is no systematic investigation of the overall benefits for children with HF.[25]

PHARMACOLOGIC THERAPY

Pharmacologic therapy is the mainstay of treatment in pediatric HF. Drug classes with primary effects on the myocardium or peripheral vasculature include cardiac glycosides, β-adrenergic receptor blockers (β-blockers), ACE inhibitors, and angiotensin-receptor blockers (ARBs). Inotropic agents are also included in this class, although their use in the outpatient setting is limited. Drug classes with primary effects on fluid balance include loop diuretics and thiazide diuretics. Drugs that combat neurohormonal activation and target remodeling include the aldosterone antagonists spironolactone and eplerenone.

ACE Inhibitors and ARBs

ACE inhibitors have been a mainstay of treatment of adults with HF since the publication of the Cooperative North Scandinavian Enalapril Survival Study (CONSENSUS) trial in 1987[26] and the Studies of Left Ventricular Dysfunction (SOLVD) trial in 1991,[27] which were among the first trials to show a survival benefit of ACE inhibition in adults with chronic HF associated with left ventricular systolic dysfunction. ACE inhibitors block the conversion of angiotensin I into angiotensin II, a key mediator in the RAA pathway. Angiotensin II is a potent vasoconstrictor with direct action on vascular smooth muscle, central effects on vascular tone, and promotion of volume expansion by enhancing the production of aldosterone and antidiuretic hormone.[28] In addition, angiotensin II is implicated as a cause of cardiac fibrosis.[29] Reversal of ventricular remodeling in chronic HF has also been shown with ACE inhibitors.[30]

ARBs are a related class of drugs that exert their effect at the angiotensin II type I receptor. Theoretical advantages of ARBs compared with ACE inhibitors include higher specificity for antiangiotensin II effect and lack of ACE escape, a phenomenon in which aldosterone and angiotensin II serum levels increase despite ACE inhibitor use.[31] In addition, a potentially beneficial synergistic effect of ACE inhibitors and ARBs in combination has been reported,[32] although the magnitude of this effect has recently been called into question.[33] In practice, the major benefit of ARBs compared with ACE inhibitors seems to be mitigation of cough, a side effect commonly seen with ACE inhibitors because of the unopposed production of bradykinin.

ACE inhibitors are recommended for all adult patients with HF with reduced left ventricular systolic function, unless specific contraindications to their use exist.[11] Studies of ACE inhibitors and ARBs in children are limited. The beneficial effects of captopril (Capoten) on hemodynamics in infants with left-to-right shunt lesions were reported as early as 1988,[34] but in 1991 the first report on the use of captopril in children with congestive and restrictive cardiomyopathies was published.[35] In this study, 16 children, predominantly with DCM, showed significant increases in cardiac index and left ventricular stroke volume, with a decrease in systemic vascular resistance following acute administration of captopril. No effects on blood pressure, heart rate, or wedge pressure were seen. More recently, Calabro and colleagues[36] reported reduction in mitral regurgitation and an increase in left ventricular ejection fraction with enalapril using echocardiography in patients with chronic mitral regurgitation.

There are few studies of ACE inhibition in pediatric patients with HF and congenital heart disease. In 1997, Kouatli and colleagues[37] published the results of a randomized, double-blinded, crossover, placebo-controlled study of the effects of enalapril on measures of exercise performance and diastolic function following the Fontan operation. The mean age of the population was 14.5 years, and all were asymptomatic. No differences were found with respect to exercise capacity or measures of diastolic function as measured by echocardiography. Potential explanations for the lack of effect in this single-ventricle population include small sample size, the use of exercise as a primary end point, as well as a potentially deleterious effect of ACE inhibition on lowering central venous pressure and therefore pulmonary blood flow.

ACE inhibitors have been studied in a prospective fashion in patients with Duchenne muscular dystrophy. In 2005, Duboc and colleagues[38] evaluated perindopril (Aceon) in a 2-phase, prospective, randomized, placebo-controlled trial in patients with Duchenne muscular dystrophy and normal left ventricular ejection fraction. In this study of 57 patients, administration of perindopril for 3 years to the treatment group, followed by an open-label phase of perindopril administration in placebo and treatment groups for 2 more years, decreased the progression of left ventricular dysfunction as measured by radionuclide scintigraphy ($P = .02$). The same group recently reported an additional 5-year follow-up, in which all-cause reduction in mortality of 27.4% was noted in the early treatment group with perindopril ($P = .02$).[39] These results have yet to be confirmed through multicenter prospective studies.

Prevention of late myocardial dysfunction following treatment of childhood cancer has also been studied with ACE inhibitors. The cardiotoxic effect of anthracycline chemotherapy has been well established.[40] Lipshultz and colleagues showed early (within the first 6 years of treatment) beneficial effects of enalapril on left ventricular dimensions and shortening fraction. However, this benefit was not sustained beyond 6 years.[41] In adults, ACE inhibitors have been studied as protective agents against the development of cardiotoxicity, with early promising results,[42] but this has not been studied in children nor has it been confirmed in larger trials.

There are no published studies regarding ARB use in pediatric patients with HF. In the absence of such evidence, no recommendations can be made for or against the use of ARBs in pediatric HF. The 2009 update to the guidelines for the treatment of HF in adults from the American College of Cardiology and the American Heart Association reserve ARB use for patients with current or prior symptoms of HF and reduced LV ejection fraction who are unable to tolerate ACE inhibitors (eg, cough, angioedema).[43]

β-blockers

β-blockers exert their primary effect on β_1 and β_2 receptors, which are present in the myocardium and in the peripheral vasculature. β_1 receptor stimulation primarily increases contractility, chronotropy, and vascular tone, whereas β_2 receptors have a vasodilatory effect. β-blockers, as a class, are grouped according to their selectivity for β_1 and β_2 receptors; however, some agents also possess α_1 receptor-blocking capabilities.

The beneficial effects of β-blockade in HF derive from their ability to counteract the maladaptive neurohormonal activation seen in chronic HF. Improvements in ejection fraction, promotion of reverse modeling, decreases in hospitalization, and decreases in mortality have all been ascribed to the use of β-blockers in adults with chronic HF.[44] Although numerous agents are available, only 3 β-blockers have been shown to reduce all-cause mortality in symptomatic chronic HF: the extended-release form of the β_1-selective agent metoprolol (Metoprolol Randomized Intervention Trial in Heart Failure [MERIT-HF]),[45] the β_1-selective agent bisoprolol (Cardiac Insufficiency Bisoprolol Study [CIBIS]-II),[46] and carvedilol, a nonselective β-blocker with α_1-blocking properties (Multicenter Oral Carvedilol Heart Failure Assessment [MOCHA], US Carvedilol, and Carvedilol Prospective Randomized Cumulative Survival [COPERNICUS] trials).[47–49] Definitive data regarding superiority of all β-blockers are not yet available in head-to-head comparison trials; however, a recent European trial of carvedilol versus short-acting metoprolol (COMET trial) found significantly less all-cause mortality with carvedilol.[50]

The rationale for the use of β-blockers in the long-term management of chronic HF in pediatric patients has largely been derived from the results of adult trials, with a contribution from small multicenter trials in pediatric patients. The first retrospective multicenter report in pediatric patients with HF reviewed the effects of metoprolol therapy in 15 patients with chronic HF of diverse causes on ventricular function, as assessed by echocardiography.[51] In this study, significant increases in left ventricular ejection fraction (27.0%–41.1%) were noted, although long-term outcome variables were not assessed.

Carvedilol has been the subject of study in pediatric patients through several trials in which improvements in symptoms and ventricular function were noted.[52–56] In 2007, results from the first prospective, randomized, placebo-controlled trial of an HF medication in children were published.[57] In this study, 161 patients less than 18 years of age with symptomatic systemic ventricular systolic dysfunction from DCM or congenital heart disease were randomized to 6 months of placebo, low-dose carvedilol, or high-dose carvedilol. A primary clinical composite end point of worsened, improved, or unchanged HF was used.

Several findings arose from this trial.[57] First, enrollment of 161 patients took 4 years, showing the difficulties of conducting an adequately powered prospective trial in children. When the combined high- and low-dose groups were compared with placebo, no differences were detected in the composite outcome of worsened, improved, or unchanged (odds ratio 0.79, 95% confidence interval 0.36–1.59, $P = .47$). A trend was noted toward improvement in the composite end point in patients with a systemic left ventricle, whereas no improvement was noted in patients whose systemic ventricle was not a left ventricle. The clinical course of the patients enrolled in the trial was better than expected, with 56% improvement in the placebo and carvedilol groups ($P = .74$). Therefore, the study was likely underpowered[58] to detect an effect of carvedilol in this group of patients with a higher than expected rate of improvement. In addition, the lack of improvement seen in patients with carvedilol may have been related to a population with fewer symptoms than anticipated in the study design (72% of the patients were in NYHA class II HF), potentially making it harder to detect a treatment effect of the medication.

Although evidence is lacking that β-blockers reduce mortality in children with HF, reports of the usage of β blocker therapy in this group of patients have been common, regardless of cause. In the prospective, randomized, multicenter pediatric carvedilol trial, there was a significant interaction between study drug and ventricular morphology, suggesting a possible differential effect of treatment between patients with a systemic left ventricle (beneficial trend) and those whose systemic ventricle was not a left ventricle.[40] Similarly, echocardiographic improvement was seen in those with a systemic left ventricle, but no such improvement could be detected in those whose systemic ventricle was not a left ventricle. This suggests that the response to carvedilol may be affected by the morphology of a patient's systemic ventricle, with a beneficial response more likely in those whose systemic ventricle is a left ventricle. There may also be an emerging role for use of carvedilol in patients at high risk for the development of DCM, such as those receiving anthracycline chemotherapy[59] or patients with DCM associated with muscular dystrophy.[60,61] β-Blockers are generally well tolerated, with important, but uncommon, side effects including bradycardia and atrioventricular block, hypoglycemia in patients with diabetes mellitus, bronchospasm in patients with asthma or reactive airway disease, constipation, and lassitude. In the prospective, randomized, multicenter pediatric carvedilol trial, no significant differences in cardiovascular adverse effects were noted between placebo and treatment groups, and the most commonly reported adverse effects of upper respiratory tract infections, vomiting, and cough were likely not related to carvedilol itself.[57]

Digoxin

Digoxin is a cardiac glycoside that increases sarcoplasmic calcium concentrations via inhibition of the myocardial sodium-potassium ATPase pump. In addition, it helps to counteract the neurohormonal activation seen in patients with HF through its sympatholytic effects. Digoxin has been in the armamentarium of cardiologists for decades, and continues to play a role in the management of symptomatic HF in adults. However, digoxin has assumed a more limited role in adult HF management following the publication of the Digitalis Investigators Group[62] (DIG) trial in 1997, which found no improvement in mortality relative to placebo. The results of this trial, combined with the narrow therapeutic window of digoxin, led to digoxin no longer being recommended for first-line treatment of HF in the most recent guidelines for the treatment of HF in adults from the American College of Cardiology and the American Heart Association.[11]

Nonetheless, digoxin use in pediatrics remains common in many centers, perhaps because of familiarity with its use in dysrhythmias as well as evidence from older studies showing potential benefit in patients with large left-to-right shunts.[63] However, no study has shown a survival benefit from digoxin in children or adults with HF.

Diuretics

Diuretics represent a mainstay of therapy for acute and chronic HF, and are effective in relieving symptoms of fluid overload and sodium retention. However no data are available regarding the long-term benefit of diuretics on mortality in adult or pediatric patients with HF. The chronic adverse effects of diuretics on serum electrolytes are well known (hyponatremia, hypochloremia, and hypokalemia leading to a metabolic alkalosis) and warrant careful surveillance of serum electrolytes during diuretic therapy. Injudicious diuretic use may lead to volume depletion, azotemia, and renal insufficiency, so meticulous attention to the physical examination and monitoring of fluid intake and output are also necessary.

Although the aldosterone antagonists spironolactone and eplerenone are often grouped in the diuretic class of medications (potassium-sparing diuretics), their effect on fluid balance is weak. The rationale for the use of aldosterone antagonists in patients with HF derives from their ability to reduce angiotensin II effect (angiotensin II stimulates aldosterone formation) as well as observations that aldosterone causes adverse effects on cardiac structure and function (remodeling).[64,65] Both drugs compete for mineralocorticoid receptors, but eplerenone is more selective for the aldosterone receptor,[66] resulting in fewer endocrine side effects (eg, gynecomastia).

The Randomized Aldactone Evaluation Study (RALES), published in 1999, was the first to show a survival benefit of low-dose spironolactone in adults with NYHA class III or IV HF with severe left ventricular dysfunction (ejection fraction <35%).[67] All patients in this trial were on an ACE inhibitor and a loop diuretic at the time of enrollment. The trial was terminated early after 24 months of follow-up by the trial's Data and Safety Monitoring Board (DSMB) because of a significantly lower incidence of all-cause and cardiac-related mortality in the spironolactone group. The only significant adverse effect of aldosterone was gynecomastia (seen in 10% of the men receiving aldosterone). In clinical practice studies, the safety of spironolactone therapy has been less impressive, with a 12% incidence of serious hyperkalemia noted in 1 study, compared with 2% in the RALES trial.[68] This finding highlights the important distinction between evaluation of a medication in a clinical trial and subsequent clinical use of the medication.

The efficacy of eplerenone in adults with HF was established through the Eplerenone Neurohormonal Efficacy and Survival Study (EPHESUS).[69] In this study, approximately 6000 patients with left ventricular dysfunction (ejection fraction <40%) following acute myocardial infarction were randomized to eplerenone versus placebo; all patients were receiving standard HF therapy. As with aldosterone, all-cause and cardiac-related mortality were significantly reduced in the eplerenone group. An important side effect of eplerenone noted in the EPHESUS trial was hyperkalemia (serum $K^+ \geq 6$ mEq/liter) in 5.5% of those receiving eplerenone ($P = .002$); hyperkalemia was more common in patients with a baseline impairment in creatinine clearance.

Neither spironolactone nor eplerenone have been rigorously studied in children with HF. Mahle and colleagues[70] recently published a preliminary report describing the effects of spironolactone on endothelial function and serum cytokine profiles (a surrogate for remodeling) at a dose of 50 mg daily in 10 patients following Fontan palliation. No changes were seen in endothelial function, nor were any significant alterations of inflammatory serum cytokines detected in association with spironolactone use.

Controversy remains in the adult literature regarding the most appropriate combination of medications to effectively block the RAA pathway: ACE inhibitor versus ARB, ACE inhibitor and ARB in combination versus either class alone, ACE inhibitor or ARB in combination with an aldosterone antagonist.[71]

Inotropic Agents

Commonly used intravenous inotropes in the acute management of HF in children and adults include dopamine, dobutamine, milrinone, epinephrine, norepinephrine, nesiritide, and vasopressin. The specific indications, mechanisms of action, and side effects of these drugs are beyond the scope of this review. These drugs are only available in intravenous preparations and are reserved for acute refractory HF symptoms; they are typically reserved for in-hospital use. However, some investigators have advocated the use of continuous or intermittent outpatient intravenous inotrope therapy (typically dobutamine or milrinone) in patients who are unable to wean from inotropes, but who are otherwise stable for hospital discharge.[72–74] Routine use of intermittent outpatient inotrope infusions is currently not rec-ommended in adults, but may offer palliation of symptoms to adults with refractory end-stage HF or as a bridge to HT.[11,43] Two case series describe home inotrope use in children[75,76]; the potential risks of catheter-related sepsis, pump malfunc-tion, and adverse events related to the inotrope (eg, proarrhythmia) must be balanced against the potential benefits.

DEVICE THERAPY

Device therapy (implantable cardioverter-defibrillators [ICDs] and cardiac resynchronization therapy [CRT] using biventricular pacing, or a combination of the two) is an emerging mode of therapy for the treatment of pediatric HF. A well-established body of evidence currently exists in the adult HF literature regarding the beneficial effects of ICDs and CRT in adults with HF and reduced ejection fraction from ischemic and noni-schemic cardiomyopathy on several outcomes. All-cause mortality has recently been shown to be decreased with these devices. ICD therapy targets the most common cause of mortality in adult patients with HF: hemodynamic collapse from ventricular dysrhythmias such as ventricular tachycardia and ventricular fibrillation. In contrast, CRT serves to reverse the ventricular remodeling conferred by chronic left ventricular dyssychrony in patients with QRS prolongation (seen in approx-imately one-third of adult patients with left ventric-ular systolic dysfunction).[77]

The development of device therapy for adults with HF was driven in part by the unsatisfactory experience with antiarrhythmic drug therapy for the prevention of ventricular dysrhythmias and sudden cardiac death.[78–80] Among the most effec-tive antiarrhythmic agents is amiodarone, a class III agent, which is widely used because of its effi-cacy, low risk of proarrhythmia, and minimal nega-tive inotropic effect. Although it is not considered to negatively affect survival in adults with HF,[81] and may confer a survival benefit in select settings,[82,83] amiodarone has been shown to be inferior to ICDs for reduction of all-cause mortality in adult patients with HF.[84]

ICDs have been shown to be of benefit for primary and secondary prevention of sudden cardiac death in adults with ischemic and noni-schemic cardiomyopathy associated with decreased ejection fraction. Primary prevention refers to the implantation of an ICD before the undesired outcome (eg, ventricular dysrhythmias leading to hemodynamic compromise); in contrast, secondary prevention involves ICD implantation in patients who have survived cardiac arrest (presumably mediated primarily by ventric-ular dysrhythmias). Data supporting the use of ICDs for the secondary prevention of sudden cardiac death first emerged in the 1990s with the Antiarrhythmics versus Implantable Defibrillators (AVID),[85] Canadian Implantable Defibrillator (CID),[86] and Cardiac Arrest Study Hamburg (CASH)[87] trials of ICD implantation in patients resuscitated from cardiac arrest. Subsequently, several large trials have shown the efficacy of ICDs for primary prevention in reducing all-cause mortality in patients with ischemic cardiomy-opathy (Multicenter Automatic Defibrillator Implanta-tion Trial [MADIT],[88] MADIT II,[89] Multicenter Unstable Tachycardia Trial [MUSTT][90] trials) and nonischemic cardiomyopathy (Sudden Cardiac Death/Heart Failure Trial [SCD-HeFT]).[84]

The survival benefit conferred by ICDs for primary prevention seems to be less substantial than that for secondary prevention,[91] and refining the indications for ICD implantation in adult patients with HF remains a source of significant controversy,[92,93] particularly when balanced against the risks of proarrhythmia and inappro-priate shocks. Current guidelines for ICD use in adults have recently been published[94] and are listed in **Box 2**.

The indications for ICD use in pediatric patients have recently been reviewed,[95] but because pedi-atric patients represent less than 1% of all ICD implants, indications for children are not clearly defined. Recently, a large retrospective multicenter study of ICD use in pediatric patients and patients with congenital heart disease was published,[96] which gives valuable insights into the current use of, and complications related to, ICDs in children. Notably, 25% of the 443 patients in this study were adults (>21 years of age), most of whom had congenital heart disease. The indications for ICD implantation in children included congenital heart disease (46%), cardiomyopathies (23%), and primary electrical disease (31%). Shocks were found to be appropriate in 26% of patients and inap-propriate in 21%, and 12% of patients experienced early device-related complications. Novel implant techniques have been described to accommodate younger children and those with abnormal or unfa-vorable venous anatomy.[97,98] The relative paucity of data regarding ICD use in children limits recom-mendations for their use in pediatric HF.[1,94] However, consideration should be given to ICD implantation in pediatric patients with HF with aborted sudden cardiac death episodes or in those with significant ventricular dysrhythmias awaiting transplantation. ICD implantation in children should be performed at experienced centers possessing the ability to manage device-related complications.

Box 2
Indications for ICD therapy in adults and children

Adults

Class I Indications (ICD Therapy is Useful or Effective)

- Survivors of cardiac arrest caused by ventricular fibrillation (VF) or unstable ventricular tachycardia (VT) in whom reversible causes have been excluded
- Patients with spontaneous sustained VT and structural heart disease
- Patients with syncope of undetermined cause in whom hemodynamically significant VT or VF can be induced at electrophysiology study
- Patients >40 days after myocardial infarction with left ventricular ejection fraction (LVEF) $\leq$35% and NYHA class II or III
- Patients >40 days after myocardial infarction with LVEF $\leq$30% and NYHA class I
- Patients with LVEF $\leq$40% and nonsustained VT following myocardial infarction in whom VT or VF can be induced at electrophysiology study
- Patients with nonischemic DCM with LVEF $\leq$35% and NYHA class II or III

Class IIa Indications (ICD Therapy is Reasonable; Weight of Evidence/Opinion is in Favor of Usefulness/Efficacy)

- Patients with unexplained syncope, significant LV dysfunction, and nonischemic dilated cardiomyopathy
- Patients with sustained VT and normal to near-normal LV function
- Patients with hypertrophic cardiomyopathy who have $\geq$1 major risk factor for sudden cardiac death
- Patients with arrhythmogenic right ventricular dysplasia/cardiomyopathy who have $\geq$1 major risk factor for sudden cardiac death
- Patients with long QT syndrome with syncope or VT despite therapy with β-blockers
- Nonhospitalized patients awaiting cardiac transplantation
- Patients with Brugada syndrome who have experienced syncope or VT
- Patients with catecholaminergic polymorphic VT who have had syncope or sustained VT despite therapy with β-blockers
- Patients with cardiac sarcoidosis, Chagas disease, or giant cell myocarditis

Children and Patients with Congenital Heart Disease

Class I Indications (ICD Therapy is Useful or Effective)

- In the survivor of cardiac arrest, provided reversible causes have been identified and excluded

- Patients with symptomatic sustained VT in association with congenital heart disease who have undergone hemodynamic and electrophysiologic evaluation; catheter ablation or surgical repair may be alternatives in carefully selected patients

Class IIa Indications (ICD Therapy is Reasonable; Weight of Evidence/Opinion is in Favor of Usefulness/Efficacy)

- Patients with congenital heart disease experiencing recurrent syncope of undetermined cause in the presence of ventricular dysfunction or inducible ventricular arrhythmias at electrophysiology study

Adapted from Epstein AE, DiMarco JP, Ellenbogen KA, et al. ACC/AHA/HRS 2008 guidelines for device-based therapy of cardiac rhythm abnormalities: a report of the American College of Cardiology/American Heart Association Task Force on Practice Guidelines (Writing Committee to Revise the ACC/AHA/NASPE 2002 Guideline Update for Implantation of Cardiac Pacemakers and Antiarrhythmia Devices) developed in collaboration with the American Association for Thoracic Surgery and Society of Thoracic Surgeons. J Am Coll Cardiol 2008;51:e36–8.

The use of CRT in adults with HF gained widespread acceptance following the publication of the Comparison of Medical Therapy, pacing and Defibrillation in Chronic Heart Failure (COMPANION)[99] and Cardiac Resynchronization-Heart Failure (CARE-HF) trials.[100] In both trials, patients with nonischemic and ischemic cardiomyopathy, NYHA class III or IV symptoms, QRS duration greater than 120 milliseconds who were in sinus rhythm showed significant reductions in all-cause mortality compared with standard HF therapy; however, all-cause mortality was significantly reduced in the COMPANION trial only when CRT was used along with an ICD. In addition to effecting reductions in all-cause mortality, these and other studies have found improvements in left ventricular ejection fraction (LVEF), quality of life, exercise tolerance, and rates of hospitalization.[101] Current indications for CRT (with or without an ICD) in adults include HF in patients in sinus rhythm with NYHA class III or IV symptoms, QRS duration 120 milliseconds or more, and LVEF 35% or less.[43,94] Two recent publications[102,103] have reported the beneficial effects of CRT in patients with HF with dyssynchrony in the setting of mild symptoms (NYHA class I or II), although reductions in all-cause mortality as a primary end point have not yet been shown in NYHA class I or II patients. An important limitation to CRT use is that from 20% to 30% of patients do not show clinical improvement, suggesting that QRS duration alone may not be sufficient to define dyssynchrony and that mechanical dyssychrony must be considered separately from electrical dyssynchrony.[77,101,104,105] Current indications for CRT use are summarized in **Box 3**.

As with ICDs, experience with CRT in children with HF or congenital heart disease is limited.[106–109] Dubin and colleagues[106] described a retrospective multicenter experience with CRT in 103 pediatric patients or adult patients with congenital heart disease; 71% had congenital heart disease and 16% had cardiomyopathy, with the remainder having congenital complete heart block. For the entire cohort, ejection fraction increased by 13 ($\pm$13) EF units (P<.05); however, when stratified by diagnosis, no significant changes in ejection fraction were noted. The complication rate was 29%, with most complications related to problems with coronary sinus leads. Five of the 6 patients on continuous inotrope infusions before CRT were able to be weaned to oral therapy following CRT, and, of

---

Box 3
Indications for CRT in adults and children

Adults

Class I Indication (CRT is Useful or Effective)

- Patients in sinus rhythm with LVEF $\leq$35%, QRS duration $\geq$120 ms with NYHA class III or IV symptoms despite optimal medical therapy, with or without an ICD

Class IIa Indication (CRT is Reasonable; Weight of Evidence/Opinion is in Favor of Usefulness/ Efficacy)

- Patients with LVEF $\leq$35% with NYHA class I or II symptoms on optimal medical therapy undergoing permanent pacemaker or ICD implantation, in whom frequent ventricular pacing is expected

Children and Patients with Congenital Heart Disease

No formal recommendations

Adapted from Epstein AE, DiMarco JP, Ellenbogen KA, et al. ACC/AHA/HRS 2008 guidelines for device-based therapy of cardiac rhythm abnormalities: a report of the American College of Cardiology/American Heart Association Task Force on Practice Guidelines (Writing Committee to Revise the ACC/AHA/NASPE 2002 Guideline Update for Implantation of Cardiac Pacemakers and Antiarrhythmia Devices) developed in collaboration with the American Association for Thoracic Surgery and Society of Thoracic Surgeons. J Am Coll Cardiol 2008;51:e18.

Box 4
Indications for HT in pediatric heart disease

Class I Indications (HT is Useful or Effective)

- Stage D HF associated with systemic ventricular dysfunction
- Stage C HF associated with severe limitation of exercise and activity (peak maximum oxygen consumption <50% predicted for age and sex)
- Stage C HF associated with systemic ventricular dysfunction when HF is associated with significant growth failure attributable to the heart disease
- Stage C HF associated with near sudden death or life-threatening arrhythmias untreatable with medication or an ICD
- Stage C HF associated with restrictive cardiomyopathy associated with reactive pulmonary hypertension

Class IIA Indications (HT is Reasonable; Weight of Evidence/Opinion is in Favor of Usefulness/ Efficacy)

- Stage C HF associated with reactive pulmonary hypertension if there is a potential risk of developing fixed, irreversible increase of pulmonary vascular resistance
- Anatomic and physiologic conditions in infants with single-ventricle congenital heart disease, all of which worsen the natural history of such disease: (1) stenoses or atresia of the proximal coronary arteries; (2) moderate to severe stenosis or insufficiency of the atrioventricular or systemic semilunar valves; (3) severe ventricular dysfunction
- Anatomic and physiologic conditions in previously repaired or palliated congenital heart disease in patients with stage C HF, all of which worsen the natural history of the repair or palliation: (1) pulmonary hypertension at risk of developing fixed, irreversible increase of pulmonary vascular resistance; (2) severe aortic or systemic atrioventricular valve insufficiency not considered amenable to surgical correction; (3) severe cyanosis not amenable to surgical correction; (4) persistent protein-losing enteropathy despite optimal therapy

Adapted from Canter CE, Shaddy RE, Bernstein D, et al. Indications for heart transplantation in pediatric heart disease: a scientific statement from the American Heart Association Council on Cardiovascular Disease in the Young; the Councils on Clinical Cardiology, Cardiovascular Nursing, and Cardiovascular Surgery and Anesthesia; and the Quality of Care and Outcomes Research Interdisciplinary Working Group. Circulation 2007; 115:668–9.

the 18 patients listed for HT before CRT, 3 showed sufficient improvement following CRT to be removed from the waiting list. In a more recent publication, Janousek and colleagues[110] evaluated response to CRT in a European cohort of 109 subjects. In this study, children with DCM and those with poor NYHA class did not show improvement from CRT.

Based on the limited available data, it is difficult to make specific recommendations for CRT use in pediatric HF. As in adults, identification of patients who will benefit the most from CRT is the primary focus of investigation. Recently, Friedberg and colleagues[111] applied a mechanical dyssynchrony index, verified in adults, to the study of children with idiopathic DCM; 65% of patients with cardiomyopathy in this study were identified as having mechanical dyssynchrony. QRS duration was not significantly different between cardiomyopathy patients with and without mechanical dyssynchrony, indicating that electrical dyssynchrony alone is likely insufficient to determine the need for CRT therapy in children. It is expected that further research will continue to refine the indications for CRT in adults and children with various forms of ventricular dysfunction.

INDICATIONS FOR HT

A frequently encountered and complex issue in the management of pediatric patients with chronic HF

regards optimal timing of listing for HT. Clearly, inotrope-dependent patients, or those in whom ventricular assist device implantation or extracorporeal membrane oxygenation is necessary to prevent imminent demise, warrant listing for HT, provided that end-organ dysfunction is not advanced and that the cause of HF is deemed irreversible. However, many patients with chronic HF in the outpatient setting experience prolonged periods of relative clinical stability that may be followed by acute deterioration; such acute changes in clinical status are difficult to predict accurately. In 2007, the American Heart Association published guidelines for the indications for HT in pediatric heart disease[112]; these recommendations are summarized in **Box 4**.

SUMMARY AND RECOMMENDATIONS

Pediatric HF is a complex entity, the cause of which is multifactorial, and treatment regimens must be individualized. In the outpatient setting, patients with HF require careful and frequent supervision to monitor for progression of disease and response to therapy. The scientific background and rationale for HF treatment in adults is discussed in detail in the guidelines from the American College of Cardiology and the American Heart Association for the Diagnosis and Management of Chronic HF in the Adult[11]; these guidelines were updated in 2009.[43] In 2004, the first

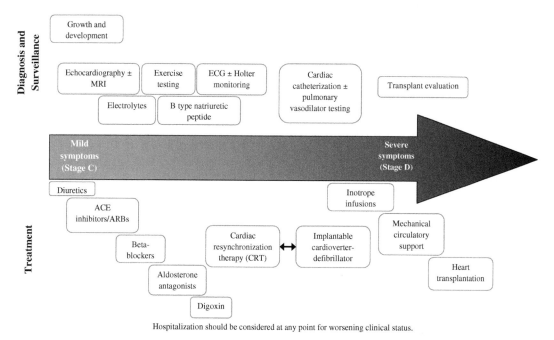

Hospitalization should be considered at any point for worsening clinical status.

Staging scheme is from the International Society of Heart and Lung Transplantation

Fig. 1. Outline of diagnostic and therapeutic strategies in pediatric HF.

pediatric-specific guidelines for the management of HF in children were published by the International Society for Heart and Lung Transplantation.[1] The authors' strategy for HF management in pediatric patients is presented in **Fig. 1**. It is hoped that ongoing prospective trials of HF medications in children will add to a small but growing body of evidence-based literature regarding optimal management of HF in children.

REFERENCES

1. Rosenthal D, Chrisant MR, Edens E, et al. International Society for Heart and Lung Transplantation: practice guidelines for management of heart failure in children. J Heart Lung Transplant 2004;23:1313–33.
2. Harmon WG, Sleeper LA, Cuniberti L, et al. Treating children with idiopathic dilated cardiomyopathy (from the Pediatric Cardiomyopathy Registry). Am J Cardiol 2009;104:281–6.
3. Wang J, Nagueh SF. Current perspectives on cardiac function in patients with diastolic heart failure. Circulation 2009;119:1146–57.
4. Lester SJ, Tajik AJ, Nishimura RA, et al. Unlocking the mysteries of diastolic function: deciphering the Rosetta Stone 10 years later. J Am Coll Cardiol 2008;51:679–89.
5. Jerosch-Herold M, Kwong RY. Magnetic resonance imaging in the assessment of ventricular remodeling and viability. Curr Heart Fail Rep 2008;5:5–10.
6. Assomull RG, Pennell DJ, Prasad SK. Cardiovascular magnetic resonance in the evaluation of heart failure. Heart 2007;93:985–92.
7. Karamitsos TD, Francis JM, Myerson S, et al. The role of cardiovascular magnetic resonance imaging in heart failure. J Am Coll Cardiol 2009; 54:1407–24.
8. Goldsmith SR. Treatment options for hyponatremia in heart failure. Heart Fail Rev 2009;14:65–73.
9. Groenveld HF, Januzzi JL, Damman K, et al. Anemia and mortality in heart failure patients: a systematic review and meta-analysis. J Am Coll Cardiol 2008;52:818–27.
10. Anand IS. Anemia and chronic heart failure: implications and treatment options. J Am Coll Cardiol 2008;52:501–11.
11. Hunt SA, Abraham WT, Chin MH, et al. ACC/AHA 2005 guideline update for the diagnosis and management of chronic heart failure in the adult. Circulation 2005;112:e154–235.
12. Heart Failure Society of America. Nonpharmacologic management and health care maintenance in patients with chronic heart failure. J Card Fail 2006;12:e29–37.
13. Maisel A, Mueller C, Adams K, et al. State of the art: using natriuretic peptide levels in clinical practice. Eur J Heart Fail 2008;10:824–39.
14. Koch A, Singer H. Normal values of B type natriuretic peptide in infants, children, and adolescents. Heart 2003;89:875–8.
15. Mir TS, Marohn S, Laer S, et al. Plasma concentrations of N-terminal pro-brain natriuretic peptide in control children from the neonatal to adolescent period and in children with congestive heart failure. Pediatrics 2002;110:e76.
16. Yoshibayashi M, Kamiya T, Saito Y, et al. Plasma brain natriuretic peptide concentrations in healthy children from birth to adolescence: marked and rapid increase after birth. Eur J Endocrinol 1995;133:207–9.
17. Ationu A, Carter ND. Brain and atrial natriuretic peptide plasma concentrations in normal healthy children. Br J Biomed Sci 1993;50:92–5.
18. Maher KO, Reed H, Cuadrado A, et al. B-type natriuretic peptide in the emergency diagnosis of critical heart disease in children. Pediatrics 2008; 121:e1484–8.
19. Tan LH, Jefferies JL, Liang JF, et al. Concentrations of brain natriuretic peptide in the plasma predicts outcomes of treatment of children with decompensated heart failure admitted to the intensive care unit. Cardiol Young 2007;17:397–406.
20. Price JF, Thomas AK, Grenier M, et al. B-type natriuretic peptide predicts adverse cardiovascular events in pediatric outpatients with chronic left ventricular systolic dysfunction. Circulation 2006; 114:1063–9.
21. Mavinkurve-Groothuis AM, Kapusta L, Nir A, et al. The role of biomarkers in the early detection of anthracycline-induced cardiotoxicity in children: a review of the literature. Pediatr Hematol Oncol 2008;25:655–64.
22. Kaski JP, Tome-Esteban MT, Mead-Regan S, et al. B-type natriuretic peptide predicts disease severity in children with hypertrophic cardiomyopathy. Heart 2008;94:1307–11.
23. Geiger M, Harake D, Halnon N, et al. Screening for rejection in symptomatic pediatric heart transplant recipients: the sensitivity of BNP. Pediatr Transplant 2008;12:563–9.
24. Bernus A, Wagner BD, Accurso F, et al. Brain natriuretic peptide levels in managing pediatric patients with pulmonary arterial hypertension. Chest 2009; 135:745–51.
25. Clark AM, Savard LA, Thompson DR. What is the strength of evidence for heart failure disease-management programs? J Am Coll Cardiol 2009; 54:397–401.
26. The CONSENSUS Trial Study Group. Effects of enalapril on mortality in severe congestive heart failure. Results of the Cooperative North Scandinavian Enalapril Survival Study (CONSENSUS). N Engl J Med 1987;316:1429–35.
27. The SOLVD Investigators. Effect of enalapril on survival in patients with reduced left ventricular

ejection fractions and congestive heart failure. N Engl J Med 1991;325:293–302.

28. Brown NJ, Vaughan DE. Angiotensin-converting enzyme inhibitors. Circulation 1998;97:1411–20.

29. Kawano H, Do YS, Kawano Y, et al. Angiotensin II has multiple profibrotic effects in human cardiac fibroblasts. Circulation 2000;101:1130–7.

30. Konstam M, Kronenberg M, Rousseau M, et al. Effects of the angiotensin converting enzyme inhibitor enalapril on the long-term progression of left ventricular dilatation in patients with asymptomatic systolic dysfunction. Circulation 1993;88:2277–83.

31. Gring CN, Francis GS. A hard look at angiotensin receptor blockers in heart failure. J Am Coll Cardiol 2004;44:1841–6.

32. McMurray JJ, Östergren J, Swedberg K, et al. Effects of candesartan in patients with chronic heart failure and reduced left-ventricular systolic function taking angiotensin-converting-enzyme inhibitors: the CHARM-added trial. Lancet 2003;362:767–71.

33. Lakhdar R, Al-Mallah MH, Lanfear DE. Safety and tolerability of angiotensin-converting enzyme inhibitor versus the combination of angiotensin-converting enzyme inhibitor and angiotensin receptor blocker in patients with left ventricular dysfunction: a systematic review and meta-analysis of randomized controlled trials. J Card Fail 2008;14:181–8.

34. Shaddy RE, Teitel DF, Brett C. Short-term hemodynamic effects of captopril in infants with congestive heart failure. Am J Dis Child 1988;142:100–5.

35. Bengur A, Beekman R, Rocchini A, et al. Acute hemodynamic effects of captopril in children with a congestive or restrictive cardiomyopathy. Circulation 1991;83:523–7.

36. Calabro R, Pisacane C, Pacileo G, et al. Hemodynamic effects of a single oral dose of enalapril among children with asymptomatic chronic mitral regurgitation. Am Heart J 1999;138:955–61.

37. Kouatli AA, Garcia JA, Zellers TM, et al. Enalapril does not enhance exercise capacity in patients after Fontan procedure. Circulation 1997;96:1507–12.

38. Duboc D, Meune C, Lerebours G, et al. Effect of perindopril on the onset and progression of left ventricular dysfunction in Duchenne muscular dystrophy. J Am Coll Cardiol 2005;45:855–7.

39. Duboc D, Meune C, Pierre B, et al. Perindopril preventive treatment on mortality in Duchenne muscular dystrophy: 10 years' follow-up. Am Heart J 2007;154:596–602.

40. Lipshultz SE, Alvarez JA, Scully RE. Anthracycline associated cardiotoxicity in survivors of childhood cancer. Heart 2008;94:525–33.

41. Lipshultz SE, Lipsitz SR, Sallan SE, et al. Long-term enalapril therapy for left ventricular dysfunction in doxorubicin-treated survivors of childhood cancer. J Clin Oncol 2002;20:4517–22.

42. Cardinale D, Colombo A, Sandri MT, et al. Prevention of high-dose chemotherapy-induced cardiotoxicity in high-risk patients by angiotensin-converting enzyme inhibition. Circulation 2006;114:2474–81.

43. Jessup M, Abraham WT, Casey DE, et al. 2009 focused update: ACCF/AHA guidelines for the diagnosis and management of heart failure in adults. Circulation 2009;119:1977–2016.

44. Jessup M, Brozena S. Heart failure. N Engl J Med 2003;348:2007–18.

45. Hjalmarson A, Goldstein S, Fagerberg B, et al. for the MERIT-HF Study Group. Effects of controlled-release metoprolol on total mortality, hospitalizations, and well-being in patients with heart failure: the metoprolol CR/XL randomized intervention trial in congestive heart failure (MERIT-HF). JAMA 2000; 283:1295–302.

46. The Cardiac Insufficiency Bisoprolol Study II (CIBIS-II): A randomised trial. Lancet 1999;353:9–13.

47. Packer M, Coats AJS, Fowler MB, et al. for the Carvedilol Prospective Randomized Cumulative Survival Study Group. Effect of carvedilol on survival in severe chronic heart failure. N Engl J Med 2001; 344:1651–8.

48. Bristow MR, Gilbert EM, Abraham WT, et al. Carvedilol produces dose-related improvements in left ventricular function and survival in subjects with chronic heart failure. Circulation 1996;94:2807–16.

49. Packer M, Bristow MR, Cohn JN, et al. The effect of carvedilol on morbidity and mortality in patients with chronic heart failure. N Engl J Med 1996; 334:1349–55.

50. Remme WJ, Poole-Wilson P, Swedberg K, et al. Comparison of carvedilol and metoprolol on clinical outcomes in patients with chronic heart failure in the Carvedilol or Metoprolol European Trial (COMET): randomised controlled trial. Lancet 2003;362:7.

51. Shaddy RE, Tani LY, Gidding SS, et al. Beta-blocker treatment of dilated cardiomyopathy with congestive heart failure in children: a multi-institutional experience. J Heart Lung Transplant 1999;18: 269–74.

52. Bruns LA, Chrisant MK, Lamour JM, et al. Carvedilol as therapy in pediatric heart failure: an initial multi-center experience. J Pediatr 2001;138:505–11.

53. Williams RV, Tani LY, Shaddy RE. Intermediate effects of treatment with metoprolol or carvedilol in children with left ventricular systolic dysfunction. J Heart Lung Transplant 2002;21:906–9.

54. Azeka E, Franchini Ramires JA, Valler C, et al. Delisting of infants and children from the heart transplantation waiting list after carvedilol treatment. J Am Coll Cardiol 2002;40:2034–8.

55. Rusconi P, Gomez-Marin O, Rossique-Gonzalez M, et al. Carvedilol in children with cardiomyopathy: 3-year experience at a single institution. J Heart Lung Transplant 2004;23:832–8.

56. Blume ED, Canter CE, Spicer R, et al. Prospective single-arm protocol of carvedilol in children with ventricular dysfunction. Pediatr Cardiol 2006;27: 336–42.

57. Shaddy RE, Boucek MM, Hsu DT, et al. Carvedilol for children and adolescents with heart failure: a randomized controlled trial. JAMA 2007;298: 1171–9.

58. Foerster SR, Canter CE. Pediatric heart failure therapy with beta-adrenoceptor antagonists. Paediatr Drugs 2008;10:125–34.

59. Kalay N, Basar E, Ozdogru I, et al. Protective effects of carvedilol against anthracycline-induced cardiomyopathy. J Am Coll Cardiol 2006; 48:2258–62.

60. Rhodes J, Margossian R, Darras BT, et al. Safety and efficacy of carvedilol therapy for patients with dilated cardiomyopathy secondary to muscular dystrophy. Pediatr Cardiol 2008;29:343–51.

61. Kajimoto H, Ishigaki K, Okumura K, et al. Beta-blocker therapy for cardiac dysfunction in patients with muscular dystrophy. Circ J 2006;70:991–4.

62. The Digitalis Investigation Group. The effect of digoxin on mortality and morbidity in patients with heart failure. N Engl J Med 1997;336:525–33.

63. Kimball TR, Daniels SR, Meyer RA, et al. Effect of digoxin on contractility and symptoms in infants with a large ventricular septal defect. Am J Cardiol 1991;68:1377–82.

64. Greenberg B, Zannad F, Pitt B. Role of aldosterone blockade for treatment of heart failure and post-acute myocardial infarction. Am J Cardiol 2006; 97:34F–40F.

65. Eapen Z, Rogers JG. Strategies to attenuate pathological remodeling in heart failure. Curr Opin Cardiol 2009;24:223–9.

66. Davis KL, Nappi JM. The cardiovascular effects of eplerenone, a selective aldosterone-receptor antagonist. Clin Ther 2003;25:2647–68.

67. Pitt B, Zannad F, Remme WJ, et al. The effect of spironolactone on morbidity and mortality in patients with severe heart failure. N Engl J Med 1999;341:709–17.

68. Bozkurt B, Agoston I, Knowlton AA. Complications of inappropriate use of spironolactone in heart failure: when an old medicine spirals out of new guidelines. J Am Coll Cardiol 2003;41:211–4.

69. Pitt B, Remme W, Zannad F, et al. Eplerenone, a selective aldosterone blocker, in patients with left ventricular dysfunction after myocardial infarction. N Engl J Med 2003;348:1309–21.

70. Mahle WT, Wang A, Quyyumi AA, et al. Impact of spironolactone on endothelial function in patients with single ventricle heart. Congenit Heart Dis 2009;4:12–6.

71. Pitt B. RAAS inhibition/blockade in patients with cardiovascular disease: implications of recent large-scale randomised trials for clinical practice. Heart 2009;95:1205–8.

72. Hauptman PJ, Mikolajczak P, George A, et al. Chronic inotropic therapy in end-stage heart failure. Am Heart J 2006;152:e1–8.

73. Young JB, Moen EK. Outpatient parenteral inotropic therapy for advanced heart failure. J Heart Lung Transplant 2000;19:S49–57.

74. Cesario D, Clark J, Maisel A. Beneficial effects of intermittent home administration of the inotrope/vasodilator milrinone in patients with end-stage congestive heart failure: a preliminary study. Am Heart J 1998;135:121–9.

75. Berg AM, Snell L, Mahle WT. Home inotropic therapy in children. J Heart Lung Transplant 2007;26:453–7.

76. Cripe LH, Barber BJ, Spicer RL, et al. Outpatient continuous inotrope infusion as an adjunct to heart failure therapy in Duchenne muscular dystrophy. Neuromuscul Disord 2006;16:745–8.

77. Abraham WT. Cardiac resynchronization therapy. Prog Cardiovasc Dis 2006;48:232–8.

78. The Cardiac Arrhythmia Suppression Trial (CAST) Investigators. Preliminary report: effect of encainide and flecainide on mortality in a randomized trial of arrhythmia suppression after myocardial infarction. N Engl J Med 1989;321:406–12.

79. Echt DS, Liebson PR, Mitchell LB, et al. Mortality and morbidity in patients receiving encainide, flecainide, or placebo. N Engl J Med 1991;324:781–8.

80. The Cardiac Arrhythmia Suppression Trial II Investigators. Effect of the antiarrhythmic agent moricizine on survival after myocardial infarction. N Engl J Med 1992;327:227–33.

81. Singh SN, Fletcher RD, Fisher SG, et al. Amiodarone in patients with congestive heart failure and asymptomatic ventricular arrhythmia. N Engl J Med 1995;333:77–82.

82. Amiodarone Trials Meta-Analysis Investigators. Effect of prophylactic amiodarone on mortality after acute myocardial infarction and in congestive heart failure: meta-analysis of individual data from 6500 patients in randomised trials. Lancet 1997;350: 1417–24.

83. Piepoli M, Villani GQ, Ponikowski P, et al. Overview and meta-analysis of randomised trials of amiodarone in chronic heart failure. Int J Cardiol 1998;66:1–10.

84. Bardy GH, Lee KL, Mark DB, et al. Amiodarone or an implantable cardioverter-defibrillator for congestive heart failure. N Engl J Med 2005;352:225–37.

85. The Antiarrhythmics versus Implantable Defibrillators (AVID) Investigators. A comparison of antiarrhythmic-drug therapy with implantable defibrillators in patients resuscitated from near-fatal ventricular arrhythmias. N Engl J Med 1997;337: 1576–84.

86. Connolly SJ, Gent M, Roberts RS, et al. Canadian Implantable Defibrillator study (CIDS): a randomized trial of the implantable cardioverter defibrillator against amiodarone. Circulation 2000;101: 1297–302.

87. Kuck K, Cappato R, Siebels J, et al. Randomized comparison of antiarrhythmic drug therapy with implantable defibrillators in patients resuscitated from cardiac arrest. Circulation 2000;102: 748–54.

88. Moss AJ, Hall WJ, Cannom DS, et al. Improved survival with an implanted defibrillator in patients with coronary disease at high risk for ventricular arrhythmia. N Engl J Med 1996;335:1933–40.

89. Moss AJ, Zareba W, Hall WJ, et al. Prophylactic implantation of a defibrillator in patients with myocardial infarction and reduced ejection fraction. N Engl J Med 2002;346:877–83.

90. Buxton AE, Lee KL, Fisher JD, et al. A randomized study of the prevention of sudden death in patients with coronary artery disease. N Engl J Med 1999; 341:1882–90.

91. Myerburg RJ. Implantable cardioverter-defibrillators after myocardial infarction. N Engl J Med 2008; 359:2245–53.

92. Epstein AE. Benefits of the implantable cardioverter-defibrillator. J Am Coll Cardiol 2008;52:1122–7.

93. Tung R, Zimetbaum P, Josephson ME. A critical appraisal of implantable cardioverter-defibrillator therapy for the prevention of sudden cardiac death. J Am Coll Cardiol 2008;52:1111–21.

94. Epstein AE, DiMarco JP, Ellenbogen KA, et al. ACC/AHA/HRS 2008 guidelines for device-based therapy of cardiac rhythm abnormalities. J Am Coll Cardiol 2008;51:e1–62.

95. Berul CI. Defibrillator indications and implantation in young children. Heart Rhythm 2008;5:1755–7.

96. Berul CI, Van Hare GF, Kertesz NJ, et al. Results of a multicenter retrospective implantable cardioverter-defibrillator registry of pediatric and congenital heart disease patients. J Am Coll Cardiol 2008;51: 1685–91.

97. Stephenson EA, Batra AS, Knilans TK, et al. A multicenter experience with novel implantable cardioverter defibrillator configurations in the pediatric and congenital heart disease population. J Cardiovasc Electrophysiol 2006;17:41–6.

98. Hsia TY, Bradley SM, LaPage MJ, et al. Novel minimally invasive, intrapericardial implantable cardioverter defibrillator coil system: a useful approach to arrhythmia therapy in children. Ann Thorac Surg 2009;87:1234–8.

99. Bristow MR, Saxon LA, Boehmer J, et al. Cardiac-resynchronization therapy with or without an implantable defibrillator in advanced chronic heart failure. N Engl J Med 2004;350:2140–50.

100. Cleland JGF, Daubert J, Erdmann E, et al. The effect of cardiac resynchronization on morbidity and mortality in heart failure. N Engl J Med 2005; 352:1539–49.

101. Jarcho JA. Biventricular pacing. N Engl J Med 2006;355:288–94.

102. Linde C, Abraham WT, Gold MR, et al. Randomized trial of cardiac resynchronization in mildly symptomatic heart failure patients and in asymptomatic patients with left ventricular dysfunction and previous heart failure symptoms. J Am Coll Cardiol 2008;52:1834–43.

103. Moss AJ, Hall WJ, Cannom DS, et al. Cardiac-resynchronization therapy for the prevention of heart-failure events. N Engl J Med 2009;361: 1329–38.

104. Nagueh SF. Mechanical dyssynchrony in congestive heart failure: diagnostic and therapeutic implications. J Am Coll Cardiol 2008;51:18–22.

105. Chung ES, Leon AR, Tavazzi L, et al. Results of the predictors of response to CRT (PROSPECT) trial. Circulation 2008;117:2608–16.

106. Dubin AM, Janousek J, Rhee E, et al. Resynchronization therapy in pediatric and congenital heart disease patients. J Am Coll Cardiol 2005;46: 2277–83.

107. Cecchin F, Frangini PA, Brown DW, et al. Cardiac resynchronization therapy (and multisite pacing) in pediatrics and congenital heart disease: five years experience in a single institution. J Cardiovasc Electrophysiol 2009;20:58–65.

108. Janousek J, Vojtovic P, Hucin B, et al. Resynchronization pacing is a useful adjunct to the management of acute heart failure after surgery for congenital heart defects. Am J Cardiol 2001;88:145–52.

109. Zimmerman FJ, Starr JP, Koenig PR, et al. Acute hemodynamic benefit of multisite ventricular pacing after congenital heart surgery. Ann Thorac Surg 2003;75:1775–80.

110. Janousek J, Gebauer RA, Abdul-Khaliq H, et al. Cardiac resynchronisation therapy in paediatric and congenital heart disease: differential effects in various anatomical and functional substrates. Heart 2009;95:1165–71.

111. Friedberg MK, Roche SL, Balasingam M, et al. Evaluation of mechanical dyssynchrony in children with idiopathic dilated cardiomyopathy and associated clinical outcomes. Am J Cardiol 2008;101: 1191–5.

112. Canter CE, Shaddy RE, Bernstein D, et al. Indications for heart transplantation in pediatric heart disease. Circulation 2007;115:658–76.

Heart Failure Treatment in the Intensive Care Unit in Children

John Lynn Jefferies, MD, MPH[a], Timothy M. Hoffman, MD[b], David P. Nelson, MD, PhD[a],*

KEYWORDS

• Heart failure • Children • Intensive care unit

In recent years, there has been a paradigm shift in our understanding of heart failure. Although heart failure was previously described as a condition in which the heart was unable to maintain an adequate cardiac output to meet the metabolic demands of the body, the definition of heart failure has been expanded to incorporate molecular and neurohormonal changes integral to the condition. Arnold Katz defined heart failure as a "clinical syndrome in which heart disease reduces cardiac output, increases venous pressures, and is accompanied by molecular abnormalities that cause progressive deterioration of the failing heart and premature myocardial cell death."[1] Stated otherwise, heart failure is a constellation of signs or symptoms, structural and functional abnormalities, increased filling pressures, and neurohormonal activation.

Although pediatric heart failure is generally a chronic, progressive disorder,[2] recovery of ventricular function may occur with some forms of cardiomyopathy. For example, left ventricular (LV) noncompaction can have an undulating phenotype with periods of improvement and/or deterioration in function.[3] Another exception is acute myocarditis, especially the fulminant form, in which patients can have complete recovery of function. Guidelines for the management of chronic heart failure in adults and children have recently been published by the International Society of Heart and Lung Transplant, the American College of Cardiology, and the American Heart Association.[4–6] The primary aim of heart failure therapy is to reduce symptoms, preserve long-term ventricular performance, and prolong survival primarily through antagonism of the neurohormonal compensatory mechanisms. Because some medications may be detrimental during an acute decompensation, physicians who manage these patients as inpatients must be knowledgeable of the medications and therapeutic goals of chronic heart failure treatment. Furthermore, understanding the mechanisms of chronic heart failure may foster improved understanding of the treatment of decompensated heart failure.

CAUSE OF HEART FAILURE IN INFANTS AND CHILDREN

Pediatric heart failure can manifest in both congenital and acquired forms with causes as disparate as structural, metabolic, and environmental in origin. In children with structural heart disease, heart failure can result from excessive pulmonary blood flow, valvar insufficiency, or

a Division of Cardiology, The Heart Institute at Cincinnati Children's Hospital Medical Center, 3333 Burnet Avenue, Cincinnati, OH 45244, USA
b Division of Pediatric Cardiology, Nationwide Children's Hospital, 700 Childrens Drive, Columbus, OH 43205, USA
* Corresponding author. Division of Cardiology, The Heart Institute at Cincinnati Children's Hospital Medical Center, 3333 Burnet Avenue, Cincinnati, OH 45244.
E-mail address: david.nelson@cchmc.org

Heart Failure Clin 6 (2010) 531–558
doi:10.1016/j.hfc.2010.06.001

obstruction of ventricular inflow or outflow. The most common cause of heart failure in infants with congenital heart disease is a large left-to-right shunt with excessive pulmonary blood flow. Symptomatic pulmonary overcirculation differs markedly from the classic forms of congestive heart failure described in adults. The respiratory distress and feeding difficulties associated with a large ventricular septal defect, truncus arteriosus, or single ventricle heart results from excessive pulmonary blood flow and volume overload of the heart. Although ventricular systolic function is normally preserved, pulmonary overcirculation still leads to increased filling pressures, compensatory activation of the neurohormonal system, and progressive symptoms, and thus deserves to be recognized within the spectrum of heart failure.

Pediatric heart failure can also be caused by a primary heart muscle disorder or cardiomyopathy. Primary cardiomyopathies are predominantly genetic disorders intrinsic to the myocardium that result from abnormalities of structural or regulatory proteins of the myocardium. Secondary cardiomyopathies can result from extrinsic myocyte injury from various insults, such as ischemia, infectious agents, environmental or toxin exposures, autoimmune reactions, arrhythmias, nutritional deficiencies, or abnormal autonomic responses. Metabolic disorders that affect substrate use or energy production within the myocardium can also lead to a cardiomyopathy. Myocarditis is the most common cause of secondary ventricular dysfunction in both children and adults. Another common secondary cause of pediatric cardiomyopathy is the treatment of cancer with anthracycline-derived chemotherapeutic agents and/or radiation.

The most common clinical heart failure scenario in the pediatric intensive care setting is the postoperative surgical patient with low cardiac output syndrome (LCOS).[7] Despite significant advances in myocardial protection and surgical techniques, approximately 25% of patients still exhibit low cardiac output and impaired systemic oxygen delivery in the early postoperative period after congenital heart surgery.[8] The transient and predictable decrease in cardiac output after cardiac surgery is due primarily to transient myocardial dysfunction, compounded by acute changes in myocardial loading conditions, including increased systemic and/or pulmonary vascular resistance (PVR). Residual cardiac abnormalities will further aggravate the underlying low output state. Surgical repair of cardiac malformations exposes the myocardium to periods of ischemia, resulting in transient myocardial stunning or damage. Cardiopulmonary bypass (CPB), which activates the complement and inflammatory cascades,[9] can contribute to myocardial injury and alterations in pulmonary and systemic vascular reactivity.[10] Although advances in myocardial protection, cardioplegia, and perfusion techniques have dramatically reduced perioperative cardiovascular injury, even relatively simple cardiac procedures are still associated with measurable myocardial dysfunction.[11]

MOLECULAR AND CELLULAR MECHANISMS OF MYOCARDIAL DYSFUNCTION

Heart failure in pediatric patients is a summation of a complex interaction between various modifiable and nonmodifiable factors, including genetic alterations, the neurohormonal axis, biochemical changes, damage to the myocardium, and inflammation. Heart failure alters the structure and function of the myocardium at molecular and cellular levels. Calcium dysregulation is central to this pathophysiologic process, resulting in maladaptive changes in the contractile apparatus as heart failure progresses.[12] In the normal heart, cellular depolarization leads to voltage-gated Ca^{2+} influx into the myocyte, which, in turn, triggers release of Ca^{2+} stores from the sarcoplasmic reticulum (SR) via a receptor-mediated Ca^{2+} channel known as ryanodine (RyR).[13] The pulse of free cytosolic Ca^{2+} interacts with sarcomeric components to activate the excitation-contraction process. Myocyte relaxation results from closure of RyR channels and rapid removal of cytosolic calcium by reuptake into the SR via the SR Ca^{2+}/adenosine triphosphatase (ATPase) pump (SERCA). The sarcolemmal Na^+/Ca^{2+} exchanger (NCX) and sarcolemmal calcium ATPase pump also contribute to Ca^{2+} efflux from the cytoplasm. These processes are meticulously balanced to ensure no net gain or loss of cellular calcium with each contraction-relaxation cycle.

This complex interplay of ion pumps, exchangers, and modulators often becomes dysregulated in patients with heart failure. The result is a reduction in SR Ca^{2+} stores, which decreases the amplitude and duration of cytosolic Ca^{2+} release, thus reducing contractile force production. One likely mechanism for depletion of SR Ca^{2+} stores in heart failure is decreased SERCA activity.[12] Decreased SERCA expression has been shown in patients with heart failure and in animal models of heart failure. Restoration of SERCA expression in animal models of heart failure improves ventricular function.[14] Other mechanisms implicated in the depletion of SR calcium in heart failure include increased NCX activity and altered function of RyR channels. Increased NCX activity enhances efflux of Ca^{2+} from the cytosol, which decreases SR Ca^{2+} uptake. Enhanced phosphorylation of RyR channels modifies channel-gating properties and induces diastolic leak of Ca^{2+}. This not only blunts Ca^{2+} mediated Ca^{2+} release during systole but also can trigger after-depolarizations and ventricular arrhythmias.[15] NCX overexpression and alterations in RyR channels have been shown in animal models of heart failure.[16] The confluence of these and other molecular maladaptations form the cellular basis for cardiac dysfunction in heart failure.

Because the structural integrity of the myocardium is integral to ventricular contractile performance, alterations in both sarcomeric and cytoskeletal proteins can cause cardiomyopathy and cardiac dysfunction.[17] Mutations in various sarcomeric and cytoskeletal proteins have been implicated in both dilated and hypertrophic phenotypes. The cytoskeletal protein, dystrophin, responsible for the muscular dystrophies and X-linked cardiomyopathy, was the first cytoskeletal gene identified to cause dilated cardiomyopathy.[18] Related cytoskeletal proteins that interact with dystrophin have subsequently been shown to also cause dilated phenotypes.[19] Acquired defects in cytoskeletal and sarcomeric proteins have also been shown to cause cardiac dysfunction. For example, protease cleavage of troponin I results in systolic dysfunction.[20,21] Similarly, protease cleavage of dystrophin has been detected in the hearts of patients with myocarditis and other forms of end-stage cardiomyopathy.[22] Mechanical unloading of the heart with a ventricular assist device (VAD) can reverse these changes in dystrophin.[23]

Ventricular hypertrophy is an integral response to stimuli such as hemodynamic overload, mechanical stress, and disruption of myocyte structure and function, all of which are common in chronic heart failure. Although myocardial remodeling is an adaptive response that is initially beneficial to cardiac function, it can result in the progression of heart failure and has been linked to the pathogenesis of cardiac arrhythmias and sudden death. A major stimulus for ventricular hypertrophy and myocardial remodeling is mechanical stress secondary to hemodynamic overload. Exposure of cardiac myocytes to mechanical stress results in activation of numerous molecular signaling cascades, including reactivation of fetal gene programs, which induce cellular growth, protein synthesis, and hypertrophic changes.[24] Because calcium signaling is central to the function of cardiomyocytes, it is not surprising that calcineurin, an intracellular Ca^{2+}-calmodulin activated phosphatase, has

been implicated in mechanisms of cardiac hypertrophy associated with heart failure.[25] Hemodynamic overload and neurohormonal activation lead to an acute increase in sarcoplasmic free Ca^{2+}, which results in the activation of calcineurin. Neurohumoral factors are also known to play key roles in the induction of cardiac hypertrophy. The renin-angiotensin and endothelin systems are both known to contribute to maladaptive ventricular remodeling.[26,27] Evidence suggests that numerous growth factors also play a role in the development of cardiac hypertrophy in the presence of heart failure. The most prominent of these is transforming growth factor B, but other growth factors such as fibroblast growth factor, insulinlike growth factor, and epidermal growth factor have also been implicated.[24]

NEUROHORMONAL ALTERATIONS IN CHILDREN WITH HEART FAILURE

Heart failure results in a baroreceptor-mediated increase in sympathetic tone, which leads to increased levels of circulating catecholamines, such as epinephrine and norepinephrine. The high catechol-state mediates various pathophysiologic responses, including tachycardia, increased cardiac contractility, and arterial and venous vasoconstriction. In the acute setting, increased catechol levels mediate the expected tachycardia and enhanced contractility, but over time, chronic cardiac stimulation leads to a relative catechol depletion phenomenon and downregulation of adrenergic receptors. This illustrates one of the ways that the chronic cardiac stimulation that accompanies heart failure results in maladaptive changes.

The renin-angiotensin-aldosterone system (RAAS), which acts in concert with the sympathetic nervous system, is also highly activated in heart failure.[28] Patients with progressive heart failure show marked increases in circulating renin, aldosterone, and angiotensin II, which increases ventricular afterload, and leads to salt and water retention, which is clearly counterproductive in the setting of heart failure.[29] In addition to these maladaptive physiologic effects, norepinephrine, angiotensin II, and aldosterone have also all been found to have direct toxicity on cardiomyocytes, likely resulting from calcium overload.[30,31] Clinical studies have corroborated these findings by showing an association between increased levels of these neurohormonal markers and poor prognosis.[32,33]

Natriuretic peptides are counterregulatory hormones that mediate beneficial effects such as vasodilation and natriuresis.[34,35] The discovery that infusion of atrial tissue extracts resulted in natriuresis in rats was first observed in 1982. Since then, 3 distinct, major natriuretic peptides have been isolated and synthesized (atrial natriuretic peptide, B-type natriuretic peptide [BNP], and C-type natriuretic peptide). Although genotypically different, all 3 have functionally been found to have potent natriuretic, diuretic, and vasorelaxant properties via their action on guanylyl cyclase linked membrane receptors.[34,35] Myocardial stretch and chamber pressure seem to be the principal mechanisms by which the natriuretic peptides are activated.

BNP is synthesized predominantly in the cardiac ventricles, and is released in response to certain pathophysiologic states such as heart failure. BNP has physiologic counterregulatory effects, which lead to systemic vasodilation and natriuresis. It suppresses RAAS and reduces the overall extracellular fluid volume.[36] It also counters sympathetic vascular tone, which leads to vasorelaxation and a blunted tachycardia response. BNP infusions in humans have been shown to promote natriuresis and inhibit RAAS in a manner independent of blood pressure changes.[36–38]

INFLAMMATION IN CHILDREN WITH HEART FAILURE

Inflammation has increasingly been recognized as critical to the development and progression of myocardial dysfunction and chronic heart failure. The initial assessment of this in adult populations was measurement of C-reactive protein (CRP).[39] CRP is an acute-phase reactant released by hepatocytes secondary to circulating interleukin 6 (IL-6).[40] Because traditional CRP assessment lacks the sensitivity to detect small variations in CRP levels in chronic subclinical inflammatory states such as heart failure, the high-sensitivity test (hsCRP) was developed as a tool for assessment and prevention of cardiovascular disease hsCRP testing has subsequently become widespread in adults.[41] In adult populations, increased CRP levels predict adverse outcome and need for readmission in acute and chronic heart failure.[42,43] There are also data implicating high CRP levels with vascular disease secondary to a reduction in production of nitric oxide (NO) release.[44] Although there are no significant data on the use of CRP in pediatric patients with heart failure, investigations are ongoing. Skrak and colleagues[45] have reported increased levels of CRP in children after CPB. However, the clinical usefulness of this information remains to be clarified.

Other inflammatory biomarkers have been identified, such as tumor necrosis factor α (TNF-α) and

members of the interleukin (IL) family, specifically IL-1, Il-6, and IL-18. TNF-α is the most widely studied of these proinflammatory cytokines, which are produced by nucleated cells in the heart.[46] Evidence suggests that these cytokines can directly depress ventricular function and mediate other detrimental effects, which supports the cytokine hypothesis, which proposes that a significant stress to the heart, such as myocarditis or ischemia, triggers an innate immune response.[47] Cytokines and their receptors are independent predictors of morbidity and mortality in adults with advanced heart failure.[48] In addition to the acute functional effects on the heart, it is becoming increasingly clear that inflammatory mediators play an important role in the process of ventricular remodeling. Cytokines have been implicated in the development of myocyte hypertrophy, activation of matrix metalloproteinases, and even myocyte apoptosis and necrosis.[24] Although it has been postulated that cytokine blockade may have a favorable effect on myocardial function and outcomes, adult studies evaluating TNF-α blockade did not observe a clinical benefit for patients with heart failure.[49,50] The pediatric assessment of these cytokines remains limited. Ratnasamy and colleagues[51] measured hsCRP, TNF-α, and soluble TNF-α receptors in 15 children and adolescents with dilated cardiomyopathy and 4 with congenital heart disease and systolic dysfunction. Levels of hsCRP and TNF-α were negatively associated with systolic function, and TNF-α was positively associated with LV dilation. Increased hsCRP also correlated with patient heart failure symptoms. There is growing interest in using markers of inflammation for pediatric patients with heart failure.

Fas (also known as APO-1) is another cytokine that is expressed on myocytes that augment the progression of heart failure. These cytokines activated by Fas ligand mediate apoptosis and the progression of heart failure. Fas is a member of the TNF-α receptor family and increased levels of the soluble form are seen in patients with heart failure. Furthermore, higher levels are associated with more severe disease. Efforts are ongoing to assess if modulation of Fas via intravenous immunoglobulin or pentoxyfilline may improve LV function.[52,53]

Another mediator thought to play a role in the inflammatory cascade of heart failure is NO.[46] NO mediates multiple signaling pathways in the heart, both beneficial and detrimental, depending on the setting. Beneficial effects of NO include improved relaxation, increased preload reserve, and decreased afterload, whereas detrimental effects include myocardial depression and β-adrenergic desensitization. Enhanced NO synthase (NOS) activity and increased systemic NO production have been detected in dilated cardiomyopathy and chronic heart failure.[54,55] Although there is speculation that NO may act directly as a negative inotrope, its exact role in the progression of heart failure, and its precise mechanism of action, have not been clearly elucidated.

Inflammation continues to be a central theme in all types of cardiovascular diseases, including coronary artery disease, peripheral vascular disease, and heart failure. Numerous adult studies and limited pediatric reports have documented increased levels of inflammatory cytokines in failing hearts, and it is well established that these cytokines have detrimental physiologic effects. The remaining clinical questions revolve around modulation of these markers. Treatment strategies directed at modulating the effects of the cytokines have been unsuccessful. Numerous ongoing adult studies are under way assessing different treatment strategies. Because of their pleiotropic effects, including antiinflammation and RAAS inhibition, statins have been widely touted as a potential therapy in heart failure.[56] Recent multicenter studies evaluating statin efficacy in patients with nonischemic heart failure have been disappointing.[57] There is undoubtedly a complex interplay between molecular mechanisms, hypertrophic changes, neurohormonal activation, and inflammatory mediators in heart failure. Although adaptive at its core, the outcome of these complex responses is maladaptive overall. With a better understanding of the underlying mechanisms, we may be able to identify new preventative and therapeutic modalities, which, in the future, may become invaluable in the treatment of children with heart failure.

INVOLVEMENT OF OTHER ORGAN SYSTEMS IN HEART FAILURE
Cardiorenal Syndrome

Many patients admitted with heart failure also have impaired kidney function. Complex interplay exists between the heart and kidneys, but a clear definition of these physiologic interactions has been lacking until recently. The cardiorenal syndrome (CRS) is pathophysiologic condition in which acute or chronic dysfunction of either the heart or the kidneys may cause acute or chronic dysfunction of the entire system. Ronco and colleagues[58] have proposed classification of CRS into 5 different subtypes. CRS type 1 (acute CRS) is a rapid worsening of cardiac function leading to acute kidney injury (AKI). Given the vast number of patients who present with acute heart failure

yearly, CRS type 1 is a common finding. Multiple mechanisms can cause renal injury, such as decreased kidney perfusion, immune-mediated damage, and activation of the sympathetic nervous system and/or RAAS.[59,60] CRS type 2 (chronic CRS) represents chronic cardiac dysfunction that leads to progressive chronic kidney disease (CKD). The mechanism of kidney injury seems to be different from that seen in acute heart failure and may be secondary to venous congestion.[61] CRS type 3 is characterized by an acute worsening of kidney function such as AKI that leads to acute cardiac dysfunction. The frequency of CRS type 3 is increasing in patients in hospital and in the intensive care unit (ICU) in part as a result of increasing vigilance for renal AKI. Children admitted to both ICU and non-ICU settings are susceptible to AKI and the associated decrease in cardiac function.[62] Cardiac effects are multifactorial but may be secondary to volume overload, systemic hypertension, electrolyte derangements, acid/base disturbances, and neurohormonal activation. CRS type 4 (chronic renocardiac syndrome) is characterized by a condition of primary CKD that leads to a cardiac condition or increased risk of adverse cardiac events. Cardiac involvement may include ventricular dysfunction, hypertrophy, or arrhythmias. More than 50% of deaths in patients with CKD are attributable to cardiovascular disease.[63] CRS type 5 (secondary CRS) is the presence of combined cardiac and renal dysfunction secondary to an acute or chronic systemic disorder. A pediatric patient with sepsis would fall into this category because the primary condition impairs both cardiac and renal function via inflammation, neurohormonal changes, hypoxia, and toxemia.

Renal impairment in adult patients with heart failure is an independent risk factor for morbidity and mortality.[29,64,65] Hillege and colleagues[64] reported renal function as a strong predictor of outcome in patients with heart failure with either systolic or diastolic dysfunction. Data in pediatric patients are growing. Dent and colleagues[66] documented the usefulness of neutrophil gelatinase-associated protein as an early predictive marker of AKI, morbidity, and mortality in 120 children undergoing CPB. Price and colleagues[67] recently investigated the incidence of renal injury in pediatric patients with heart failure, and found that worsening renal function during hospitalization, defined as an increase in serum creatinine of 0.3 mg/dL or greater, was independently associated with a combined end-point of in-hospital death or need for mechanical circulatory support.

The scope of CRS in pediatrics remains to be defined. Part of the limitation to diagnosing renal injury has been the use of creatinine as a marker of renal dysfunction. Increases in creatinine are delayed and lack sensitivity as a marker of AKI.[68] Newer diagnostic modalities are being used to detect AKI earlier and more reliably.[68,69] Studies are ongoing to assess the utility of these novel biomarkers as prognostic tools in pediatric heart failure.

HEPATIC DERANGEMENTS IN HEART FAILURE

Hepatic dysfunction is common with heart failure and correlates with poor outcomes.[70] The prevalence may be as high as 65%. Liver dysfunction results from impaired cardiac output and increased central venous pressure (CVP), and worsens with worsening heart failure, especially when CVP is greater than 10 mm Hg and cardiac index (CI) is less than 1.5 L/min/m^2.[71,72] van Deursen and colleagues[73] evaluated liver function abnormalities and hemodynamic profiles in 323 patients with heart failure, and reported that liver dysfunction correlates with CVP, whereas total bilirubin, alanine aminotransferase, and aspartate aminotransferase (AST) were related to both increased CVP and decreased CI. In addition, univariate analysis showed that AST and lactate dehydrogenase levels were predictors of all-cause mortality.

Acute and chronic heart failure can lead to other hepatic complications. In the setting of low cardiac output, ischemic hepatitis may occur.[74] As much as a third of the total cardiac output is directed to the mesenteric circulation during a normal hemodynamic state. However, during times of cardiogenic shock, selective mesenteric vasoconstriction can result in mesenteric ischemia.[75] Furthermore, mesenteric vessels exhibit a disproportionate vasoconstrictive response to RAAS activation.[76] This situation can lead to hepatocellular necrosis, characterized by increased hepatic transaminases.[77] By contrast, the chronic hepatopathy and resultant cirrhosis associated with long-standing heart failure is characterized by an increase in cholestatic markers with only minimal or no changes in transaminases. In addition, patients with chronic heart failure and cirrhosis may have impaired albumin synthesis and hypoalbuminemia. This situation can exacerbate fluid accumulation and worsen heart failure symptoms. Other parameters of hepatic synthetic function may be altered in the setting of acute and chronic heart failure, leading to coagulation disturbances that may require targeted intervention, depending on the clinical status of the patient. Primary cirrhotic patients may have associated ventricular dysfunction as well as electrophysiological abnormalities, specifically prolonged QT intervals. This condition is termed cirrhotic cardiomyopathy and is typically managed medically or with liver transplantation.[78]

Hematologic Abnormalities in Heart Failure

Hematologic derangements are frequently seen in heart failure. Increased white blood cell and platelet counts are common in acute decompensated heart failure (ADHF), and thought to be secondary to the inflammatory changes described earlier. Perhaps the most important hematologic abnormality is anemia. Anemia is a frequent finding in adults with chronic heart failure, with a prevalence as high as 60%.[79] Anemia is not isolated to patients with systolic dysfunction, but is also seen frequently in patients with abnormal diastolic function and preserved systolic function.[80] Although anemia is an independent predictor of death and hospitalization of adults with acute or chronic heart failure, data in pediatric heart failure are lacking.[81]

Although mechanisms of anemia in patients with heart failure remain poorly defined, factors thought to contribute include: (1) iron deficiency, (2) renal impairment, (3) chronic disease/inflammation, (4) neurohormonal activation, and (5) hemodilution.[82] Iron deficiency is common in heart failure, presumably because of reduced uptake of iron, vitamin B$_{12}$, and folic acid.[83] Nutrition is often poor in patients with chronic heart failure because of decreased appetite, malabsorption as a result of hypoperfusion, and increased TNF-α and other cytokines that cause cachexia. Patients with heart failure may also be on antiplatelet or anticoagulation therapy, which can lead to intestinal blood loss. The diagnosis of iron-deficiency anemia can be challenging because traditional markers, such as ferritin, may not be increased.[84] As noted earlier, renal insufficiency is common in patients with heart failure. Decreases in glomerular filtration rate less than 60 mL/min result in diminished production of erythropoeitin and a resultant decrease in hemoglobin.[85] The chronic disease state of heart failure with persistent inflammation and neurohormonal activation may also contribute to anemia. Upregulation of TNF-α and other cytokines decreases bioavailability of iron stores and suppresses activity of erythropoietin in the bone marrow.[86] In addition, experimental models of heart failure have documented a decrease in the number and activity of marrow progenitor cells.

Neurologic Abnormalities in Heart Failure

Patients with heart failure frequently exhibit neurologic abnormalities such as altered states of alertness, cognitive impairment, and behavioral abnormalities. Neurologic findings may include hypotonia, asterixis, and diffuse slowing on electroencephalogram. Although limited data exist on neurologic findings in heart failure, impairment in memory and visual tactile perception have been observed in patients with end-stage heart failure undergoing cardiac transplant evaluation.[87] These cognitive impairments often improve when patients are supported with an LV assist device (LVAD).[88]

Causes of brain dysfunction in heart failure are multifactorial. Hypoxia resulting from pulmonary edema can cause neurocognitive impairment.[89] Electrolyte and acid-base disturbances associated with heart failure may alter brain function. RAAS-mediated fluid expansion increases venous pressure, which is transmitted to the dural venous sinuses and intracranial veins, resulting in fluid accumulation of the cisterns and subarachnoid spaces of the brain. Increases in CVP may also decrease brain perfusion by reducing cerebral perfusion pressure, especially in the face of hypotension or low cardiac output.

MEDICAL MANAGEMENT OF ADHF

When children with chronic heart failure require intensive care, they are usually in some form of ADHF, which refers to acute cardiovascular failure along with exacerbation of the preexisting molecular abnormalities and symptoms of heart failure. Most patients with heart failure experience repeat bouts of acute or chronic decompensation. There are an estimated 1 million hospitalizations annually for ADHF in adults, and this is the most common reason for hospital admission in patients older than 65 years.[90] As in adults, most admissions because of heart failure in children are for acute exacerbations of chronic heart failure. Although the burden of disease in the pediatric population is not known, ADHF in children has become more common as survival of children with congenital heart disease and primary myocardial disease has increased. In contrast to adult patients, ischemic cardiomyopathy is rare in children and idiopathic dilated cardiomyopathy is common. When decompensated heart failure persists, mechanical circulatory support and/or cardiac transplantation are usually required. At present, the leading diagnosis resulting in pediatric transplantation is primary myocardial disorders, but palliated congenital heart disease is quickly becoming more common, emphasizing the evolving demographics of this patient population.

Irrespective of cause, heart failure is thought to occur after an index event produces an initial decline in heart function. As noted earlier, this situation leads to compensatory mechanisms including an activation of RAAS and the sympathetic nervous system, resulting in salt and water preservation, and production of inflammatory cytokines. These compensatory mechanisms often delay onset of symptoms for months or even years. The compensatory mechanisms are generally counterproductive over time, although they contribute to progressive myocardial damage, LV remodeling, and eventual cardiac decompensation.[2] Because the symptoms of heart failure seem to progress independent of the patient's hemodynamic status,[2] heart failure therapy should not be guided by echocardiographic and/or catheterization results.

Clinical Presentation of Decompensated Heart Failure

Clinical manifestations of ADHF in children are dependent on age of presentation. Common neonatal causes include perinatal asphyxia, toxemia, incessant tachyarrhythmias, neonatal myocarditis, severe anemia, or hyperviscosity syndrome. These neonates present with respiratory distress, venous congestion (hepatomegaly, jugular venous distension, hydrops) and sometimes shock. After the immediate perinatal period, causes of heart failure in infants can be divided into 2 groups: those that occur in the first few weeks of life and those that occur at 1 to 3 months of life. In the absence of fetal diagnosis, congenital heart anomalies dependent on ductal blood flow typically present in the first few weeks of life as the ductus begins to close. Defects with ductal-dependent systemic perfusion (eg, hypoplastic left heart syndrome, critical aortic stenosis, critical coactation) present with shock and respiratory distress, whereas defects with ductal-dependent pulmonary perfusion present with progressive and marked cyanosis. As PVR falls after the first few weeks of life, infants with significant shunt lesions typically present with heart failure at 1 to 3 months of life because of the increasing pulmonary blood flow and volume overload. These infants typically present with respiratory symptoms and feeding difficulties, although systemic perfusion is usually preserved. Other important causes of ADHF in infants include primary myocardial diseases, myocarditis, and anomalous left coronary artery from the pulmonary artery (ALCAPA). Infants with ALCAPA typically present with ventricular dysfunction and heart failure secondary to myocardial ischemia. These infants often present with unique symptoms of intense irritability and presumed angina, particularly during feeding. Older children are more likely to develop heart failure from acquired heart disease or palliated structural heart disease. Myocarditis, the most common cause of acquired heart disease, can present at any age. Other potential causes of acquired heart failure in older children include rheumatic heart disease, hypothyroidism, or Kawasaki disease. Patients with palliated structural heart disease may develop progressive heart failure as a consequence of chronic pressure or volume overload.

Dysrhythmias in ADHF

Dysrhythmias are commonly associated with heart failure, but the cause and effect can be difficult to discern. Although poor cardiac function can lead to rhythm disturbances, tachycardia can also be the primary cause of myocardial dysfunction (tachycardia-induced cardiomyopathy). All forms of incessant tachycardias (atrial junctional, accessory pathway, and ventricular) can result in tachycardia-mediated cardiomyopathy. Although the minimal heart rate necessary to develop cardiomyopathy is not known, studies suggest that patients who develop ventricular dysfunction typically have persistent heart rates in excess of 140 beats per minute.[91]

Children with heart failure may develop atrial or ventricular arrhythmias, increasing the risk of sudden death. The maladaptive remodeling and sarcomeric changes of heart failure can predispose the myocardium to after-depolarizations, which may initiate ventricular arrhythmias. In adults, multiform premature ventricular contractions, ventricular couplets, and ventricular tachycardia were observed in 80% to 90% of patients with chronic heart failure. The frequency and complexity of ventricular ectopy increase as ventricular function worsens.[92]

Laboratory Evaluation of ADHF

Assessment of the child with ADHF should include comprehensive laboratory evaluation, chest radiograph, electrocardiography, and echocardiography. Classic findings on blood work include metabolic and respiratory acidemia caused by tissue hypoperfusion and pulmonary congestion, hyponatremia, and hypochloremia caused by free water retention, and increased creatinine caused by poor renal perfusion and compromised renal function. Hemoglobin should be assessed because any degree of anemia can accentuate heart failure.

Assessment of the neurohormonal activation of heart failure has important prognostic value, and may ultimately be useful to guide therapy.

Increased norepinephrine, aldosterone, angiotensin II, and vasopressin have all been linked to outcomes.[32,33] Measurement of serum BNP has taken a particularly prominent role in the assessment of heart failure. Since its approval in 2000 by the US Food and Drug Administration (FDA), the BNP assay has subsequently been shown to be effective in diagnosing heart failure in numerous clinical scenarios.[93,94] Measurement of serum BNP is clinically useful in differentiating pulmonary causes of dyspnea from cardiac causes of dyspnea.[95] In children, BNP levels correlate with a clinical heart failure score and negatively correlate with ejection fraction.[96,97] More importantly, increased BNP levels in heart failure correlate with morbidity and mortality.[32]

Algorithm for Rapid Assessment of ADHF

A useful tool to guide management of the patient with ADHF is the rapid assessment algorithm proposed by Grady.[98] Patients are classified by the presence or absence of pulmonary or systemic congestion (ie, increased filling pressure) and the adequacy of perfusion. As shown in **Fig. 1**, patients are classified according to signs of increased filling pressures (wet or dry) and adequacy of perfusion (warm or cold). The goal is to maintain or transfer a patient to the warm and dry category. Patients who present as warm and wet or cold and wet generally respond well to medical management. The cold and dry state is usually a dire condition, which may warrant more aggressive treatment, such as mechanical support. This conceptual framework was designed for adults with heart failure. Although the benefit of this approach for children with heart failure has not been validated, it is a useful conceptual framework to approach patient management.

Increased filling pressures with adequate perfusion: warm and wet

The patient with congestion but adequate perfusion is the most common presentation requiring hospitalization, and the group that responds best to medial therapy. Diuresis is the first-line treatment and may be the only therapy needed to improve symptoms in patients with adequate perfusion. In adult patients, diuretics increase stroke volume, decrease pulmonary capillary wedge pressure, and decrease systemic vascular resistance.[99] Diuretics combined with a vasodilator can reduce mitral regurgitation and increase forward ejection fraction.[100] Overdiuresis should be avoided as it may cause kidney injury and lead to the CRS.[67]

Assessment of systemic perfusion is essential to determine whether chronic therapy for heart failure

	No Congestion	Congestion
Adequate perfusion	**"Warm and Dry"** A Optimal profile: focus on prevention of disease progression and decompensation	**"Wet and Warm"** B Diuresis with continuation of standard therapy
Critical hypoperfusion	**"Cold and Dry"** L Limited further options for therapy	**"Wet and Cold"** C Diuresis and redesign of regimen with other standard therapies

Fig. 1. Profile of resting hemodynamics. Patients frequently progress from profile A to profile B or profile C. Profile L refers to patients presenting with low output and no congestion. The letter L was chosen rather than the letter D to avoid the implication that this profile necessarily follows profile C or is a less desirable profile than C. (*From* Grady KL, Dracup K, Kennedy G, et al. Team management of patients with heart failure: a statement for healthcare professionals from the cardiovascular Nursing Council of the American Heart Association. Circulation 2000;102:2443–56; with permission.)

should be continued during an acute exacerbation. β-Blockers and angiotensin-converting enzyme (ACE) inhibitors can be continued if perfusion is adequate, but the negative inotropic effects of β-blockade may necessitate discontinuation or dose reduction if perfusion is marginal. Some patients may not tolerate acute withdrawal from β-blockade. In adults, continuance of chronic β-blocker therapy during hospitalization is associated with a decreased risk of death or rehospitalization.[101] Initiation of β-blocker is usually contraindicated while the patient is in a decompensated state of heart failure. Delaying initiation of a β-blocker until the patient has been transitioned back to the warm and dry state is prudent.

Increased filling pressures with poor perfusion: cold and wet

The next most common presentation of ADHF is the patient with congestion and poor perfusion. Nohria and colleagues[102] reported that 20% of adult patients admitted for heart failure were in this group. Compared with patients with adequate perfusion, the risk of death or need for heart transplant is greater in these patients. Although the approach to these patients depends on the degree of circulatory compromise, the cornerstone of therapy is afterload reduction. Vasodilation is the best way to increase cardiac output in a failing heart, as opposed to whipping it with an inotropic agent. Vasodilators and diuretics alone are often adequate therapy, especially if blood pressure is adequate.[60,103] Other inotropic agents may be needed if a patient is hypotensive, but mounting evidence indicates that high-dose inotropic agents are detrimental to long-term survival and should be avoided whenever possible. A review of over 15,000 adults hospitalized for heart failure

observed higher in-hospital mortality in patients treated with dobutamine or milrinone compared with patients treated with nitroglycerin or nesiritide.[37] Long-term therapy with positive inotropic agents has never been shown to improve outcomes in patients with heart failure. Because positive inotropic agents have been repeatedly shown to be associated with increased morbidity and mortality, these agents should be used cautiously.

There are no pediatric data to support the use of one vasodilator over another for acute heart failure. Although it is commonly used in adult patients, there is minimal pediatric experience with nitroglycerin for heart failure treatment. Nitroprusside is an effective vasodilator that has been used in the treatment of heart failure for decades.[104] Because of its rapid half-life, it can be quickly titrated to effect. Cyanide toxicity is an important potential side effect, especially with chronic use, high doses, or renal impairment. The human recombinant BNP, nesiritide, is a new vasodilator agent that also has positive lusitropic properties and promotes natriuresis. Although it can rapidly improve symptoms in adults with ADHF, long-term data are lacking, and concerns have been raised about renal toxicity and long-term survival.[105,106] There is limited experience with use of nesiritide in children. Jefferies and colleagues[38] assessed the use of nesiritide in 26 children ranging from 3 weeks to 12 years of age, and observed increased urine output and decreased CVP. No episodes of hypotension were noted, despite a maximum dose of 0.03 µg/kg/min.

Inotropic agents may be required for hypotension or to improve perfusion in the cold and wet patient. The decision to use inotropic agents should be based on clinical assessment of perfusion and not on echocardiographic results. Patients with severe ventricular dysfunction often remain compensated; they do not need and are potentially harmed by inotropic agents.

Among the most commonly used inotropic agents for pediatric heart failure is milrinone, a phosphodiesterase (PDE) inhibitor with inotropic, lusitropic, and vasodilatory properties. Milrinone inhibits breakdown of cyclic adenosine monophosphate (cAMP) to enhance calcium influx and improve myocyte contractility.[107] Because calcium reuptake is also cAMP dependent, these agents may also enhance diastolic myocardial relaxation. PDE inhibitors increase contractility and promote vasodilation without increasing myocardial oxygen consumption or ventricular afterload.[108] Although milrinone improves symptoms and decreases filling pressure in adult patients with heart failure, mounting evidence suggests that it may not improve long-term survival.[109–112] In a study of nearly 1000 patients randomized to short-term milrinone or placebo, there was no difference in mortality, hospital length of stay, or hospital readmission, but there was an increased incidence of hypotension and arrhythmias in milrinone-treated patients.[110] In a retrospective analysis of ischemic cardiomyopathy patients, short-term milrinone was associated with increased hospital mortality, and a higher rate of rehospitalization.[111] Milrinone-treated patients with nonischemic cardiomyopathy had reduced rates of death and rehospitalization. Other studies have also failed to show the long-term benefit of milrinone. A prospective study of outpatient oral milrinone for chronic heart failure observed that patients treated with milrinone had increased hospitalization, and higher cardiovascular mortality.[113] It is unclear whether these data from adult patients can be translated to pediatric patients with heart failure. At our centers, milrinone is still first-line therapy for patients with decompensated heart failure in the cold and wet state, and use of β-adrenergic agonists is avoided, especially at higher doses. Although there are no trials of milrinone use in pediatric patients with ADHF, the multicenter PRIMACORP trial observed a dose-dependent reduction in the incidence of LCOS after surgery.[8]

Other traditional inotropic agents used for decompensated heart failure include dobutamine, dopamine, and epinephrine. Dobutamine is an adrenergic agonist that stimulates both β_1 and β_2 receptors. Stimulation of cardiac β_1 receptors increases intracellular cAMP to promote SR calcium release and enhance contractility. Activation of β_2 receptors mediates vasodilation to decrease systemic vascular resistance. Dobutamine has been shown to improve symptoms, lower filling pressures, increase ejection fraction, and improve exercise tolerance, but undesired effects include tachycardia, arrhythmias, and increased myocardial oxygen consumption.[114–116] As noted earlier, dobutamine was associated with increased mortality in adult patients with heart failure, compared with nesiritide or nitroglycerin. The CASINO trial also found dobutamine was associated with higher mortality, compared with levosimendan or placebo. For reasons given earlier, routine use of dobutamine for heart failure has fallen out of favor.

Although other inotropes have not been studied as extensively as dobutamine, they are likely to be equally detrimental for treatment of decompensated heart failure, which explains why afterload reduction is the cornerstone of treatment rather than inotropic therapy. Dopamine is an endogenous catecholamine that stimulates β_1-adrenergic receptors in the heart, increasing contractility and heart rate. At low doses (2–5 μg/kg/min), it also stimulates dopamine receptors in the renal, cerebral, coronary, mesenteric, and pulmonary vasculature, although there is no evidence to support use of renal dose dopamine. At higher doses ($\geq$ 10 μg/kg/min), α-adrenergic receptors are stimulated to mediate vasoconstriction of the systemic and pulmonary vasculature. The side effect profile is similar to dobutamine, including the propensity for tachycardia, arrhythmias, and increased myocardial oxygen consumption. There are no clinical trials of dopamine use for treatment of ADHF in adult or pediatric patients. A trial of ibopamine, an oral dopaminergic drug, was prematurely stopped because of increased mortality in patients treated with ibopamine.[117] Dopamine continues to be a common inotropic agent in children, so studies to evaluate its role in heart failure would be valuable. Epinephrine has dose-dependent actions on α- and β-adrenergic receptors. At low doses, β-adrenergic responses predominate, resulting in vasodilation and increased heart rate and contractility. At higher doses, α-receptor stimulation mediates vasoconstriction and increased systemic vascular resistance. Although acute increases in contractility may initially improve perfusion, this may occur at the expense of tachycardia, arrhythmias, and increases in systemic vascular resistance, myocardial oxygen consumption, and myocardial work. For this reason, use of epinephrine should optimally be time limited to allow initiation of other vasodilator agents such as milrinone or nitroprusside. Prolonged use of epinephrine is poorly tolerated by the failing myocardium and will exacerbate cardiomyocyte and sarcomeric injury, thus aggravating diastolic and systolic ventricular dysfunction.[30,31] If a patient with heart failure requires prolonged use of high-dose epinephrine (>0.03 µg/kg/min) or its equivalent, mechanical circulatory support should be considered.

A continuous infusion of calcium chloride is a good alternative to β-adrenergic agonists in patients with depressed systolic function or hypotension. Calcium chloride has been used to increase myocardial contractility in the postarrest setting.[118] In the adult heart, calcium released from the SR accounts for most of the calcium that binds to troponin C. In the neonate, the SR is sparse and undifferentiated, so the neonatal myocardium is more dependent on extracellular calcium stores for contractile function.[119] Contractility is proportional to the level of ionized calcium in the blood.[120] In contrast to cathecholamines, calcium chloride does not induce tachycardia or arrhythmias. In adult patients, calcium chloride infusions have been discouraged as a result of studies implicating calcium with increased myocardial necrosis and worsening diastolic dysfunction.[121] There are no studies evaluating the use of chronic calcium chloride in pediatric patients for decompensated heart failure, but it has been used extensively in perioperative patients with congenital heart disease. The use of calcium chloride can acutely improve myocardial contractility and cardiac output without excessive tachycardia, especially in younger patients. The long-term safety and efficacy of calcium infusions in children have not been studied.

The use of arginine vasopressin as an inotropic agent has increased in recent years. When used during and after cardiac arrest, it has been shown to improve return of spontaneous circulation and survival in some series.[122] Vasopressin levels are increased in children with heart failure,[123] but depressed in patients after CPB. Vasopressin acts directly on vascular smooth muscle to increase systemic vascular resistance, but without the associated tachycardia observed with catecholamines. Vasopressin may also have direct effects on the myocardium by increasing cytosolic calcium via V1 receptors.[124] Studies of its use in vasodilatory shock showed an improvement in stroke volume, an unexpected finding if arginine vasopressin acts only to increase afterload.[125] Vasopressin has been shown to improve low cardiac output in children with catecholamine resistant shock after cardiac surgery.[126] Even if vasopressin has direct myocardial effects, prolonged increases in afterload with vasopressin may not be well tolerated in patients with heart failure.

Levosimendan is a promising new agent in a new class of medications known as calcium sensitizers. As previously noted, calcium dysregulation and reduced calcium sensitivity are common in the failing myocardium.[127] Traditional inotropic agents that increase intracellular calcium are associated with increased oxygen consumption, impaired myocardial relaxation, and arrhythmias.[128] Levosimendan is a novel agent that increases both inotropy and vasodilation without increasing intracellular calcium or myocardial oxygen demand.[129] Enhancement of contractility occurs by binding to troponin C and increasing myofilament sensitivity to calcium. Levosimendan causes vasodilatation via opening of potassium dependent adenosine triphosphate channels. The unique property of improving cardiac function without increasing intracellular calcium may prove to be a major breakthrough in the treatment of acute and chronic heart failure. Levosimendan has been used safely and effectively in adults, with recent studies showing improved long-term outcomes. There are isolated case reports of its use in children with postoperative cardiac dysfunction and in a patient with decompensated heart failure.[130,131] The drug is not currently available in the United States.

Normal filling pressures with poor perfusion: cold and dry

Patients with inadequate perfusion and normal filling pressures represent a tenuous patient population. Vasodilators may not be tolerated in patients with marginal blood pressure, so inotropic agents are often necessary. In the setting of cardiogenic shock, infusion of multiple agents is often necessary. Although prolonged use of these agents alone will not likely return the patient to an asymptomatic state, titration of vasodilator therapy may become feasible if perfusion and blood pressure can be improved transiently by aggressive inotropic therapy. If this is not possible, these agents may be acutely life saving, but they may decrease long-term ventricular function and worsen mortality. In the setting of increasing inotropic requirements to maintain adequate perfusion and lack of response to vasodilation therapy, it is our practice to consider mechanical support.

Assessment of Therapeutic Efficacy

Because all inotropic agents and other heart failure therapies have unwanted side effects, it is imperative to assess efficacy of interventions following initiation or dosage adjustment. In adult patients, relief of symptoms correlates well with decreased filling pressures, but it is unclear whether the use of a pulmonary artery catheter can improve outcome over clinical assessment. As illustrated in **Fig. 2**, we advocate use of central venous/superior vena cava (SVC) oxygen saturation for goal-directed therapy in patients with decompensated heart failure. Clinical assessment should include determinants of overall cardiac output, pulmonary congestion, and systemic perfusion. Laboratory parameters such as BNP levels and high-resolution CRP have been shown to correlate with heart failure severity. It is not clear that following these levels improves outcome when managing ADHF.

Use of Mechanical Circulatory Support for Patients with ADHF

In the setting of increasing inotropic requirements for the failing myocardium, the situation is dire. Medical therapy is unlikely to return the patient to an asymptomatic state and continuation of therapy will likely increase the stress on the failing myocardium. At this point, mechanical support should be considered to rest the myocardium. In children, mechanical support in this setting has generally been used as a bridge to cardiac transplantation.

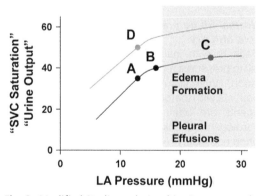

Fig. 2. Modified Starling relationship. Because stroke volume is not easily monitored, indirect measures of cardiac output (such as SVC saturation) or measures of end-organ perfusion (such as urine output) may be plotted against atrial pressure to attain a modified Starling relationship. Fluid administration augments preload and leads to improvement in SVC saturation and end-organ perfusion (point A to point B). Preload augmentation is limited, however; progressive fluid administration leads to excessive atrial pressures, with resultant edema formation, (point C). Alternative ways to improve SVC saturation or urine output include afterload reduction or improvements in lusitropy or inotropy, which all shift the Starling relationship leftward (point D). The therapeutic goal of enhanced lusitropy, increased contractility or afterload reduction is improvement in systemic blood flow for a comparable preload (reflected as improved SVC saturation and enhanced organ perfusion).

In the setting of a potentially reversible process, such as myocarditis, mechanical support has been used as a bridge to recovery. Reducing the chronic mechanical stress of a failing heart may reverse some of the pathologic molecular changes characteristics of heart failure. For example, mechanical support has been associated with reversal of cytoskeletal abnormalities, including dystrophin proteolytic cleavage.[23]

Because a broader discussion of mechanical circulatory support can be found elsewhere in this issue, we discuss briefly the indications and current strategies for the use of mechanical circulatory support in heart failure. Use of VADs in adults and children entails one of 3 treatment strategies: (1) bridge to transplantation, (2) bridge to recovery, or (3) destination therapy. All of these strategies are used currently in adult patients with end-stage heart failure. Although VAD support as a bridge to transplant is an established practice in children, pediatric use of VADs as a bridge to recovery or as destination therapy remains poorly defined. In pediatric myocarditis, both LVADs and biventricular VADs (biVADs) have been used successfully as bridge to recovery and bridge to transplant. The HeartMate XVE LVAD (Thoratec, Pleasanton, CA, USA) is approved by the FDA in the United States for destination therapy in adults with class IV heart failure who are on optimal medical therapy, have a life expectancy of less than 2 years, and who are ineligible for transplant, but use of a VAD as destination therapy in children has not been approved in the United States. Durability of current devices limit this option at present. There is increasing use of VADs in the outpatient setting in both adolescents and adults. Given the rapidly advancing field of VADs, new questions arise regarding the type of pump (continuous vs pulsatile), the degree of support (single ventricle vs biventricular), and the expected time of support. All of these important questions weigh heavily on the device chosen and the concurrent management of end-organ surveillance and hematologic management. Pending approval by the FDA, current pediatric strategies are limited given size requirements of existing devices. The ongoing Berlin EXCOR study in pediatrics may expand pediatric support options.

Use of extracorporeal membrane oxygenation (ECMO) may also be used in ADHF but has recognized limitations of duration of therapy. Patients with an acute, reversible insult may be considered candidates for ECMO. However, if longer periods of support are anticipated, transition to LVAD or biVAD support should be considered. These topics are discussed in more depth elsewhere.

TREATMENT OF LOW CARDIAC OUTPUT AFTER CONGENITAL HEART SURGERY

Morbidity and mortality associated with LCOS following cardiac surgery are high. During the earlier days of infant cardiac surgery, surgical mortality approached 20%.[132] Although LCOS is less common and less likely to lead to mortality in the current era, it results in increased hospital stay, resource use, and possible long-term cognitive dysfunction.[133] Prompt recognition, diagnosis, and management of LCOS are fundamental to optimal cardiac intensive care and essential for optimal patient outcome. The standard management of postoperative LCOS entails the following fundamentals: minimizing O_2 consumption, optimization of preload and afterload, prompt diagnosis of residual cardiac lesions, prevention of hypoxia, anemia, and acidosis, and administration of pharmacologic agents to improve myocardial contractile function.

Minimize Oxygen Consumption

Reduced cardiac output and increased systemic oxygen consumption can adversely alter the systemic oxygen balance after CPB. Oxygen consumption may be increased following CPB procedures, especially if a patient is febrile.[134] Fever in the setting of LCOS should be treated aggressively with antipyretic medication or surface cooling, but shivering should be avoided because it may increase oxygen consumption. Total oxygen consumption can be decreased by the induction of heavy sedation, paralysis, or mild hypothermia that reduces the metabolic rate.[135] Case reports of moderate hypothermia for patients with refractory LCOS suggest this may be a rescue therapy for LCOS.[136,137]

Ensure Adequate Preload

Inadequate preload is common in postoperative cardiac surgical patients. Potential causes of postoperative hypovolemia include bleeding, excessive ultrafiltration, and vasodilation from rewarming or afterload reduction. Cardiac tamponade or pneumothorax, which impair preload by altering diastolic compliance, should always be considered in patients with LCOS. Myocardial swelling, which may limit myocardial filling and prevent adequate output, may necessitate sternal reopening. Patients with low cardiac output as a result of right heart failure may benefit from creation or enlargement of an atrial shunt to allow right-to-left shunting to maintain the preload of the systemic ventricle.

Although true preload is end-diastolic volume of a ventricle, preload assessment can be estimated from right and left atrial pressures. Continual reassessment of the optimal preload is essential, as ventricular compliance and subsequent preload needs often change postoperatively. The top panel of **Fig. 3** shows how preload determination is predominantly a trial-and-error process. When atrial pressure is low, fluid administration augments end-diastolic volume and increases stroke volume. With successive fluid administration, however, increases in stroke volume become limited because of the nonlinear nature of the ventricular diastolic compliance. Preload augmentation is also limited by increases in end-diastolic pressure, which results in clinically significant edema formation. Interpretation of hemodynamic pressure monitoring data should always be made with an understanding of the patient's underlying physiology. Patients with diastolic dysfunction, such as with right ventricular (RV) dysfunction after tetralogy of Fallot repair, may require higher filling pressures than normal to generate an adequate output. These patients may also benefit from lusitropic therapy intended to improve diastolic ventricular filling. **Fig. 3**, panel ii illustrates how a change in ventricular diastolic compliance affects atrial pressure. Enhanced lusitropy should result in a greater stroke volume for a comparable atrial pressure.

Prompt Recognition of Arrhythmias

Early recognition of postoperative arrhythmias is imperative; therefore, a baseline postoperative surface electrocardiogram is essential for comparison with preoperative and subsequent postoperative tracings. Continuous electrocardiographic monitoring during the postoperative period is standard. Sinus bradycardia, bundle branch block, and atrioventricular block can occur after many cardiac surgical procedures; temporary atrial and ventricular pacing wires are typically placed to facilitate pacing. Arrhythmias are common in postoperative patients, and may require overdrive pacing, cardioversion, or pharmacologic intervention.[138] Hoffman and colleagues[138] reviewed the incidence of arrhythmias in postoperative cardiac surgical patients, and found that nonsustained ventricular and supraventricular tachycardia were most common, with incidences of 22% and 12%. Sustained ventricular, junctional, and supraventricular arrhythmias were slightly less common. Loss in atrioventricular synchrony can compromise preload, increase pulmonary congestion, and significantly diminish cardiac output, thus maintenance of atrioventricular synchrony is critical (via pacing, if necessary).

Junctional tachycardia (JET) usually occurs in the first 48 hours following surgery, especially after procedures involving closure of a ventricular septal defect.[139] It is poorly tolerated, especially in patients with unstable hemodynamics. Early recognition of arrhythmias may be aided by surveillance of atrial pressure waveforms; loss of the distinct a and v waves, indicating loss of atrioventricular synchrony, is often the first indication of arrhythmia and/or atrioventricular dyssynchrony. Once diagnosed, reestablishment of atrioventricular synchrony via atrial or atrioventricular

i. Preload Recruitment

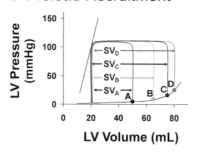
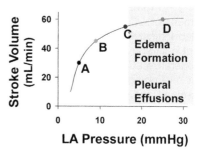

ii. Improve Diastolic Function (Positive Lusitropy)

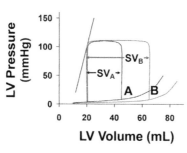
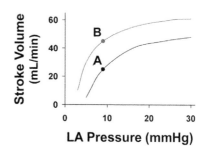

iii. Increase Contractility (Positive Inotropy)

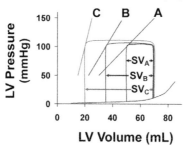
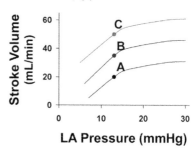

iv. Afterload Reduction

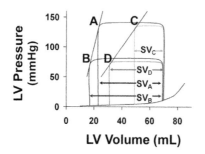
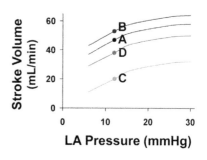

sequential pacing is the key to the treatment of JET. When possible, adrenergic agents should be reduced or discontinued, because they play a role in initiation and/or progression of JET. If the junctional rate is too fast to allow pacing, pharmacologic therapy is needed to provide rate control so that atrial or dual-chamber pacing can be performed. Both amiodarone and procainamide administration (in combination with induction of hypothermia) have been shown effective for rate control in JET.[140,141] Because the risk of JET increases in the presence of low output ("low cardiac output begets JET"), the diagnosis of JET should prompt the cardiac intensivist to search for other causes of LCOS, including other residual cardiac lesions.

Prompt Diagnosis of Residual Cardiac Lesions

Residual cardiac lesions in the postoperative patient can lead to LCOS and result in increased morbidity and mortality. Careful evaluation for residual cardiac abnormalities is indicated especially when patients do not follow their expected postoperative course after heart surgery. Data from indwelling intracardiac catheters and transesophageal or transthoracic echocardiography should be used to rule out residual structural lesions in patients with LCOS following cardiac surgery. Catheterization should be considered if LCOS persists and the cause remains elusive.

Prompt diagnosis of residual structural lesions can help direct medical management optimally, or may prompt surgical or catheter-based intervention.

Treatment of Depressed Myocardial Contractility

Because low cardiac output after pediatric heart surgery is often associated with some level of contractile dysfunction, inotropic support in the early postoperative period is usually necessary. Panel iii of **Fig. 3** shows the beneficial effects of positive inotropy on the pressure-volume and Starling relationships. At constant preload, increased contractility should enhance ejection to increase stroke volume. As noted earlier, because inotropic agents have unwanted side effects, it is important to assess efficacy of these agents following initiation or dosage adjustment. **Fig. 2** illustrates the potential utility of Starling curves to assess efficacy of most hemodynamic interventions. The Starling relationship specifies the therapeutic goal of all inotropic agents: enhanced contractility should result in a greater stroke volume for a comparable preload. Measurement of stroke volume is not routine in postoperative patients, so an alternative to the true Starling relationship is illustrated in **Fig. 2**. Because stroke volume is not easily monitored, indirect measures of

---

Fig. 3. Paired changes in pressure-volume and Starling relationships with isolated manipulations in preload (*i*), lusitropy (*ii*), contractility (*iii*), and afterload (*iv*). End-diastolic point A and stroke volume A (SV$_A$) for each pair of graphs represent the initial baseline hemodynamic condition. (*i*) The effect of preload recruitment on the pressure-volume and Starling relationships. Fluid volume administration augments end-diastolic volume (EDV) from points A to B, with the increase in stroke volume represented as the difference between SV$_A$ and SV$_B$. Because diastolic compliance is nonlinear, increases in stroke volume are progressively less with further fluid administration (SV$_C$ and SV$_D$). End-diastolic volumes A, B, C, and D define the diastolic compliance relationship. Preload augmentation is limited by increases in LV end-diastolic pressure (EDP), which can lead to impaired myocardial perfusion and increases in atrial pressure, with resultant transcapillary leak and edema formation. (*ii*) The beneficial effects of positive lusitropy on the pressure-volume and Starling relationships. Enhanced ventricular compliance corresponds to an increased EDV for the same EDP, thereby augmenting stroke volume without increasing atrial pressure. Enhanced lusitropy results in a greater stroke volume for a comparable atrial pressure. (*iii*) The beneficial effects of positive inotropy on the pressure-volume and Starling relationships. Increases in contractility are shown as enhancement of the end-systolic pressure-volume relationship (ESPVR), shown by increases in the slopes of line A to line C on the left-hand graph. At constant preload, increased contractility enhances ejection during isovolumic contraction, decreasing the end-systolic volume and increasing stroke volume (from SV$_A$ to SV$_B$ to SV$_C$). Enhanced contractility results in a greater stroke volume for a comparable preload. (*iv*) The beneficial effects of afterload reduction on the pressure-volume and Starling relationships. From baseline conditions A or C, afterload reduction allows the heart to eject to a lower systolic pressure and volume (points B and D), enhancing ejection and augmenting stroke volume (SV$_A$ to SV$_B$ and SV$_C$ to SV$_D$). At normal contractility (slope AB), the ventricle responds to altered afterload with only small changes in stroke volume (SV$_A$ to SV$_B$). On the other hand, neonatal and failing hearts are particularly sensitive to alterations in afterload. Benefits of afterload reduction are therefore more pronounced in neonatal hearts and in the setting of poor contractility. With reduced contractility (as shown by the reduced slope of ESPVR CD), the increase in stroke volume is greater for a comparable change in afterload. Afterload reduction results in a greater stroke volume for a comparable preload.

cardiac output (such as SVC saturation) or measures of end-organ perfusion (such as urine output) may be plotted against atrial pressure to attain a modified Starling relationship. Points A-C of **Fig. 2** illustrate how preload recruitment is used to increase SVC saturation or urine output. Because preload recruitment is limited, however, inotropic agents are used to improve SVC saturation or urine output by shifting the Starling relationship leftward (point D). Using the modified Starling relationship, the therapeutic goal of enhanced contractility is improvement in systemic blood flow for a comparable preload (reflected as improved SVC saturation and enhanced organ perfusion).

Inotropic agents and vasodilators are routinely used in pediatric cardiac surgical patients to help reestablish adequate myocardial function during and after surgery. Support is often initiated with low-dose infusions of a β-agonist catecholamine. The infusion rate is usually titrated to optimize systemic blood flow and pressure. High-dose dopamine (>10 μg/kg/min) is rarely used because of increasing vasoconstrictor and chronotropic effects with higher doses. Although some centers use higher doses of dobutamine, we advocate adding another agent if more support is necessary. Epinephrine is a more potent inotrope than dopamine or dobutamine because of its greater myocardial α_1- and β_1-adrenergic effects and is preferred for treatment of severe ventricular dysfunction. High-dose epinephrine (≥ 0.1 μg/kg/min) frequently results in tachycardia and systemic vasoconstriction. Epinephrine is often used in combination with intravenous vasodilators such as milrinone, sodium nitroprusside, or phenoxybenzamine to treat ventricular dysfunction and decrease systemic afterload (or at least attenuate the unwanted α_1-effects of epinephrine). Because norepinephrine has more potent vasoconstrictor effects than epinephrine, it is usually avoided in children after congenital heart surgery.

Because PDE inhibitors do not share many of the shortcomings of catecholamine agents, their use has increased considerably in recent years. PDE inhibitors improve CI by enhancing systolic and diastolic function, and by reducing systemic and PVR. In the pediatric population, milrinone is used more frequently than inamrinone because of its shorter half-life and lower incidence of thrombocytopenia.[107,142] The multicenter PRIMACORP study reported a dose-dependent reduction in the incidence of LCOS with milrinone use in children after congenital heart surgery.[8] For patients at high risk for LCOS, many centers prefer to load with milrinone during bypass to avoid potential hypotension associated with loading. Because renal dysfunction results in delayed clearance of both milrinone and inamrinone, patients with renal insufficiency are at risk for toxicity from excessive drug levels.[143] Infusion rates should be reduced as creatinine clearance falls to avoid excessive and prolonged vasodilation, especially in neonates.[144]

Alterations in cardiomyocyte calcium regulation and calcium sensitivity also occur after cardiac surgery, especially in neonates. Hypocalcemia is common in the postoperative period and may be pronounced in patients with 22q11 deletion syndrome or in neonates with transient hypoparathyroidism. Transfusion of citrate-treated blood products and administration of loop diuretics may exacerbate the hypocalcemia. Ionized calcium, the physiologically active form of calcium, should be monitored frequently in the postoperative period and maintained at normal or supernormal levels with supplementation. Many centers routinely use calcium infusions in neonates after CPB to augment and stabilize extracellular ionized calcium, especially in patients with 22q11 deletion syndrome. Calcium-sensitizing agents, as described earlier, have many potential advantages over traditional inotropic agents. Levosimendan has been shown to be hemodynamically beneficially in children after congenital heart surgery.

Although the mechanism remains unclear, investigators have advocated thyroid hormone therapy as a potential treatment of LCOS.[145,146] During CPB, circulating levels of the thyroid hormones triiodothyronine (T_3) and thyroxine (T_4) are reduced; these deficiencies can persist for several days and may play a role in postoperative myocardial depression.[145,146] One small study reported hemodynamic improvement in infants with refractory LCOS when treated with T_3.[147] Another randomized study reported children given postoperative T_3 supplementation had significantly higher cardiac output after surgery than those given placebo.[145]

Arginine vasopressin has been advocated as a therapeutic option for pediatric patients with LCOS and/or refractory hypotension after cardiac surgery, especially when conventional therapies are ineffective. CPB leads to decreased arginine vasopressin levels. Arginine vasopressin has also been shown to be effective for refractory hypotension in patients on mechanical circulatory support,[148,149] and also reverses phenoxybenzamine-related hypotension.[150]

Both pre- and postoperative patients can develop persistent low cardiac output that requires escalating inotropic support that is refractory to other therapy. Recent data suggest adrenal dysfunction contributes to morbidity in critically ill adult patients, and low-dose corticosteroid administration has been suggested as an option for patients with refractory LCOS. In a retrospective study of neonates receiving escalating, high-dose epinephrine, inotrope requirements were observed to decrease significantly within 24 hours of corticosteroid treatment.[151] Some patients showed low random cortisol levels with a normal adrenocorticotrophic hormone stimulation test, suggesting adrenal dysfunction. These data suggest stress-dose hydrocortisone (50 mg/m^2/d) may help reduce inotropic requirements in pediatric patients with LCOS refractory to conventional therapy. The physiologic basis for the reduction in inotropic support after both arginine vasopressin and corticosteroid therapy remains obscure, but they may share a similar mechanism, because arginine vasopressin serves as a potent stimulus for adrenocorticotropin.[152]

Afterload Reduction for Systemic Ventricular Failure

Increased afterload is particularly detrimental to the neonatal heart, especially when compounded by postoperative myocardial dysfunction. Afterload reduction is thus often beneficial in postoperative patients showing signs of LCOS. Furthermore, if high-dose catecholamines are necessary, vasodilator therapy should be considered to counter catecholamine vasoconstrictor effects. The lower panel of **Fig. 3** shows beneficial effects of afterload reduction on pressure-volume and Starling relationships. This panel also shows an important principle: benefits of afterload reduction are particularly pronounced in neonatal hearts and in the setting of poor contractility. With neonatal hearts or impaired contractility, afterload reduction is particularly useful to augment stroke volume and improve cardiac output. As with inotropic agents, it is important to assess efficacy of these agents following initiation or dosage adjustment because vasodilator agents also have unwanted side effects. The therapeutic goal of afterload reduction should be a greater stroke volume for a comparable preload. As noted earlier, however, because measurement of stroke volume is not routine in postoperative patients, the modified Starling relationship can be used to assess efficacy of most hemodynamic interventions, including afterload reduction. As shown in **Fig. 2**, the therapeutic goal of afterload reduction is improvement in systemic blood flow for a comparable preload (reflected as improved SVC saturation and enhanced organ perfusion).

Some centers advocate use of the potent vasodilator phenoxybenzamine, an α-adrenergic blocking agent, in selected pediatric patients after cardiac surgery.[153] Because phenoxybenzamine is a potent vasodilator with a prolonged half-life (>24 hours), its use may be complicated by severe hypotension. For this reason, many centers prefer the use of nitroprusside for afterload reduction and vasodilator therapy after heart surgery. Although nitroprusside may be a slightly less effective vasodilator than phenoxybenzamine, its therapeutic effects are easier to titrate. Nitroprusside may be especially useful in patients after single ventricle palliation with excessive pulmonary blood flow.[154] In such patients, the dual effects of nitroprusside include afterload reduction for improvement of myocardial performance and reduction of systemic vascular resistance to balance pulmonary and systemic blood flow. PDE inhibitors also provide afterload reduction in pediatric patients with congenital heart disease. In patients who require high doses of adrenergic agents, one or more vasodilator agents should be considered.

Management of RV Failure

Right heart failure is a common complication of congenital heart surgery that can lead to LCOS. Factors contributing to postoperative RV dysfunction may include RV hypertrophy, a ventriculotomy and difficulties with right heart myocardial protection. Patients undergoing right heart procedures, including tetralogy of Fallot and Fontan procedures may exhibit restrictive physiology (diastolic RV dysfunction), characterized by antegrade diastolic pulmonary arterial flow coinciding with atrial systole.[155] Children with restrictive physiology have a decreased CI because the stiff right ventricle has impaired diastolic filling.[155] These patients typically have a slower postoperative recovery and a prolonged stay in the ICU with longer periods of inotropic and ventilatory support. Alterations in LV filling may also occur if the RV is hypertensive and thus impedes LV filling. Because alterations in ventricular compliance make patients with RV failure more sensitive to alterations in venous return caused by intrathoracic pressure changes, these patients benefit from ventilation strategies that minimize intrathoracic pressure.[156–158] Patients with RV failure may benefit from manipulation of PVR to minimize RV afterload. PDE inhibitors are particularly beneficial in these patients, because of the combined lusitropic and pulmonary vasodilatory effects.

The ability to maintain a right-to-left atrial shunt is beneficial in patients with RV dysfunction because this preserves the preload of the systemic ventricle. In patients undergoing the modified Fontan procedure, a Fontan fenestration is associated with reduced pleural effusion and significantly shorter hospital stays.[159] In patients who undergo tetralogy of Fallot repair, a right-to-left atrial shunt can be similarly facilitated by maintaining the patency of the foramen ovale or by creating a small fenestration in the atrial septum.

Ventilation Strategies in Patients with Heart Failure

As noted earlier, the ventilation strategy depends upon whether RV or LV dysfunction predominates. Positive intrathoracic pressure is typically beneficial in patients with systemic ventricular dysfunction because this reduces LV afterload. In addition to optimal lung recruitment, higher levels of positive end-expiratory pressure (PEEP) may thus be hemodynamically beneficial in these patients. Tidal volumes should be maintained in the range of 8 to 10 mL/kg to avoid overdistension, which could increase PVR and RV afterload.[160] Furthermore, there is evidence that shorter inspiratory times may augment LV filling in patients with systemic ventricular dysfunction.[161] Because alterations in thoracic pressure may have opposing hemodynamic effects, hemodynamic effects of ventilatory maneuvers must be carefully evaluated with respect to systemic oxygen delivery.

As noted earlier, alterations in ventricular compliance make patients with RV failure particularly sensitive to changes in venous return caused by adjustments in intrathoracic pressure. Spontaneous inspiration enhances diastolic flow in these patients, so early extubation can be particularly beneficial. Because of the detrimental effects of positive pressure ventilation on RV dynamics, alternative modes of ventilation, such as negative-pressure or high-frequency jet ventilation (HFJV) have been advocated in patients with RV dysfunction and in patients with Fontan circulations. Because HFJV reduces mean airway pressure and PVR while maintaining a similar $Paco_2$, it may be ideally suited for postoperative Fontan patients, or patients with RV dysfunction or pulmonary hypertension.[162] Similarly, negative-pressure ventilation has been shown to augment cardiac output in patients with restrictive physiology after tetralogy of Fallot repair,[158] and those with Fontan physiology.[156] Although the technical challenges associated with HFJV and negative-pressure ventilation in postoperative patients have limited use of these modes, the ventilation strategy for patients with RV failure should aim to minimize mean airway pressure while maintaining lung volume at functional residual capacity, when lung function, PVR, and RV afterload are optimal.

TREATMENT OF HEART FAILURE IN CHILDREN WITH COMPLEX CONGENITAL HEART DISEASE

Heart Failure in Patients with Single Ventricle Hearts

Understanding the potential heart failure issues surrounding patients with single ventricle hearts requires knowledge of the physiology of the non-palliated state and of the different staged palliations. In turn, the treatment of heart failure in those with a single ventricle is dependent on the stage of surgical intervention and the associated hemodynamic and physiologic effects of the palliative procedure.

Single ventricle physiology may be defined in many ways depending on the status of the patient, before intervention or after intervention. The type of intervention affects the hemodynamics and the balance of Qp:Qs. Neonates who have not had an intervention often have heart failure as a result of an imbalance of the Qp:Qs, with excessive pulmonary blood flow at the expense of systemic blood flow, and resultant decreased oxygen delivery and impaired end-organ function. Tabbutt and colleagues[163] investigated the effect of subambient oxygen and inhaled CO_2 to balance Qp:Qs in this clinical setting. Both interventions reduced Qp:Qs, but inhaled CO_2 appeared to be more beneficial to systemic oxygen delivery overall. Although inspired CO_2 may be a more effective intervention, subambient oxygen can be used with a natural airway, thus avoiding the necessity of controlled ventilation necessary to use inspired CO_2. Patients require such interventions only if signs of poor cardiac output and/or end-organ damage are present. In patients with a balanced circulation, maneuvers that lower PVR or increase systemic vascular resistance should be avoided. For example, excessively high Fio_2 or hyperventilation can drop PVR and reduce systemic perfusion by increasing Qp:Qs. Although it has not been studied, milrinone is often used in this setting to augment stroke volume and optimize systemic vascular resistance. The only predictable way to balance the circulation in a patient with excessive Qp:Qs is through surgical intervention to mechanically limit pulmonary flow.

The stage I procedure for hypoplastic left heart syndrome has been modified and improved since the initial reports by Norwood.[164–166] Individual centers have reported improved outcomes based on perioperative care protocols.[153,167] Stage I palliation can be accomplished by the conventional Norwood procedure, the Sano procedure, or the hybrid procedure, which avoids use of CPB. Each procedure results in hemodynamic derangements, which require careful intensive care management to assure optimal cardiac output and systemic oxygen delivery. Because pulmonary blood flow is provided by a right ventricle to pulmonary artery conduit with the Sano procedure and by a Blalock-Taussig shunt in the conventional Norwood procedure, the resultant postoperative hemodynamics are different. Specifically, mean diastolic pressure is higher after Sano palliation than with Norwood palliation. Pulmonary blood flow is thought to be more stable after the Sano procedure and hence Qp:Qs is typically easier to balance.[168] There is a strong evidence supporting use of phenoxybenzamine postoperatively as an α-antagonist to balance Qp:Qs and afford optimal afterload reduction.[153] Other institutions prefer milrinone and nitroprusside to provide inotropic support, afterload reduction and balance Qp:Qs.[144,169] Studies comparing short-term and long-term survival and morbidity after Sano and Norwood procedures have not found significant differences in survival between the operative techniques.[170] Compared with Norwood palliation, there was a trend toward increased need for catheter-based or surgical interventions after the Sano operation.[170]

Hybrid stage I hemodynamics are not characterized so well in all populations.[171–173] Comprehensive data of the hemodynamics after the hybrid operation were recently published by the Toronto group.[173] They found that hemodynamics and Qp:Qs were less predictable after hybrid procedure than after the conventional Norwood palliation. These data included hybrid patients who required a reverse shunt to assure coronary perfusion.[173] Comprehensive data of the postoperative hemodynamics of the hybrid stage I without a reverse shunt are lacking, but reports to date describe use of catecholamines without need for afterload reduction. Theoretically, there has been concern about use of afterload reduction after the hybrid procedure because of fixed anatomic obstructions (ie, at the level of the pulmonary artery bands, ductus stent, or possible retrograde arch obstruction). Speculation exists about use of milrinone transiently to afford afterload reduction and inotropic support for patients after the hybrid procedure who exhibit increased systemic vascular resistance regardless of the use of a reverse shunt. Although reported outcomes are comparable with results of the Norwood and Sano stage 1 palliation, further investigation is necessary to elucidate the optimal management strategies after the hybrid stage 1 palliation.[172]

Outcomes after the second stage of palliation, the cavopulmonary anastomosis or bidirectional Glenn, depend on many factors, including good systolic and diastolic ventricular performance with low filling pressures and low PVR. Postoperative issues include cyanosis, ventricular dysfunction, and hypertension. Low PVR is an important factor for short-term survival, arterial saturation, and to minimize risk of perioperative morbidities such as pleural effusions. The cavopulmonary connection (either bidirectional Glenn shunt or hemi-Fontan procedure) results in volume unloading of the single ventricle, which is thought to be important for the long-term preservation of ventricular function. This volume unloading is an age-dependent phenomenon that positively affects ventricular mass, ejection fraction, and contractility.

The single ventricle morphology affects the muscle response to loading conditions. Compared with a morphologic left ventricle, the morphologic right ventricle does not exhibit the same increase in muscle mass with volume loading. This attenuated response of the right ventricle may compromise its ability to respond to physiologic challenges and thus may increase the risk of heart failure in the long-term. For example, the relative reduction in muscle mass of the morphologic right ventricle means that the ventricular afterload is greater than with a morphologic left ventricle.[174,175] Over time, this may limit exercise and functional capacity. This may be one of the reasons that protein-losing enteropathy is seen more frequently in patients with a morphologic right ventricle. Patients with a morphologic right ventricle also have an increased frequency of wall motion abnormalities and interventricular conduction delays, which may lead to impaired lusitropy.[176]

Improving survival with the Fontan procedure over the last few decades is likely because of improvements in surgical technique, perioperative care, and pattern recognition concerning expected outcomes and adverse events.[177,178] Morbidity after the Fontan operation is well characterized and includes heart failure, persistent effusions, thromboembolism, and arrhythmias.[179] The incidence of heart failure after the Fontan procedure increases with each year after palliation. By univariate analysis, independent risk factors for the development of heart failure after Fontan palliation included protein-losing enteropathy, a morphologic right ventricle, increased right atrial pressure at follow-up, thrombus in the Fontan pathway, and cerebral vascular accident. Multivariate analysis identified protein-losing enteropathy, increased right atrial pressure, and a morphologic RV as predictive of eventual heart failure.[179] Patients with single ventricle hearts also exhibit impaired lusitropy as is evidenced by abnormal intraventricular relaxation times. In a large study of patients after the Fontan palliation, a normal ejection fraction was observed in 73% of the patients, but abnormal diastolic function was present in 72% of the patients.[174,175] Those with a morphologic RV exhibited diastolic dysfunction more often than those with a morphologic LV.

Paramount to the care of children after Fontan palliation is the anticipation, prompt recognition, and treatment of arrhythmias. The type of Fontan pathway has evolved from direct anastomosis of the right atrium to the pulmonary artery to the lateral tunnel and extracardiac Fontan pathways.[180,181] Despite significant speculation that the extracardiac Fontan pathway would result in reduced incidence of arrhythmias, the incidence of atrial tachycardia and sinus node dysfunction seems to be comparable with the lateral tunnel and extracardiac Fontan procedures.[178,182,183] Prompt treatment of arrhythmias is especially important in patients with Fontan physiology who may have limited ability to compensate for loss of atrioventricular synchrony. Assuring atrioventricular synchrony and a good chronotropic response may be paramount to successful Fontan physiology and to a satisfactory quality of life. For these reasons, pacemaker placement may be necessary in a subset of patients after Fontan palliation. Atrial re-entrant tachycardia is a common problem after Fontan palliation and freedom from dysrhythmias lessens as time from Fontan operation increases.[178] Patients who develop persistent arrhythmias after Fontan palliation have an increased risk of heart failure and thromboembolic complications.[184] Medical management to treat the tachycardia and restore sinus rhythm promotes optimal hemodynamics. Medical therapy also attempts to prevent recurrences and/or provide rate control. Patients who are recalcitrant to medical therapy usually require cardioversion. Before cardioversion, imaging to assure thrombus is not present in the Fontan pathway or other intracardiac structures is necessary to avoid embolism and stroke.

Speculation exists regarding the importance of afterload reduction for acute and long-term management of the patient with a single ventricle heart, but evidence for this is lacking. Outpatient studies have failed to note any short- or long-term effect of angiotensin-converting enzyme inhibitors or β-blocking agents. During acute episodes of decompensation, milrinone is often used for afterload reduction, pulmonary vasodilation, and enhanced lusitropy, but evidence to support such inpatient therapies in this patient population is lacking.

Heart Failure in Patients with 2 Ventricle Hearts

Heart failure in those with previously palliated congenital heart disease follows a similar pattern to those with primary heart failure, but the pathophysiology is usually different.[174,175] After palliative or corrective surgery, the pediatric cardiologist should monitor a patient's potential for heart failure from residual lesions such as pressure or volume overload, valvar insufficiency, or residual shunts. For example, a volume-loaded ventricle is predisposed to morphologic alterations that may lead to systolic or diastolic dysfunction. This situation may lead to symptoms and require heart failure therapies, but surgical or catheter interventions to reduce or eliminate the volume load should always be considered. Similarly, many congenital heart lesions are associated with pressure overload of the ventricle. Although the focus of heart failure care in these patients is symptomatic relief, the treatment strategy must also consider surgical or catheter intervention to reduce the pressure load and the resultant ventricular hypertrophy. Patients with a morphologic right ventricle as their systemic ventricle, such as the patient with corrected transposition, are at increased risk for ventricular dysfunction over their lifetime and must be monitored appropriately for the development of heart failure. As stated earlier, the morphologic right ventricle seems to have an attenuated response to pressure and volume loading.

NOVEL THERAPIES FOR PEDIATRIC HEART FAILURE

Significant interest is increasing in novel medical and device therapies for treatment of heart failure in adults and children. However, treatment of pediatric heart failure is challenging secondary to the heterogeneity of the population and causes of myocardial disease as well as the absence of extensive, standardized guidelines.[174,175] Because of the growing population, the need for established medical therapies has never been greater. Novel therapies for pediatric heart failure may include experimental therapies, but often rely on adopting existing therapies in a more consistent manner (ie, ACE inhibitors, β-blockers, potassium-sparing diuretics such as spironolactone) as well as validation of advanced adult therapies such as cardiac resynchronization therapy.[185–187] Progress is being made in these areas but remains difficult given the limitations on performing robust multicenter pediatric heart failure trials.

Evidence supporting therapies for ADHF in the ICU setting are limited but increasing. The safety and efficacy of nesiritide has been reported.[38,188] Nesiritide has favorable actions on urine output, serum creatinine, and serum aldosterone without significant hypotension. Widespread use of nesiritide has been limited by concerns of increased renal dysfunction and mortality in adults. The ongoing Acute Study of Clinical Effectiveness of Nesiritide in Decompensated Heart Failure Trial (ASCEND-HF) will answer these questions and may lead to further pediatric investigation.[189] Two new vasodilators, relaxin and ularitide, are under investigation but may have favorable effects on pediatric heart failure.[190] The use of levosimendan as an inotropic agent has been the topic of significant investigation. This drug exerts its effects by binding to cardiac troponin C, thereby increasing sensitivity of contractile proteins to calcium. Although not currently available in the United States, levosimendan has been studied extensively and has promise in the pediatric population secondary to its ability to enhance myocardial contractility and improve symptoms.[191–193] However, there have also been concerns for increased mortality in the adult population.[194] These concerns may be secondary to the inotropic classification of the drug and the appropriate use of this class of drugs for heart failure (for patients who have evidence of low cardiac output and poor perfusion). Further pediatric studies are warranted to determine the optimal population for these and other new drugs. The treatment of volume overload is one that can be modified as well. Traditional therapy revolves around the use of intravenous diuretics. However, this approach has associated unfavorable effects on renal function and many patients with advanced heart failure are refractory. Ultrafiltration has become an accepted strategy for use in this setting with favorable outcome.[59,195]

Areas of future study are broader than direct interventions on the cardiovascular system. As stated earlier, therapies directed at treatment of other organ systems that are critically involved in the development and progression of heart failure may offer survival benefit. A greater understanding of the CRS may have a significant effect on heart failure management. In addition, treatment of anemia may offer therapeutic benefits that have not previously been pursued in pediatric heart failure. To answer these questions, a more dedicated effort at multicenter investigation is paramount. Tremendous research questions remain unanswered in heart failure. Pediatric heart failure offers the unique opportunity to study this complex syndrome without the confounding conditions seen in adults such as hypertension or atherosclerotic disease. More importantly, the numbers of these patients will continue to increase, requiring thoughtful and available diagnostic and treatment options.

REFERENCES

1. Katz AM. Overview, definition, historical aspects. Philadelphia: Lippincott Williams and Wilkins; 2003.
2. Mann DL. 1st edition. Heart failure as a progressive disorder, vol. 1. Philadelphia: Saunders; 2004.
3. Pignatelli RH, McMahon CJ, Dreyer WJ, et al. Clinical characterization of left ventricular noncompaction in children: a relatively common form of cardiomyopathy. Circulation 2003;108:2672.
4. Hunt SA. ACC/AHA 2005 Guideline Update for the Diagnosis and Management of Chronic Heart Failure in the Adult: a report of the American College of Cardiology/American Heart Association Task Force on Practice Guidelines (Writing Committee to Update the 2001 Guidelines for the Evaluation and Management of Heart Failure). J Am Coll Cardiol 2005;46:e1.
5. Hunt SA, Abraham WT, Chin MH, et al. ACC/AHA 2005 Guideline Update for the Diagnosis and Management of Chronic Heart Failure in the Adult: a report of the American College of Cardiology/American Heart Association Task Force on Practice Guidelines (Writing Committee to Update the 2001 Guidelines for the Evaluation and Management of Heart Failure): developed in collaboration with the American College of Chest Physicians and the International Society for Heart and Lung Transplantation: endorsed by the Heart Rhythm Society. Circulation 2005;112:e154.
6. Rosenthal D, Chrisant MR, Edens E, et al. International Society for Heart and Lung Transplantation: practice guidelines for management of heart failure in children. J Heart Lung Transplant 2004;23:1313.
7. Wernovsky G, Wypij D, Jonas RA, et al. Postoperative course and hemodynamic profile after the arterial switch operation in neonates and infants. A comparison of low-flow cardiopulmonary bypass and circulatory arrest. Circulation 1995;92:2226.
8. Hoffman TM, Wernovsky G, Atz AM, et al. Efficacy and safety of milrinone in preventing low cardiac output syndrome in infants and children after corrective surgery for congenital heart disease. Circulation 2003;107:996.
9. Hall RI, Smith MS, Rocker G. The systemic inflammatory response to cardiopulmonary bypass: pathophysiological, therapeutic, and pharmacological considerations. Anesth Analg 1997;85:766.
10. Schermerhorn ML, Tofukuji M, Khoury PR, et al. Sialyl lewis oligosaccharide preserves cardiopulmonary and endothelial function after hypothermic circulatory arrest in lambs. J Thorac Cardiovasc Surg 2000;120:230.

11. Chaturvedi RR, Lincoln C, Gothard JW, et al. Left ventricular dysfunction after open repair of simple congenital heart defects in infants and children: quantitation with the use of a conductance catheter immediately after bypass. J Thorac Cardiovasc Surg 1998;115:77.

12. Piacentino V 3rd, Weber CR, Chen X, et al. Cellular basis of abnormal calcium transients of failing human ventricular myocytes. Circ Res 2003;92:651.

13. Fill M, Copello JA. Ryanodine receptor calcium release channels. Physiol Rev 2002;82:893.

14. Miyamoto MI, del Monte F, Schmidt U, et al. Adenoviral gene transfer of SERCA2a improves left-ventricular function in aortic-banded rats in transition to heart failure. Proc Natl Acad Sci U S A 2000;97:793.

15. Hersel J, Jung S, Mohacsi P, et al. Expression of the L-type calcium channel in human heart failure. Basic Res Cardiol 2002;97(Suppl 1):I4.

16. Ahmmed GU, Dong PH, Song G, et al. Changes in Ca(2+) cycling proteins underlie cardiac action potential prolongation in a pressure-overloaded guinea pig model with cardiac hypertrophy and failure. Circ Res 2000;86:558.

17. Towbin JA, Bowles NE. The failing heart. Nature 2002;415:227.

18. Hoffman EP, Brown RH Jr, Kunkel LM. Dystrophin: the protein product of the Duchenne muscular dystrophy locus. Cell 1987;51:919.

19. Towbin JA, Bowles KR, Bowles NE. Etiologies of cardiomyopathy and heart failure. Nat Med 1999; 5:266.

20. Gao WD, Atar D, Liu Y, et al. Role of troponin I proteolysis in the pathogenesis of stunned myocardium. Circ Res 1997;80:393.

21. Schwartz SM, Duffy JY, Pearl JM, et al. Glucocorticoids preserve calpastatin and troponin I during cardiopulmonary bypass in immature pigs. Pediatr Res 2003;54:91.

22. Chang AN, Potter JD. Sarcomeric protein mutations in dilated cardiomyopathy. Heart Fail Rev 2005;10:225.

23. Vatta M, Stetson SJ, Jimenez S, et al. Molecular normalization of dystrophin in the failing left and right ventricle of patients treated with either pulsatile or continuous flow-type ventricular assist devices. J Am Coll Cardiol 2004; 43:811.

24. Hefti MA, Harder BA, Eppenberger HM, et al. Signaling pathways in cardiac myocyte hypertrophy. J Mol Cell Cardiol 1997;29:2873.

25. Molkentin JD, Lu JR, Antos CL, et al. A calcineurin-dependent transcriptional pathway for cardiac hypertrophy. Cell 1998;93:215.

26. Ito H, Hirata Y, Hiroe M, et al. Endothelin-1 induces hypertrophy with enhanced expression of muscle-specific genes in cultured neonatal rat cardiomyocytes. Circ Res 1991;69:209.

27. Miyada S, Haneda T, Osaki J. Renin-angiotensin system in stretch-induced hypertrophy of cultured neonatal rat heart cells. Eur J Pharmacol 1996; 307:81.

28. Brunner-La Rocca HP, Vaddadi G, Esler MD. Recent insight into therapy of congestive heart failure: focus on ACE inhibition and angiotensin-II antagonism. J Am Coll Cardiol 1999;33:1163.

29. Hillege HL, Girbes AR, de Kam PJ, et al. Renal function, neurohormonal activation, and survival in patients with chronic heart failure. Circulation 2000;102:203.

30. Colucci WS, Sawyer DB, Singh K, et al. Adrenergic overload and apoptosis in heart failure: implications for therapy. J Card Fail 2000;6:1.

31. Singh K, Communal C, Sawyer DB, et al. Adrenergic regulation of myocardial apoptosis. Cardiovasc Res 2000;45:713.

32. Anand IS, Fisher LD, Chiang YT, et al. Changes in brain natriuretic peptide and norepinephrine over time and mortality and morbidity in the Valsartan Heart Failure Trial (Val-HeFT). Circulation 2003; 107:1278.

33. Maron BJ, Tholakanahalli VN, Zenovich AG, et al. Usefulness of B-type natriuretic peptide assay in the assessment of symptomatic state in hypertrophic cardiomyopathy. Circulation 2004;109:984.

34. Abassi Z, Karram T, Ellaham S, et al. Implications of the natriuretic peptide system in the pathogenesis of heart failure: diagnostic and therapeutic importance. Pharmacol Ther 2004;102:223.

35. McCullough PA, Sandberg KR. Sorting out the evidence on natriuretic peptides. Rev Cardiovasc Med 2003;4(Suppl 4):S13.

36. de Lemos JA, McGuire DK, Drazner MH. B-type natriuretic peptide in cardiovascular disease. Lancet 2003;362:316.

37. Abraham WT, Adams KF, Fonarow GC, et al. In-hospital mortality in patients with acute decompensated heart failure requiring intravenous vasoactive medications: an analysis from the Acute Decompensated Heart Failure National Registry (ADHERE). J Am Coll Cardiol 2005;46:57.

38. Jefferies JL, Price JF, Denfield SW, et al. Safety and efficacy of nesiritide in pediatric heart failure. J Card Fail 2007;13:541.

39. Elster SK, Braunwald E, Wood HF. A study of C-reactive protein in the serum of patients with congestive heart failure. Am Heart J 1956;51:533.

40. Castell JV, Gomez-Lechon MJ, David M, et al. Acute-phase response of human hepatocytes: regulation of acute-phase protein synthesis by interleukin-6. Hepatology 1990;12:1179.

41. Ridker PM. High-sensitivity C-reactive protein: potential adjunct for global risk assessment in the

primary prevention of cardiovascular disease. Circulation 2001;103:1813.

42. Alonso-Martinez JL, Llorente-Diez B, Echegaray-Agara M, et al. C-reactive protein as a predictor of improvement and readmission in heart failure. Eur J Heart Fail 2002;4:331.

43. Anand IS, Latini R, Florea VG, et al. C-reactive protein in heart failure: prognostic value and the effect of valsartan. Circulation 2005;112:1428.

44. Venugopal SK, Devaraj S, Jialal I. Effect of C-reactive protein on vascular cells: evidence for a proinflammatory, proatherogenic role. Curr Opin Nephrol Hypertens 2005;14:33.

45. Skrak P, Kovacikova L, Kunovsky P. Procalcitonin, neopterin and C-reactive protein after pediatric cardiac surgery with cardiopulmonary bypass. Bratisl Lek Listy 2007;108:501.

46. Anker SD, von Haehling S. Inflammatory mediators in chronic heart failure: an overview. Heart 2004; 90:464.

47. Seta Y, Shan K, Bozkurt B, et al. Basic mechanisms in heart failure: the cytokine hypothesis. J Card Fail 1996;2:243.

48. Deswal A, Petersen NJ, Feldman AM, et al. Cytokines and cytokine receptors in advanced heart failure: an analysis of the cytokine database from the Vesnarinone trial (VEST). Circulation 2001; 103:2055.

49. Mann DL. Targeted anticytokine therapy and the failing heart. Am J Cardiol 2005;95:9C.

50. Mann DL, McMurray JJ, Packer M, et al. Targeted anticytokine therapy in patients with chronic heart failure: results of the Randomized Etanercept Worldwide Evaluation (RENEWAL). Circulation 2004;109:1594.

51. Ratnasamy C, Kinnamon DD, Lipshultz SE, et al. Associations between neurohormonal and inflammatory activation and heart failure in children. Am Heart J 2008;155:527.

52. Gullestad L, Aukrust P. Review of trials in chronic heart failure showing broad-spectrum anti-inflammatory approaches. Am J Cardiol 2005;95:17C.

53. Sliwa K, Woodiwiss A, Kone VN, et al. Therapy of ischemic cardiomyopathy with the immunomodulating agent pentoxifylline: results of a randomized study. Circulation 2004;109:750.

54. de Belder AJ, Radomski MW, Why HJ, et al. Myocardial calcium-independent nitric oxide synthase activity is present in dilated cardiomyopathy, myocarditis, and postpartum cardiomyopathy but not in ischaemic or valvar heart disease. Br Heart J 1995;74:426.

55. Satoh M, Nakamura M, Tamura G, et al. Inducible nitric oxide synthase and tumor necrosis factor-alpha in myocardium in human dilated cardiomyopathy. J Am Coll Cardiol 1997;29:716.

56. Patel R, Nagueh SF, Tsybouleva N, et al. Simvastatin induces regression of cardiac hypertrophy and fibrosis and improves cardiac function in a transgenic rabbit model of human hypertrophic cardiomyopathy. Circulation 2001;104:317.

57. Tavazzi L, Maggioni AP, Marchioli R, et al. Effect of rosuvastatin in patients with chronic heart failure (the GISSI-HF trial): a randomised, double-blind, placebo-controlled trial. Lancet 2008;372:1231.

58. Ronco C, Haapio M, House AA, et al. Cardiorenal syndrome. J Am Coll Cardiol 2008;52:1527.

59. Liang KV, Williams AW, Greene EL, et al. Acute decompensated heart failure and the cardiorenal syndrome. Crit Care Med 2008;36:S75.

60. Mebazaa A, Gheorghiade M, Pina IL, et al. Practical recommendations for prehospital and early in-hospital management of patients presenting with acute heart failure syndromes. Crit Care Med 2008;36:S129.

61. Mullens W, Abrahams Z, Francis GS, et al. Importance of venous congestion for worsening of renal function in advanced decompensated heart failure. J Am Coll Cardiol 2009;53:589.

62. Goldstein SL. Overview of pediatric renal replacement therapy in acute kidney injury. Semin Dial 2009;22:180.

63. Foley RN, Parfrey PS, Sarnak MJ. Clinical epidemiology of cardiovascular disease in chronic renal disease. Am J Kidney Dis 1998;32:S112.

64. Hillege HL, Nitsch D, Pfeffer MA, et al. Renal function as a predictor of outcome in a broad spectrum of patients with heart failure. Circulation 2006;113:671.

65. Shlipak MG, Smith GL, Rathore SS, et al. Renal function, digoxin therapy, and heart failure outcomes: evidence from the digoxin intervention group trial. J Am Soc Nephrol 2004;15:2195.

66. Dent CL, Ma Q, Dastrala S, et al. Plasma neutrophil gelatinase-associated lipocalin predicts acute kidney injury, morbidity and mortality after pediatric cardiac surgery: a prospective uncontrolled cohort study. Crit Care 2007;11:R127.

67. Price JF, Mott AR, Dickerson HA, et al. Worsening renal function in children hospitalized with decompensated heart failure: evidence for a pediatric cardiorenal syndrome? Pediatr Crit Care Med 2008;9:279.

68. Devarajan P. The future of pediatric acute kidney injury management–biomarkers. Semin Nephrol 2008;28:493.

69. Nickolas TL, Barasch J, Devarajan P. Biomarkers in acute and chronic kidney disease. Curr Opin Nephrol Hypertens 2008;17:127.

70. Allen LA, Felker GM, Pocock S, et al. Liver function abnormalities and outcome in patients with chronic heart failure: data from the Candesartan in Heart Failure: Assessment of Reduction in Mortality and

Morbidity (CHARM) program. Eur J Heart Fail 2009;11:170.

71. Kubo SH, Walter BA, John DH, et al. Liver function abnormalities in chronic heart failure. Influence of systemic hemodynamics. Arch Intern Med 1987; 147:1227.

72. Lau GT, Tan HC, Kritharides L. Type of liver dysfunction in heart failure and its relation to the severity of tricuspid regurgitation. Am J Cardiol 2002;90:1405.

73. van Deursen VM, Damman K, Hillege HL, et al. Abnormal liver function in relation to hemodynamic profile in heart failure patients. J Card Fail 2010;16:84.

74. Ceppa EP, Fuh KC, Bulkley GB. Mesenteric hemodynamic response to circulatory shock. Curr Opin Crit Care 2003;9:127.

75. Reilly PM, Toung TJ, Miyachi M, et al. Hemodynamics of pancreatic ischemia in cardiogenic shock in pigs. Gastroenterology 1997;113:938.

76. Gunther S, Gimbrone MA Jr, Alexander RW. Identification and characterization of the high affinity vascular angiotensin II receptor in rat mesenteric artery. Circ Res 1980;47:278.

77. Myers RP, Cerini R, Sayegh R, et al. Cardiac hepatopathy: clinical, hemodynamic, and histologic characteristics and correlations. Hepatology 2003;37:393.

78. Baik SK, Fouad TR, Lee SS. Cirrhotic cardiomyopathy. Orphanet J Rare Dis 2007;2:15.

79. Tang YD, Katz SD. Anemia in chronic heart failure: prevalence, etiology, clinical correlates, and treatment options. Circulation 2006;113:2454.

80. Felker GM, Shaw LK, Stough WG, et al. Anemia in patients with heart failure and preserved systolic function. Am Heart J 2006;151:457.

81. He SW, Wang LX. The impact of anemia on the prognosis of chronic heart failure: a meta-analysis and systemic review. Congest Heart Fail 2009;15: 123.

82. Drakos SG, Anastasiou-Nana MI, Malliaras KG, et al. Anemia in chronic heart failure. Congest Heart Fail 2009;15:87.

83. Witte KK, Desilva R, Chattopadhyay S, et al. Are hematinic deficiencies the cause of anemia in chronic heart failure? Am Heart J 2004;147:924.

84. Nanas JN, Matsouka C, Karageorgopoulos D, et al. Etiology of anemia in patients with advanced heart failure. J Am Coll Cardiol 2006;48:2485.

85. McCullough PA, Lepor NE. Anemia: a modifiable risk factor for heart disease. Introduction. Rev Cardiovasc Med 2005;6(Suppl 3):S1.

86. Weiss G, Goodnough LT. Anemia of chronic disease. N Engl J Med 2005;352:1011.

87. Schall RR, Petrucci RJ, Brozena SC, et al. Cognitive function in patients with symptomatic dilated cardiomyopathy before and after cardiac transplantation. J Am Coll Cardiol 1989;14:1666.

88. Petrucci RJ, Wright S, Naka Y, et al. Neurocognitive assessments in advanced heart failure patients receiving continuous-flow left ventricular assist devices. J Heart Lung Transplant 2009;28:542.

89. Caplan LR. Cardiac encephalopathy and congestive heart failure: a hypothesis about the relationship. Neurology 2006;66:99.

90. Thom T, Haase N, Rosamond W, et al. Heart disease and stroke statistics–2006 update: a report from the American Heart Association Statistics Committee and Stroke Statistics Subcommittee. Circulation 2006;113:e85.

91. Gelb BD, Garson A Jr. Noninvasive discrimination of right atrial ectopic tachycardia from sinus tachycardia in "dilated cardiomyopathy". Am Heart J 1990;120:886.

92. Doval HC, Nul DR, Grancelli HO, et al. Randomised trial of low-dose amiodarone in severe congestive heart failure. Grupo de Estudio de la Sobrevida en la Insuficiencia Cardiaca en Argentina (GESICA). Lancet 1994;344:493.

93. Dao Q, Krishnaswamy P, Kazanegra R, et al. Utility of B-type natriuretic peptide in the diagnosis of congestive heart failure in an urgent-care setting. J Am Coll Cardiol 2001;37:379.

94. Maisel AS, Krishnaswamy P, Nowak RM, et al. Rapid measurement of B-type natriuretic peptide in the emergency diagnosis of heart failure. N Engl J Med 2002;347:161.

95. McCullough PA, Nowak RM, McCord J, et al. B-type natriuretic peptide and clinical judgment in emergency diagnosis of heart failure: analysis from Breathing Not Properly (BNP) Multinational Study. Circulation 2002;106:416.

96. Mir TS, Marohn S, Laer S, et al. Plasma concentrations of N-terminal pro-brain natriuretic peptide in control children from the neonatal to adolescent period and in children with congestive heart failure. Pediatrics 2002;110:e76.

97. Westerlind A, Wahlander H, Lindstedt G, et al. Clinical signs of heart failure are associated with increased levels of natriuretic peptide types B and A in children with congenital heart defects or cardiomyopathy. Acta Paediatr 2004;93:340.

98. Grady KL, Dracup K, Kennedy G, et al. Team management of patients with heart failure: a statement for healthcare professionals from the Cardiovascular Nursing Council of the American Heart Association. Circulation 2000;102:2443.

99. Wilson JR, Reichek N, Dunkman WB, et al. Effect of diuresis on the performance of the failing left ventricle in man. Am J Med 1981;70:234.

100. Stevenson LW, Brunken RC, Belil D, et al. Afterload reduction with vasodilators and diuretics decreases mitral regurgitation during upright exercise in advanced heart failure. J Am Coll Cardiol 1990;15:174.

101. Butler J, Young JB, Abraham WT, et al. Beta-blocker use and outcomes among hospitalized heart failure patients. J Am Coll Cardiol 2006;47:2462.

102. Nohria A, Tsang SW, Fang JC, et al. Clinical assessment identifies hemodynamic profiles that predict outcomes in patients admitted with heart failure. J Am Coll Cardiol 2003;41:1797.

103. Sackner-Bernstein JD. Management of diuretic-refractory, volume-overloaded patients with acutely decompensated heart failure. Curr Cardiol Rep 2005;7:204.

104. Guiha NH, Cohn JN, Mikulic E, et al. Treatment of refractory heart failure with infusion of nitroprusside. N Engl J Med 1974;291:587.

105. Sackner-Bernstein JD, Kowalski M, Fox M, et al. Short-term risk of death after treatment with nesiritide for decompensated heart failure: a pooled analysis of randomized controlled trials. JAMA 2005;293:1900.

106. Sackner-Bernstein JD, Skopicki HA, Aaronson KD. Risk of worsening renal function with nesiritide in patients with acutely decompensated heart failure. Circulation 2005;111:1487.

107. Bailey JM, Miller BE, Lu W, et al. The pharmacokinetics of milrinone in pediatric patients after cardiac surgery. Anesthesiology 1999;90:1012.

108. Chang AC, Atz AM, Wernovsky G, et al. Milrinone: systemic and pulmonary hemodynamic effects in neonates after cardiac surgery. Crit Care Med 1995;23:1907.

109. Anderson JL. Hemodynamic and clinical benefits with intravenous milrinone in severe chronic heart failure: results of a multicenter study in the United States. Am Heart J 1991;121:1956.

110. Cuffe MS, Califf RM, Adams KF Jr, et al. Short-term intravenous milrinone for acute exacerbation of chronic heart failure: a randomized controlled trial. JAMA 2002;287:1541.

111. Felker GM, Benza RL, Chandler AB, et al. Heart failure etiology and response to milrinone in decompensated heart failure: results from the OPTIME-CHF study. J Am Coll Cardiol 2003;41:997.

112. Seino Y, Momomura S, Takano T, et al. Multicenter, double-blind study of intravenous milrinone for patients with acute heart failure in Japan. Japan Intravenous Milrinone Investigators. Crit Care Med 1996;24:1490.

113. Packer M, Carver JR, Rodeheffer RJ, et al. Effect of oral milrinone on mortality in severe chronic heart failure. The PROMISE Study Research Group. N Engl J Med 1991;325:1468.

114. Adamopoulos S, Piepoli M, Qiang F, et al. Effects of pulsed beta-stimulant therapy on beta-adrenoceptors and chronotropic responsiveness in chronic heart failure. Lancet 1995;345:344.

115. Biddle TL, Benotti JR, Creager MA, et al. Comparison of intravenous milrinone and dobutamine for congestive heart failure secondary to either ischemic or dilated cardiomyopathy. Am J Cardiol 1987;59:1345.

116. Schulz R, Rose J, Martin C, et al. Development of short-term myocardial hibernation. Its limitation by the severity of ischemia and inotropic stimulation. Circulation 1993;88:684.

117. Hampton JR, van Veldhuisen DJ, Kleber FX, et al. Randomised study of effect of ibopamine on survival in patients with advanced severe heart failure. Second Prospective Randomised Study of Ibopamine on Mortality and Efficacy (PRIME II) Investigators. Lancet 1997;349:971.

118. Kay JH, Blalock A. The use of calcium chloride in the treatment of cardiac arrest in patients. Surg Gynecol Obstet 1951;93:97.

119. Schwartz SM, Duffy JY, Pearl JM, et al. Cellular and molecular aspects of myocardial dysfunction. Crit Care Med 2001;29:S214.

120. Lang RM, Fellner SK, Neumann A, et al. Left ventricular contractility varies directly with blood ionized calcium. Ann Intern Med 1988;108:524.

121. Katz AM. Potential deleterious effects of inotropic agents in the therapy of chronic heart failure. Circulation 1986;73:III184.

122. Wenzel V, Krismer AC, Arntz HR, et al. A comparison of vasopressin and epinephrine for out-of-hospital cardiopulmonary resuscitation. N Engl J Med 2004;350:105.

123. Price JF, Towbin JA, Denfield SW, et al. Arginine vasopressin levels are elevated and correlate with functional status in infants and children with congestive heart failure. Circulation 2004;109:2550.

124. Xu YJ, Gopalakrishnan V. Vasopressin increases cytosolic free [Ca^{2+}] in the neonatal rat cardiomyocyte. Evidence for V1 subtype receptors. Circ Res 1991;69:239.

125. Luckner G, Dunser MW, Jochberger S, et al. Arginine vasopressin in 316 patients with advanced vasodilatory shock. Crit Care Med 2005;33:2659.

126. Rosenzweig EB, Starc TJ, Chen JM, et al. Intravenous arginine-vasopressin in children with vasodilatory shock after cardiac surgery. Circulation 1999;100:II182.

127. Gwathmey JK, Copelas L, MacKinnon R, et al. Abnormal intracellular calcium handling in myocardium from patients with end-stage heart failure. Circ Res 1987;61:70.

128. Felker GM, O'Connor CM. Inotropic therapy for heart failure: an evidence-based approach. Am Heart J 2001;142:393.

129. Ukkonen H, Saraste M, Akkila J, et al. Myocardial efficiency during levosimendan infusion in congestive heart failure. Clin Pharmacol Ther 2000;68:522.

130. Braun JP, Schneider M, Dohmen P, et al. Successful treatment of dilative cardiomyopathy in a 12-year-old girl using the calcium sensitizer

levosimendan after weaning from mechanical bi-ventricular assist support. J Cardiothorac Vasc Anesth 2004;18:772.

131. Braun JP, Schneider M, Kastrup M, et al. Treatment of acute heart failure in an infant after cardiac surgery using levosimendan. Eur J Cardiothorac Surg 2004;26:228.

132. Parr GV, Blackstone EH, Kirklin JW. Cardiac performance and mortality early after intracardiac surgery in infants and young children. Circulation 1975;51:867.

133. Bellinger DC, Wypij D, Kuban KC, et al. Developmental and neurological status of children at 4 years of age after heart surgery with hypothermic circulatory arrest or low-flow cardiopulmonary bypass. Circulation 1999;100:526.

134. Li J, Schulze-Neick I, Lincoln C, et al. Oxygen consumption after cardiopulmonary bypass surgery in children: determinants and implications. J Thorac Cardiovasc Surg 2000;119:525.

135. Moat NE, Lamb RK, Edwards JC, et al. Induced hypothermia in the management of refractory low cardiac output states following cardiac surgery in infants and children. Eur J Cardiothorac Surg 1992;6:579.

136. Dalrymple-Hay MJ, Deakin CD, Knight H, et al. Induced hypothermia as salvage treatment for refractory cardiac failure following paediatric cardiac surgery. Eur J Cardiothorac Surg 1999; 15:515.

137. Deakin CD, Knight H, Edwards JC, et al. Induced hypothermia in the postoperative management of refractory cardiac failure following paediatric cardiac surgery. Anaesthesia 1998;53:848.

138. Hoffman TM, Wernovsky G, Wieand TS, et al. The incidence of arrhythmias in a pediatric cardiac intensive care unit. Pediatr Cardiol 2002;23:598.

139. Hoffman TM, Bush DM, Wernovsky G, et al. Postoperative junctional ectopic tachycardia in children: incidence, risk factors, and treatment. Ann Thorac Surg 2002;74:1607.

140. Raja P, Hawker RE, Chaikitpinyo A, et al. Amiodarone management of junctional ectopic tachycardia after cardiac surgery in children. Br Heart J 1994; 72:261.

141. Walsh EP, Saul JP, Sholler GF, et al. Evaluation of a staged treatment protocol for rapid automatic junctional tachycardia after operation for congenital heart disease. J Am Coll Cardiol 1997;29:1046.

142. Ramamoorthy C, Anderson GD, Williams GD, et al. Pharmacokinetics and side effects of milrinone in infants and children after open heart surgery. Anesth Analg 1998;86:283.

143. Lindsay CA, Barton P, Lawless S, et al. Pharmacokinetics and pharmacodynamics of milrinone lactate in pediatric patients with septic shock. J Pediatr 1998;132:329.

144. Zuppa AF, Nicolson SC, Adamson PC, et al. Population pharmacokinetics of milrinone in neonates with hypoplastic left heart syndrome undergoing stage I reconstruction. Anesth Analg 2006;102:1062.

145. Bettendorf M, Schmidt KG, Grulich-Henn J, et al. Tri-iodothyronine treatment in children after cardiac surgery: a double-blind, randomised, placebo-controlled study. Lancet 2000;356:529.

146. Portman MA, Fearneyhough C, Ning XH, et al. Triiodothyronine repletion in infants during cardiopulmonary bypass for congenital heart disease. J Thorac Cardiovasc Surg 2000;120:604.

147. Carrel T, Eckstein F, Englberger L, et al. Thyronin treatment in adult and pediatric heart surgery: clinical experience and review of the literature. Eur J Heart Fail 2002;4:577.

148. Argenziano M, Choudhri AF, Oz MC, et al. A prospective randomized trial of arginine vasopressin in the treatment of vasodilatory shock after left ventricular assist device placement. Circulation 1997;96(Suppl 9):II286–90.

149. Morales DL, Gregg D, Helman DN, et al. Arginine vasopressin in the treatment of 50 patients with postcardiotomy vasodilatory shock. Ann Thorac Surg 2000;69:102.

150. O'Blenes SB, Roy N, Konstantinov I, et al. Vasopressin reversal of phenoxybenzamine-induced hypotension after the Norwood procedure. J Thorac Cardiovasc Surg 2002;123:1012.

151. Shore S, Nelson DP, Pearl JM, et al. Usefulness of corticosteroid therapy in decreasing epinephrine requirements in critically ill infants with congenital heart disease. Am J Cardiol 2001;88:591.

152. Liu JP, Robinson PJ, Funder JW, et al. The biosynthesis and secretion of adrenocorticotropin by the ovine anterior pituitary is predominantly regulated by arginine vasopressin (AVP). Evidence that protein kinase C mediates the action of AVP. J Biol Chem 1990;265:14136.

153. Tweddell JS, Hoffman GM, Fedderly RT, et al. Phenoxybenzamine improves systemic oxygen delivery after the Norwood procedure. Ann Thorac Surg 1999;67:161.

154. Rossi AF, Sommer RJ, Lotvin A, et al. Usefulness of intermittent monitoring of mixed venous oxygen saturation after stage I palliation for hypoplastic left heart syndrome. Am J Cardiol 1994;73:1118.

155. Chaturvedi RR, Shore DF, Lincoln C, et al. Acute right ventricular restrictive physiology after repair of tetralogy of Fallot: association with myocardial injury and oxidative stress. Circulation 1999;100:1540.

156. Shekerdemian LS, Bush A, Shore DF, et al. Cardiopulmonary interactions after Fontan operations: augmentation of cardiac output using negative pressure ventilation. Circulation 1997;96:3934.

157. Shekerdemian LS, Bush A, Shore DF, et al. Cardio-respiratory responses to negative pressure ventilation after tetralogy of Fallot repair: a hemodynamic tool for patients with a low-output state. J Am Coll Cardiol 1999;33:549.

158. Shekerdemian LS, Shore DF, Lincoln C, et al. Negative-pressure ventilation improves cardiac output after right heart surgery. Circulation 1996;94:II49.

159. Bridges ND, Mayer JE Jr, Lock JE, et al. Effect of baffle fenestration on outcome of the modified Fontan operation. Circulation 1992;86:1762.

160. Cheifetz IM, Craig DM, Quick G, et al. Increasing tidal volumes and pulmonary overdistention adversely affect pulmonary vascular mechanics and cardiac output in a pediatric swine model. Crit Care Med 1998;26:710.

161. Meliones J, Kocis K, Bengur AR, et al. Diastolic function in neonates after the arterial switch operation: effects of positive pressure ventilation and inspiratory time. Intensive Care Med 2000;26:950.

162. Meliones JN, Bove EL, Dekeon MK, et al. High-frequency jet ventilation improves cardiac function after the Fontan procedure. Circulation 1991;84:III364.

163. Tabbutt S, Ramamoorthy C, Montenegro LM, et al. Impact of inspired gas mixtures on preoperative infants with hypoplastic left heart syndrome during controlled ventilation. Circulation 2001;104:I159.

164. Norwood WI, Kirklin JK, Sanders SP. Hypoplastic left heart syndrome: experience with palliative surgery. Am J Cardiol 1980;45:87.

165. Norwood WI, Lang P, Casteneda AR, et al. Experience with operations for hypoplastic left heart syndrome. J Thorac Cardiovasc Surg 1981;82:511.

166. Norwood WI, Lang P, Hansen DD. Physiologic repair of aortic atresia-hypoplastic left heart syndrome. N Engl J Med 1983;308:23.

167. Tweddell JS, Hoffman GM, Mussatto KA, et al. Improved survival of patients undergoing palliation of hypoplastic left heart syndrome: lessons learned from 115 consecutive patients. Circulation 2002;106:I82.

168. Malec E, Januszewska K, Kolcz J, et al. Right ventricle-to-pulmonary artery shunt versus modified Blalock-Taussig shunt in the Norwood procedure for hypoplastic left heart syndrome–influence on early and late haemodynamic status. Eur J Cardiothorac Surg 2003;23:728.

169. Nelson DP, Schwartz SM, Chang AC. Neonatal physiology of the functionally univentricular heart. Cardiol Young 2004;14(Suppl 1):52.

170. Scherurer M. Survival and clinical course at Fontan after stage one palliation with either a modified Blalock-Taussig shunt or a right ventricle to pulmonary artery conduit. J Am Coll Cardiol 2008;52:52.

171. Galantowicz M, Cheatham JP. Lessons learned from the development of a new hybrid strategy for the management of hypoplastic left heart syndrome. Pediatr Cardiol 2005;26:190.

172. Galantowicz M, Cheatham JP, Phillips A, et al. Hybrid approach for hypoplastic left heart syndrome: intermediate results after the learning curve. Ann Thorac Surg 2008;85:2063.

173. Li J, Zhang G, Benson L, et al. Comparison of the profiles of postoperative systemic hemodynamics and oxygen transport in neonates after the hybrid or the Norwood procedure: a pilot study. Circulation 2007;116:I179.

174. Hsu DT, Pearson GD. Heart failure in children: part I: history, etiology, and pathophysiology. Circ Heart Fail 2009;2:63.

175. Hsu DT, Pearson GD. Heart failure in children: part II: diagnosis, treatment, and future directions. Circ Heart Fail 2009;2:490.

176. Cheung YF, Penny DJ, Redington AN. Serial assessment of left ventricular diastolic function after Fontan procedure. Heart 2000;83:420.

177. Gentles TL, Mayer JE Jr, Gauvreau K, et al. Fontan operation in five hundred consecutive patients: factors influencing early and late outcome. J Thorac Cardiovasc Surg 1997;114:376.

178. Weipert J. Occurrence and management of atrial arrhythmia after long-term Fontan circulation. J Thorac Cardiovasc Surg 2004;127:457.

179. Khairy P. Long-term survival, modes of death, and predictors of mortality in patients with Fontan surgery. Circulation 2008;117:85.

180. Fiore AC, Turrentine M, Rodefeld M, et al. Fontan operation: a comparison of lateral tunnel with extracardiac conduit. Ann Thorac Surg 2007;83:622.

181. Giannico S, Hammad F, Amodeo A, et al. Clinical outcome of 193 extracardiac Fontan patients: the first 15 years. J Am Coll Cardiol 2006;47:2065.

182. Cohen MI, Bridges ND, Gaynor JW, et al. Modifications to the cavopulmonary anastomosis do not eliminate early sinus node dysfunction. J Thorac Cardiovasc Surg 2000;120:891.

183. Shirai LK, Rosenthal DN, Reitz BA, et al. Arrhythmias and thromboembolic complications after the extracardiac Fontan operation. J Thorac Cardiovasc Surg 1998;115:499.

184. Ghai A, Harris L, Harrison DA, et al. Outcomes of late atrial tachyarrhythmias in adults after the Fontan operation. J Am Coll Cardiol 2001;37:585.

185. Abraham WT, Fisher WG, Smith AL, et al. Cardiac resynchronization in chronic heart failure. N Engl J Med 2002;346:1845.

186. Bristow MR, Saxon LA, Boehmer J, et al. Cardiac-resynchronization therapy with or without an implantable defibrillator in advanced chronic heart failure. N Engl J Med 2004;350:2140.

187. Dubin AM, Janousek J, Rhee E, et al. Resynchronization therapy in pediatric and congenital heart

disease patients: an international multicenter study. J Am Coll Cardiol 2005;46:2277.

188. Jefferies JL, Denfield SW, Price JF, et al. A prospective evaluation of nesiritide in the treatment of pediatric heart failure. Pediatr Cardiol 2006;27:402.

189. Hernandez AF, O'Connor CM, Starling RC, et al. Rationale and design of the Acute Study of Clinical Effectiveness of Nesiritide in Decompensated Heart Failure Trial (ASCEND-HF). Am Heart J 2009;157:271.

190. Gheorghiade M, Pang PS. Acute heart failure syndromes. J Am Coll Cardiol 2009;53:557.

191. Follath F, Cleland JG, Just H, et al. Efficacy and safety of intravenous levosimendan compared with dobutamine in severe low-output heart failure (the LIDO study): a randomised double-blind trial. Lancet 2002;360:196.

192. Nawarskas JJ, Anderson JR. Levosimendan: a unique approach to the treatment of heart failure. Heart Dis 2002;4:265.

193. Slawsky MT, Colucci WS, Gottlieb SS, et al. Acute hemodynamic and clinical effects of levosimendan in patients with severe heart failure. Study Investigators. Circulation 2000;102:2222.

194. Cleland JG, McGowan J. Levosimendan: a new era for inodilator therapy for heart failure? Curr Opin Cardiol 2002;17:257.

195. Costanzo MR. Ultrafiltration in the management of heart failure. Curr Opin Crit Care 2008;14:524.

Mechanical Support in Childhood Heart Failure

John Lynn Jefferies, MD, MPH[a,b,]*, Jack F. Price, MD[c],
David L.S. Morales, MD[d,e]

KEYWORDS

- Pediatric • Mechanical support
- Ventricular assist devices • Heart failure

Despite optimization of standard medical therapy, some patients with chronic heart failure (HF) will deteriorate clinically to a point that they require hospitalization for intravenous therapies and inpatient monitoring. The clinical spectrum of decompensated HF ranges from the outpatient who is seen in clinic with subtle signs such as worsening peripheral edema to the child presenting to the emergency department in life-threatening cardiogenic shock. Once the condition is recognized, the fundamental therapeutic goals are the same when managing patients with this very challenging clinical syndrome: reverse hemodynamic derangements, correct metabolic abnormalities, and provide symptomatic relief.

Achievement of these goals requires individualized care and a familiarity with the risks and benefits of particular therapies. Most of the data and insight relied upon for managing patients with advanced HF have been derived from studies and experience in adults, most of whom have an ischemic etiology for their left ventricular (LV) dysfunction. Because there are no formal recommendations for the treatment of advanced HF in children, one must heed the findings of adult trials, reflect on reliable anecdotal experience, and respect the principle that one should first do no harm.

Intravenous loop diuretics are considered first-line therapy for decompensated HF. Frequently, patients will require a combination of diuretic and intravenous afterload reduction (eg, nitroprusside or nitroglycerin) to lower filling pressures and achieve symptomatic relief. Patients with decompensated HF and reduced blood pressure with normal or low systemic vascular resistance may not benefit from vasodilators and should therefore be considered for inotropic therapy. In these patients, inotropic agents may be necessary to maintain circulatory function, relieve symptoms, and improve end-organ function. The Heart Failure

Dr David Morales serves as the Director of the North American Training and Reference Center for the Berlin Heart Pediatric EXCOR VAD (0% effort) and as the coinvestigator for the Berlin Heart Pediatric EXCOR VAD IDE trial, for which Texas Children's Hospital is the coordinating center. Berlin Heart, Incorporated (Berlin Heart Inc, Berlin, Germany) provides compensation to Baylor College of Medicine for Dr Morale's services as a Reference and Training Center Faculty Member. Berlin Heart, Incorporated also provides administrative support for the trial and offsets travel expenses related to the trial and reference center. Dr Morales receives no direct personal compensation.

[a] Cardiomyopathy and Heart Failure, Cardiovascular Genetics Service, Pediatric Cardiology, Texas Children's Hospital, Baylor College of Medicine, Houston, TX, USA
[b] Adult Cardiovascular Diseases, Texas Heart Institute at St Luke's Episcopal Hospital, Baylor College of Medicine, Houston, TX, USA
[c] Texas Children's Hospital, Baylor College of Medicine, Houston, TX, USA
[d] Mechanical Circulatory Support, Clinical and Industrial Research, Congenital Heart Surgery, Congenital Heart Surgery Service, Texas Children's Hospital, Baylor College of Medicine, Houston, TX, USA
[e] Surgery and Pediatrics, Baylor College of Medicine Houston, TX, USA
* Corresponding author. Adult Cardiovascular Diseases, Texas Heart Institute at St Luke's Episcopal Hospital, Baylor College of Medicine, Houston, TX.
E-mail address: jlj@bcm.tmc.edu

Heart Failure Clin 6 (2010) 559–573
doi:10.1016/j.hfc.2010.06.004
1551-7136/10/$ – see front matter © 2010 Elsevier Inc. All rights reserved.

Society of America states that intravenous inotropes are not recommended unless left heart filling pressures are known to be elevated based on direct measurement or clear clinical signs.[1]

Despite optimal medical therapy, some children progress to refractory end-stage HF and low cardiac output syndrome. Mechanical circulatory support may be the only therapeutic option remaining for those patients who are considered good candidates for heart transplantation.

INDICATIONS FOR MECHANICAL SUPPORT

Appropriate application of mechanical circulatory support (MCS) in children requires an understanding of the unique pathologic features of pediatric HF as compared with adult HF. For example, pediatric patients in systemic ventricular failure with congenital heart disease have a much higher incidence of concomitant right-sided failure and pulmonary hypertension. Unlike the right HF and pulmonary hypertension seen in adults, which is most often secondary to left HF, the pediatric pathology often can be intrinsic or anatomic. Therefore, support of the systemic ventricle in congenital heart surgery patients may not consistently translate into improvement in right heart function. Another challenge in pediatric MCS of patients with congenital heart disease can be cannulation. One must consider how the patient can be cannulated, not only in regards to what vessels or chambers to use, but how the cannulae, which at times are on opposite sides than normal (ie, patients with situs inversus), can be attached to the assist devices. Further consideration of the internal cardiac anatomy with respect to septal defects, hypoplastic chambers, and anomalous systemic and venous connections, as well as extra-cardiac anatomy (ie, aortic interruption or coarctation), must be taken into account. Some of the congenital heart defects also can complicate these patients' options in terms of support configuration (ie, biventricular assist device [BiVAD], left ventricular assist device [LVAD] extracorporeal membrane oxygenation [ECMO]) and postoperative management because of significant hypoxemia. The identification and management of systemic-to-pulmonary shunts, both surgically created (ie, Blalock-Taussig shunt) and pathologic (ie, aorto-pulmonary collateral arteries) are other necessary and often difficult steps in the MCS of patients with coronary heart disease (CHD).

Bridge to Transplantation

Most patients who undergo mechanical circulatory support as a bridge to transplantation have end-stage congenital heart disease or dilated cardiomyopathy with advanced HF. Such patients have been supported primarily with ECMO with relatively high mortality rates.[2–4] The inability of ECMO to safely bridge patients to transplant for periods longer than 2 weeks limits its applicability to the patient with end-stage HF awaiting transplant. Accordingly, there has been a shift in management of these patients from ECMO to long-term MCS when such devices are available. Use of long-term MCS in these patients has yielded favorable results, with 1- and 5-year survival rates after heart transplant of over 75% and 70%, respectively.[5–7] In Berlin, Hetzer and colleagues[8] demonstrated that bridging such patients to transplant with MCS resulted in statistically similar survival rates at 1 and 5 years in patients treated with inotropes before transplant or in those electively awaiting transplant. The Pediatric Heart Transplant Study Investigators recently reported multi-institutional data for 99 pediatric patients supported with ventricular assist devices (VADs) with the intent to bridge to transplant.[9] They found that 77% survived to transplant; 5% gained sufficient myocardial recovery to be weaned from support, and 17% died while supported.

Bridge to Recovery

Bridge to recovery has long been an indication for MCS in children. The strategy is to support the myocardium through the acute process to achieve sufficient recovery to allow for device removal. Acute viral myocarditis, transplant graft rejection, and postcardiotomy shock are examples of potentially recoverable causes of myocardial injury. The authors have reported our use of MCS in children with acute graft rejection while treating with vigorous immunosuppressive therapies.[10] Eight children received MCS for graft rejection with hemodynamic instability for a mean duration of support of 7.5 days. Five patients were weaned from MCS to recovery, and two were bridged to transplant. Unfortunately, late survival for this cohort was poor, with a 1-year mortality rate of 50%. Mechanical support in the form of ECMO or VAD also may be used in the setting of acute myocardial inflammation such as myocarditis. The authors have successfully supported patients with viral myocarditis in their institution, with a survival rate of 80%.

An indication on the periphery of the specialty is the treatment of cardiopulmonary arrest with rapid resuscitation ECMO. The authors feel obliged to mention this indication, which initially was described by del Nido and colleagues,[11] because many have championed its use. It comprises nearly 25% of all indications for ECMO in children with cardiac disease.[12] Most feel that the successful application of MCS to resuscitate these patients is directly proportional to the timing of EMCO institution. Most centers concentrating on this effort have developed different strategies to streamline ECMO initiation, including an organized team, an ECMO circuit that is portable and easily primed, and defined clinical protocols.

The rapid resuscitation ECMO team is mobilized after 10 minutes of failed standard cardiopulmonary resuscitation. The primary goal is to establish cardiac output, which often necessitates the institution of ECMO with a crystalloid prime.[13] Others have modified the ECMO circuit by decreasing the priming volume to 250 cubic centimeters (cc) by using a hollow-fiber oxygenator, a centrifugal pump, and short tubing lengths.[14] Novel approaches such as these have resulted in more than 60% of cardiac arrest patients surviving to hospital discharge. These series have demonstrated that if institution of MCS with modified ECMO circuits is rapid and aggressive, it can be lifesaving in most pediatric cardiac patients who arrest. In those situations where it appears that myocardial recovery is unlikely to occur and transplantation is necessary, it is not unusual for a patient to be transitioned to a more long-term device several days after placement on ECMO.

CONTRAINDICATIONS TO MECHANICAL SUPPORT

Although it is important to consider each patient individually, extreme prematurity, very low birth weight (<1.5 kg), severe neurologic injury, a constellation of congenital anomalies with poor prognosis, and chromosomal aberrations are widely accepted as contraindications for MCS. Other considerations are multisystem organ failure, sepsis, and severe lung disease, although, successful support has been demonstrated in all of these scenarios.[15,16] Reversal of multisystem organ failure has been demonstrated in the adult population on VAD support many times with the reversal of liver and renal dysfunction.[17–20] In regards to pulmonary insufficiency, the etiology of the insufficiency will help determine the suitability of MCS and type of support. Severe lung disease resulting in respiratory failure should prompt consideration for ECMO, whereas cardiogenic shock-induced pulmonary edema can at times be treated with VAD support. Entertaining the use of MCS in patients with certain congenital heart diagnoses such as single-ventricle physiology and pulmonary atresia, VSD, and major aorto-pulmonary collaterals should include careful consideration for whether the patients are eventual candidates for surgical correction, transplant, or are even capable of benefiting from MCS. As the field of MCS matures, the use of terminology such as absolute and relative contraindications has begun to fade as experience, data-driven medical management, and the consideration of medical feasibility, resource allocation, and ethical issues have begun to guide the use of MCS in challenging clinical situations.

CANDIDATE SELECTION

It should be emphasized that improved results are only possible if application of MCS is early, that is, before the patient is in extremis or end-organ dysfunction is significant. That being said, appropriate timing for institution of support is particularly challenging in this group, because it is often governed by which devices are available for supporting pediatric patients and institutional experience. Careful consideration must be given to cases on an individual basis before committing to long-term support, as the surgical and postoperative management experiences with these patients and devices remain in their infancy.

No standardized candidate selection criteria have been established for MCS. Lietz and colleagues[21] have identified several preoperative clinical variables that predict postimplant mortality in adults who receive VADs as destination therapy. Thrombocytopenia (platelet count <148 K), hypoalbuminemia (<3.3 g/dL), international normalized ratio (INR) greater than 1.1, requirement for vasodilator therapy, and a mean pulmonary artery pressure less than 25 mm Hg (indicating right HF) were some of the strongest predictors of in-hospital mortality. The authors have found that among children who are hospitalized with decompensated HF, worsening renal function, as defined as a rise in serum creatinine by 0.3 mg/dL, and need for mechanical ventilation are associated with death or requirement of MCS.[22] Based on these data and anecdotal experience, the authors have created candidate selection guidelines for bridging children to transplant with MCS. Patients who are considered acceptable transplant candidates and who have demonstrated inotrope dependency are monitored closely for end-organ injury. The authors will consider instituting MCS in these patients if they demonstrate any one of the following: requirement for mechanical ventilation, inability to ambulate due to HF symptoms, inability to tolerate enteral feeds, hepatic insufficiency, or acute kidney injury. Any patient with cardiogenic shock or impending shock also is considered for MCS.

DEVICE SELECTION

The selection of a device is mainly guided by what needs to be supported (right ventricle, left ventricle, or respiratory system), the length of support anticipated, the destination of the MCS, and the devices available. Unlike the adult population, the device options for pediatric MCS are limited and thus dominate much of the decision making of when to institute MCS and in what capacity. Devices usually are categorized by the expected length of support. Short-term denotes extracorporeal MCS in the intensive care unit (ICU) with only occasional opportunities to extubate. These devices are placed for acute processes such as myocarditis, postcardiotomy ventricular dysfunction, or acute cardiac graft rejection. They are placed with the hope of bridging to cardiac recovery and LVAD explant. Long-term denotes para- or intracorporeal MCS with expected extubation, physical rehabilitation in a hospital setting, and for some devices, the potential for outpatient support. The latter allows patients the freedom to return to their lives and reduces the substantial financial and psychological burden associated with long-term inpatient management.[23] These long-term devices in children for now are used as a bridge to cardiac transplantation. The term destination therapy is used to describe the long-term support of patients who are not candidates for heart transplantation whose cardiac function is not thought to be amenable to recovery, and devices for this strategy are exclusively intracorporeal. This application is currently not an option with a pediatric-specific VAD. There is also an emerging use of devices as a bridge to decision, in which a patient presents who is not well known to an institution or has question of significant end-organ dysfunction (ie, neurologic injury) but clearly needs MCS. These patients may be supported with short-term devices (ie, RotaFlow [MAQUET GmbH and Company, Rastatt, Germany]) to resuscitate their end organs and determine if they are indeed candidates for recovery or transplant. If they are transplant candidates, these patients may be converted to a long-term device. The use of a short-term device to bridge a patient to a long-term device is termed a bridge-to-bridge strategy.

In the past, device options for pediatric patients were essentially adult VADs placed in oversized adolescents, and only very recently have there been pediatric VADs, which are devices specifically designed for children. However, the direction and subsequent progress made in adult VAD technology to reduce the size of the pump (ie, axial flow and centrifugal flow pumps) have allowed more appropriate-sized devices to be used in children. This is especially true in short-term devices such as the RotaFlow, TandemHeart (CardiacAssist, Incorporated, Pittsburgh, PA, USA), and Levitronix CentriMag (Levitronix, Waltham, MA, USA). Also, smaller long-term devices such as the HeartMate II (Thoratec Corporation, Pleasanton, CA, USA) have been used in many adolescents. Most importantly, in 2004, the Berlin Heart EXCOR (BerlinHeart GmbH, Berlin, Germany) became the first pediatric-specific long-term VAD to gain widespread use throughout North America as a bridge to transplant for infants and small children. Currently, an Investigational device exemption (IDE) multi-institutional clinical trial is underway to access the efficacy and safety profile of the Berlin Heart EXCOR as a bridge to transplant.

Important in device selection is the decision whether a child requires right ventricular assist device (RVAD) support, LVAD support, or BiVAD support. This decision is critical, since it is well accepted that placement of an LVAD and the need to return to the operating room for RVAD placement result in significantly higher mortality than if a BiVAD was placed at the initial procedure. Many of the parameters studied in adults to determine the need for RVAD do not necessarily apply to children, and almost all noncongenital heart disease children can be managed with LVAD therapy only. There are two growing pediatric cohorts that have proven difficult to manage with LVAD therapy alone: patients with chronic or unremitting acute cardiac graft rejection and those with failing Fontan circulations. The experience supporting these patients is sparse, and the results are inconsistent.[3,24] The authors have supported over seven patients with acute rejection; however, the patients in whom the authors have not been able to control the rejection, have done poorly. The authors feel that both of these cohorts may be better served by a total artificial heart such as the smaller version of the CardioWest Total Artificial Heart (**Fig. 1**) being developed by SynCardia Systems, Incorporated (Tucson, AZ, USA). This device will hopefully support patients down to a body surface area (BSA) of 1 or 1.2 m^2.

The current device selection strategy at Texas Children's Hospital is illustrated in **Fig. 2**.

Short-Term Devices

ECMO

ECMO has been applied over 10,000 times since the early 1970s in newborns and has become the mainstay of MCS for the pediatric population. This type of MCS not only provides biventricular and complete respiratory support (ie, oxygenation

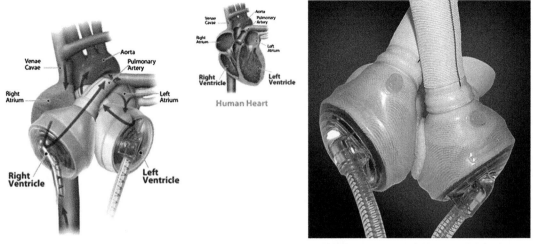

Fig. 1. CardioWest Total Artificial Heart. (*Courtesy of* SynCardia Systems, Incorporated, Tucson, AZ.)

and ventilation), but can also be easily and rapidly employed through central or peripheral cannulation to a child of almost any size.

The authors' belief is that ECMO is for cardiopulmonary support, which should only be used for patients with severe cardiac and respiratory failure. Therefore, the authors only employ ECMO in primary cardiac patients if they are arresting or present late to the authors' institution with respiratory failure that cannot be managed with a ventilator. Therefore, even if a patient is initially managed on ECMO, the authors will convert them to a short- or long-term VAD as soon as their lungs will permit, especially if they are being bridged to transplant. The authors firmly believe that ECMO should not be used to support children with HF. A more complete description of ECMO in pediatric populations can be found elsewhere.

Centrifugal VADs

Centrifugal pumps are the most commonly used cardiac assist devices, owing to their wide availability, relative simplicity of operation,

accommodation of all patient sizes, and low cost. The same centrifugal pump models used in pediatric VAD support are routinely used for ECMO and cardiopulmonary bypass as well, creating a need for clarity when analyzing outcomes of centrifugal pump support. Centrifugal VADs are extracorporeal and almost always require central cannulation via thoracotomy or sternotomy; however, a percutaneous system does exist. The pumping mechanism for centrifugal pumps involves channeling blood axially through a vortex created by a rotating component.[6] The blood exits the pump peripherally in a nonpulsatile fashion. The mode of operation is asynchronous; that is, the pumps are programmed to pump per unit time regardless of volume or native heart contraction. The centrifugal pump design reduces the risk of trauma to blood cells and generates less of an inflammatory response than pneumatic-chamber or pusher-plate VADs.[25,26] As with ECMO, a major shortcoming of centrifugal VADs available for children is their inability to support patients outside of the ICU

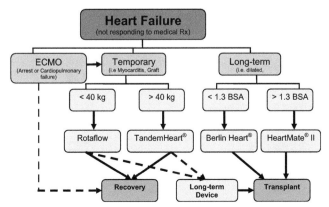

Fig. 2. Device selection strategy. (*Courtesy of* Texas Children's Hospital, Houston, TX.)

setting. These devices certainly do not allow the freedom of long-term devices to rehabilitate or be discharged from hospital, lacking durability much beyond 14 to 16 days.[27]

The following is a list of three short-term VADs that we have used at the authors' institution over the past 5 years, as well as the Levitronix, which is quite similar to the RotaFlow and has been used by others especially in Europe for supporting children.

BioMedicus BP-50 The BioMedicus Bio-Pump (Medtronic, Minneapolis, MN, USA) (**Fig. 3**) is the most common centrifugal pump used for VAD support in children. It can be used for left, right, or biventricular assistance. It is uniquely suited for the smallest of the pediatric population owing to a small-caliber pump featured in the BioMedicus line, the BP-50, so named for the volume of blood the pump head accommodates, 50 cc. Heparin-coated tubing is available with this system, reducing some of the burden of systemic anticoagulation. Thuys and colleagues[27] reported their experience with infants and children below 6 kg body weight. The weaning rate was 63%. Of those weaned, 64% were discharged from the hospital (40% of total), and 79% of these were alive 1 year later (31% overall). Survivors suffered no permanent renal, neurologic, or vascular injury.

Levitronix CentriMag The Levitronix CentriMag (**Fig. 4**) is a centrifugal pump marketed commercially in Europe but available in the United States as an investigational device only. It has been used in many pediatric patients as temporary support especially in Europe. It can be used as a left, right, or biventricular assist device. The pump employs a magnetically levitated spinning impeller to create the centrifugal force. A lack of rotating bearings reduces turbulent flow, stagnation, and potential thrombus formation as well as hemolysis. There have been reports of 100% (five patients) survival (80% to transplant) with the use of Levitronix CentriMag in the pediatric population for bridge to decision or recovery.[12]

Jostra RotaFlow Centrifugal Pump The RotaFlow (**Fig. 5**) is the next-generation temporary centrifugal VAD that can support patients of all sizes. The diameter of the pump is 50 mm, and it can provide flow rates ranging from 0 to 10 L/min and be used for as an LVAD, RVAD, or BiVAD. The pump's rotating mechanism is levitated in three magnetic fields with one point bearing, similar technology to the Levitronix. This enables laminar flow immediately and reduces wear. This combination of mechanical and magnetic bearings reduces mechanical friction, heat production, and the potential for clotting. Bennett and colleagues[28] demonstrated that when evaluated for short-term

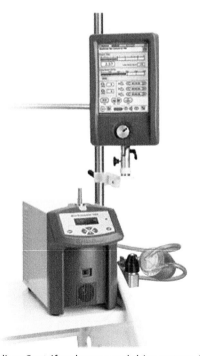
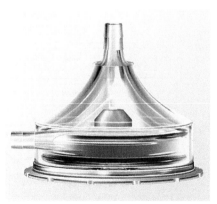

Fig. 3. BioMedicus Centrifugal pump and drive system. (*Courtesy of* Medtronic, Incorporated, Minneapolis, MN.)

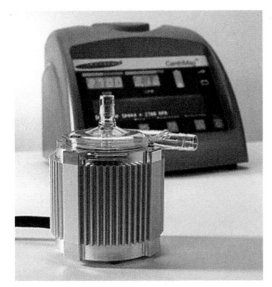

Fig. 4. Levitronix CentriMag pump in a bearing less motor system. (*Courtesy of* Levitronix LLC, Waltham, MA.)

VAD support, RotaFlow pumps show significantly less hemolysis compared with BioMedicus BP-50 starting from day sixth of support.

TandemHeart TandemHeart (**Fig. 6**) is a centrifugal extra corporeal pump with a minimal priming volume (10 mL) and a flow range from 0 to 5 L/min. It has a hydrodynamic fluid bearing system that supports the spinning rotor, and there are no mechanical roller bearings. The TandemHeart has an added advantage of percutaneous cannulation, which is particularly helpful in patients with multiple prior sternotomies. Percutaneous cannulation limits use of the device to children greater than 40 kg. In the catheterization laboratory, a trans-septal extended flow cannula is placed into the left atrium via the femoral vein. This inflow cannula unloads the left heart. The outflow cannula is placed in the femoral artery either directly or via a polytetrafluroethylene (PTFE) graft sewn to the femoral artery. The latter method allows one to avoid lower extremity vascular complications, and the authors strongly recommend it for all children less than 80 kg. Recently, Pitsis and colleagues[24] reported in adults a 73% weaning rate following a TandemHeart support and a survival to discharge of 55%. Some institutions also used the pump to support patients centrally using cardiopulmonary bypass cannulae.

Long-Term

Thoratec pVAD
The Thoratec percutaneous ventricular assist device (pVAD) (**Fig. 7**) is a paracoporeal LVAD designed for adults, but until recently, it was the most common VAD placed in pediatric patients. The Thoratec pVAD has sustained a patient for over 3 years. It is US Food and Drug Administration (FDA) approved for use as a bridge to recovery and as a bridge to transplantation. The device has tilting disc valves to ensure unidirectional flow. This system features three modes of operation, asynchronous, volume-dependent (or fill mode), and synchronous. Hospital discharge and full outpatient support are possible. Regarding voluntary feedback from 184 pediatric patients placed on the pVAD, Thoratec reported that 91 were bridged to transplant, and 15 were explanted secondary to myocardial recovery for a weaning rate of 58% (67). This is an adult device used in children and not a pediatric-specific LVAD.

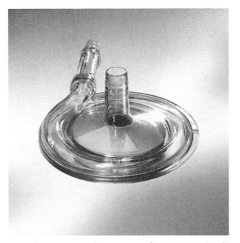

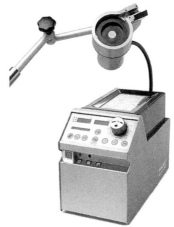

Fig. 5. Jostra RotaFlow system. (*Courtesy of* MAQUET Cardiovascular, Wayne, NJ.)

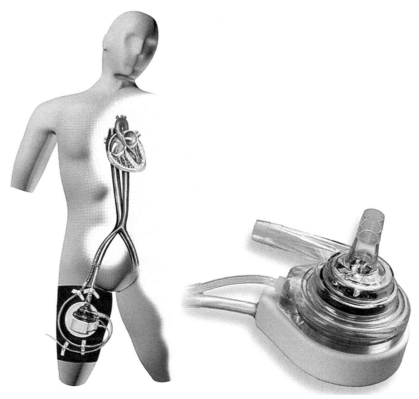

Fig. 6. TandemHeart Assist system; percutaneous device application on the left. (*Courtesy of* CardiacAssist, Incorporated, Pittsburgh, PA.)

Therefore, it is not used in small children and when used in smaller adolescents and preadolescents, it does cause significant hypertension because of the large stroke volume of 65 mL. Also, when used in smaller adolescents, the necessary decreased rate of the device heightens the concern of thromboemboic events.

Medos HIA VAD

The Medos HIA VAD (**Fig. 8**) is manufactured by Medos Medizintechnik AG (Stolberg, Germany). It has been used as MCS for 140 pediatric patients worldwide, 89 under 35 kg. The Medos system features eight different pump sizes, ranging in volume from 9 to 80 cc, making it attractive for

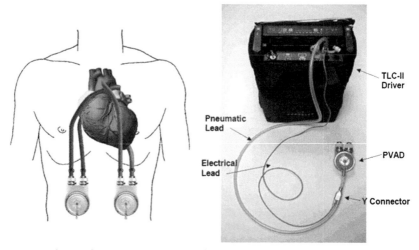

Fig. 7. Thoratec pVAD. (*From* Thoratec Corportation, Pleasanton, CA; with permission.)

the pediatric population. Regarding a European multicenter experience with 56 pediatric patients supported on the Medos HIA VAD, Reinhartz and colleagues[29] reported 11 patients were bridged to transplant, and 10 were explanted secondary to myocardial recovery, with an overall survival rate of 37.5%. This device presently is not available in the United States.

EXCOR VAD

The EXCOR VAD (**Fig. 9**) is a German-born, pneumatic-chamber pump available for use as a bridge to recovery or as a bridge to transplant. This pump was previously called the Berlin Heart, after its manufacturer, Berlin Heart AG, but now, for clarity, is generally referred to as EXCOR, to distinguish it from the Berlin Heart axial flow pump, the INCOR. The EXCOR has been placed in over 600 patients younger than 18 years of age worldwide and is the most common VAD being placed in children. There have been over 250 implantations in North America, with 85 placed in 2009. Its use in North America has gone up sharply since 2004. The EX-COR is not currently FDA approved. (**Fig. 10**) The pump is produced in eight different volumes, ranging from 10 to 80 cc, giving it a distinct advantage with respect to the pediatric population. This system can operate in asynchronous, volume-dependent, or synchronous mode. Currently, the EXCOR is undergoing a multi-institutional IDE study that started in May of 2007 to assess its efficacy as a bridge to transplant and its safety profile. There are two study groups: patients with a BSA less 0.7 m^2 and those with a BSA greater than 0.7 m^2. The study group of smaller patients is completed, and the application for humanitarian device exemption approval will most likely be filed this year.

Axial Flow VADs

For many years, the pusher-plate adult VADs (ie, Thoratec IVAD, HeartMate IP, XVE LVAS, and Novacor LVAS][WorldHeart Incorporated, Salt Lake City, UT, USA) (**Fig. 11**) had been the only choice for intracorporeal support of children. Unfortunately, all of these pumps are quite large. The Thoratec IVAD has been placed in three patients 18 years of age or younger, with the youngest being 14 years old and all over 40 kg body weight. The HeartMate LVAS has been placed in 58 pediatric patients, the youngest of whom was 8 years old. The Novacor LVAS has been placed in 42 pediatric patients worldwide, all over 40 kg. All of these devices are adult devices, which were placed in children because no pediatric intracorporeal LVAD system exists. However, the emergence of axial flow technology for adult VADs is a milestone in the evolution of pediatric VADs, because this technology represents industry's first success at developing a smaller, lighter, and quieter implantable LVADs. Axial flow pumps were engineered to assist LV function as a bridge to transplant or as destination therapy. The pump engages a magnetically levitated impeller that rotates within a cylindrical chamber, usually 7–11.5 cm (3–5 in) in length. Before exiting the chamber, blood passes through a diffuser to neutralize the rotation of the flow. Axial flow VADs are valveless, and most operate in an asynchronous mode. These devices have a small and flexible motor cable supplying power to the implanted pump that generates less of an inflammatory response than the vent drivelines used to supply the pneumatically driven pumps; additionally, they are more resistant to infection.[23]

Axial flow VADs are somewhat difficult to classify in terms of flow pulsatility. They clearly differ from the conventional pulsatile pumps that have an ejection cycle comparable to that of the native heart. Nevertheless, in the adult population, it has been consistently observed that after several days of support, pulsatility often develops in the arterial tracing. This phenomenon is explained by the fact that the preload-dependent output of axial

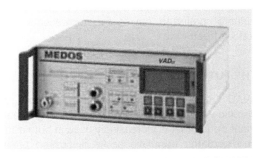
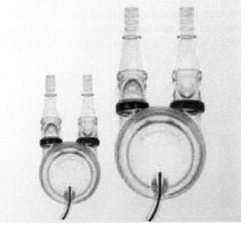

Fig. 8. Medos blood pump and drive unit. (*Courtesy of* MEDOS Medizintechnik AG, Stolberg, Germany.)

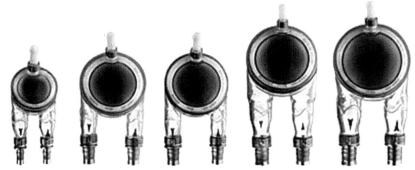

Fig. 9. Berlin Heart EXCOR – Pump sizes from 10 mL up to 50 mL for pediatric patients. (*Courtesy of* Berlin Heart, Incorporated, The Woodlands, TX.)

flow VADs may be altered by the pressure difference in the inflow and outflow cannulae during the cardiac cycle.

MicroMed DeBakey VAD/MicroMed DeBakey VAD Child Two versions of the MicroMed DeBakey VAD (MicroMed Cardiovascular, Incorporated, Houston, TX, USA) (**Fig. 12**) exist, one designed for use in patients with a BSA greater than 1.5 m^2, the MicroMed DeBakey VAD, and one tailored for use in patients with a BSA 0.7 to 1.5 m^2, the MicroMed DeBakey VAD Child, the first pediatric-specific VAD to get FDA approval. The MicroMed DeBakey VAD Child was modified to suit smaller patients by decreasing both the angle of the inflow cannula and the size of the flow probe. The pump itself was not modified and is identical in size and function to the adult version. Early outcome data regarding the MicroMed DeBakey VAD Child (<20 patients) were discouraging because of issues with thrombosis and emboli, and thus it did not gain widespread use. Presently, there have been modifications made to the DeBakey VAD Child to address these thrombosis issues, and the company is trying to introduce this improved version to the field.

HeartMate II LVAS The HeartMate II LVAS (**Fig. 13**) is the Thoratec axial flow VAD, which got FDA approval as a bridge to transplantation in April 2008 and for destination therapy in January of 2010. The inflow and outflow cannulae feature textured internal surfaces, while the internal pump surfaces are smooth. The textured surfaces promote endothelialization of the blood-contacting surfaces; however, unlike the other devices in the HeartMate line, there is a need for systemic anticoagulation. The incidence of thrombo-embolic events and device-related infections with the HeartMate II has been notably less compared with previous VADs. The low morbidity, reliability, and functional design of the HeartMate II encourage patient independence, rehabilitation, and patient discharge. The HeartMate II is the authors' preferred device for adolescents with a BSA greater than 1.3 m^2.

THE FUTURE OF VADS

LVAD implantation in patients with acute or chronic advanced HF is a life-saving treatment option that is increasingly used in both adult and pediatric populations. As discussed previously, these devices initially were implanted as a bridge to cardiac transplantation in HF patients who had had worsening clinical status. Given the static supply of donor organs available for

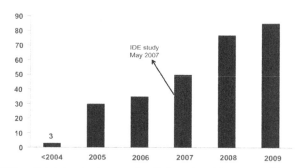

Fig. 10. Berlin Heart EXCOR pediatric implant across North America. (*Courtesy of* Texas Children's Hospital, Houston, TX.)

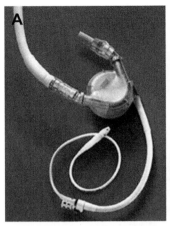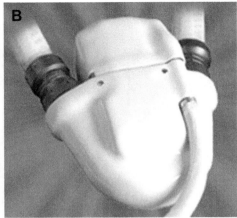

Fig. 11. Pusher-plate adult VADs. (*A*) HeartMate XVE. (*Courtesy of* Thoratec Corportation, Pleasanton, CA.) (*B*) Novacor LVAS. (*Courtesy of* World Heart Corporation, Salt Lake City, UT.)

transplantation, however, these devices have evolved into a bridge to possible recovery and as possible destination therapy. The past decade has resulted in a transformation of VADs, and the next decade will most likely hold even more favorable improvements for pediatric patients. VADs have been developed in stages, with rapidly improving changes in size and efficiency. As described previously, initial or first-generation devices were pulsatile volume displacement pumps, making them bulky and difficult to use. These pumps provided well documented hemodynamic support, but their size greatly limited their use in children and adolescents. Additionally, their durability made long-term support potentially problematic. Improvements in these pulsatile pumps such as the Berlin EXCOR device have led to use in pediatric patients as small as 3 kg in weight. The ongoing Berlin Heart EXCOR Pediatric Ventricular Assist Device Trial may result in the FDA approval of this device for pediatric use as a bridge to cardiac transplantation. Are axial flow pumps are second-generation. This allows for

a smaller device with smaller drivelines that result in less infection and require less extensive dissection for implantation.[30] These devices are nonpulsatile with only one moving part, and quiet, allowing for greater patient comfort. Initial animal studies suggested that nonpulsatile flow might not deliver optimal perfusion to distal vascular beds.[31] However, pulsatile devices face several engineering obstacles that limit long-term use. Axial flow devices only have one moving part and are more durable. The Heartmate II device is a widely used example of a second-generation device that is a continuous-flow axial pump that has an internal rotor with helical blades that curve around the central shaft. This device received FDA approval in 2008 for clinical use as a bridge to transplant. Over 3000 of these devices have been implanted. Given their smaller size and durability, the Heartmate II is now being used more widely in pediatrics. And, given that these devices do not completely unload the left ventricle, the native heart still ejects some blood, allowing for some pulsatility that is sufficient to allow

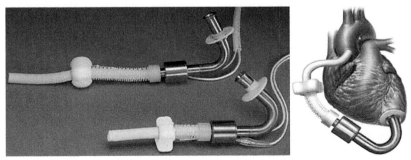

Fig. 12. MicroMed DeBakey VAD Adult and Pediatric. (*Courtesy of* MicroMed Cardiovascular, Incorporated, Houston, TX.)

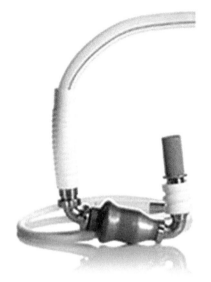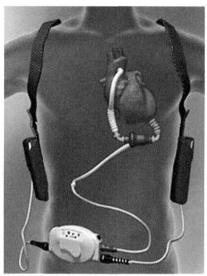

Fig. 13. Thoratec HeartMate II LVAS. (*Courtesy of* Thoratec Corporation, Pleasanton, CA.)

end-organ recovery in HF patients. At the authors' institution, five adolescents have been successfully implanted with this device and bridged to transplantation. Interestingly, two of these patients were discharged from the hospital and managed as outpatients with their VADs without significant complication. Other second-generation devices that are used in clinical practice include the Jarvik 2000 (Jarvik Heart Inc, Manhattan, NY, USA), the Berlin Heart Incor (Berlin Heart Inc, Berlin, Germany), and the MicroMed-Debakey device (MicroMed Cardiovascular Inc, Houston, TX, USA). These devices have been used only sparingly in pediatrics with limited success. The third-generation devices are magnetic levitation pumps that are being evaluated for clinical use. These include the Terumo Heart (Terumo Heart Inc, Ann Arbor, MI, USA) and HeartWare devices (HeartWare Inc, Framingham, MA, USA) that have had no pediatric applications thus far. These devices may be even more durable and afford greater ease of implantation than the previous generation devices. The DuraHeartTM LVAS (Terumo Heart, Incorporated) has been investigated since 2004 and received European commercial launch in 2006. In 2008, the FDA approved a clinical trial "Evaluating the Safety and Effectiveness of the DuraHeartTM LVAS in Patients Awaiting Transplant." An initial report of the first six implantations is favorable, but final results are pending.[32]

An evolving area of clinical interest is the use of percutaneous MCS. Historically, the use of intra-aortic balloon pumps (IABPs) has been the most widely used strategy for short-term support, as they are widely available and easily placed. The use of IABP in children has been limited but is perhaps an underutilized modality. Use of the device has been limited in the pediatric cohort, largely because the balloon's inflation cycle does not synchronize well with faster heart rates. Furthermore, the pediatric aorta is more elastic than that of the adult, which renders the reduction in afterload minimal, as the aorta forcefully recoils upon deflation. Recently manufacturers (ie, Maquet Inc, Wayne, NJ, USA) have created pediatric systems with balloon volumes down to 2.5 cc (6 mm diameters inflated) and catheters ranging from 4.5 to 7.0 Fr, respectively. Pinkney and colleagues[33] reported in their review of 29 infants and children who received IABP support for all indications a 62% survival rate overall. It should be noted that in the infant subgroup, the mortality rate was 50%. Akomea-Agyin and colleagues,[34] regarding their experience with 14 children placed on IABP support after cardiotomy, reported a 71% weaning rate with a 80% long-term survival of those weaned. Accordingly, the IABP should be regarded as a viable option for adjunct mechanical support in children with low cardiac output syndrome.

Newer MCS devices have been developed that show promise for short-term support including the Impella (Abiomed, Danvers, MA, USA), the Capiox (Terumo), and the TandemHeart pVAD (Cardiac Assist, Pittsburgh, PA, USA). Desirable features have been suggested and include easy access to the device, the ability to ensure adequate hemodynamic support across wide ranging patient sizes, safety and ease of insertion, the possibility of leaving the device in for multiple days without significant morbidity, and easy removal without significant bleeding or vascular injury.[35] The Impella device has been used extensively in adults for support of cardiogenic shock of varying etiologies and has been used in pediatrics for recovery of acute myocarditis in a 13-year-old boy.[36–38] This device can be placed quickly in retrograde fashion sitting across the aortic valve where it aspirates blood and expels it in the ascending aorta. The Impella device can provide up to 2.5 L/min of cardiac output and is continuously purged with heparin during use. The TandemHeart is a device that can be placed either percutaneously or surgically and can provide flow rates of up to 4 L/min. The TandemHeart is an extracorporeal, axial-flow device that aspirates blood from a left atrial catheter (placed transseptally) and returns blood to the body via a catheter in the femoral artery as described previously. This device provides excellent support in multiple clinical settings and can be used as a bridge both to recovery and to more long-term support. The authors have successfully used the Tandem-Heart in their institution for fulminant acute viral myocarditis in two adolescent boys. Both were decannulated and recovered normal systolic function. These devices are not without potential complications including bleeding, thromboembolism, infection, arteriovenous fistula formation, and cannula dislodgement.[39] Close monitoring is essential to ensure successful use of pVADs. The concept of superimposing continuous flow via a percutaneous device on native pulsatile flow or aortic flow therapy (AFT) has been studied recently in adults, with improvement in cardiac performance independent of changes in preload or afterload.[40] This support strategy involves the use of two arterial catheters. An inflow catheter is placed in the iliac artery, and the outflow catheter terminates in the descending thoracic aorta. No pediatric use has been documented.

The development of a total artificial heart (TAH) has undergone numerous changes since the initial implantation by Dr Cooley and colleagues[41] in 1969. Given the limited donor organs available, the development of a functional, durable TAH would have significant impacts on HF patients world-wide. Currently there are two TAH devices available. These are the AbioCor device (Abiomed) and the CardioWest device (SynCardia, Tucson, AZ, USA).[42,43] These devices are pulsatile and large in nature, greatly limiting their ability to be used in smaller males and most females. However, Syncardia within the year will be starting clinical testing in a smaller version of its TAH that will support patients down to a BSA of 0.8 or 1 m^2, which will allow its application in most adolescents. In addition, they contain valves that are subject to wear over time and may promote thrombus formation.[42] Newer innovations in TAH are applying the concept of continuous flow as seen in the Heart Mate II device to TAH. The Cleveland Clinic has recently developed a TAH (CFTAH) that is a pulsatile, continuous flow device that is valveless and that balances left heart and right heart circulation without any electronic intervention.[44] This device is much smaller and durable than the AbioCor or CardioWest and requires no external driver. No reports exist of use of any of these devices in pediatric populations, but as these devices become smaller, pediatric implantations will most likely be pursued.

The future of VAD use in pediatrics does not only involve the development of smaller devices. The success of VADs in pediatrics as in adults revolves on appropriate patient selection and pre- and postdevice implantation management. Preimplantation management must be focused on end organ preservation. This involves appropriate use of medical therapies and adequate surveillance of function. Identification of patients at risk for complication from MCS would offer great benefit to care givers and may allow for more timely and aggressive interventions. The Interagency Registry For Mechanical Circulatory Support (INTERMACS) is a collaborative effort between the National Heart, Lung, and Blood Institute (NHLBI), FDA, Centers for Medicare and Medical Services (CMS), and the HF professional community that requires mandatory data submission on all durable mechanical circulatory devices.[45] A recent report from INTERMACS characterized the causes of death based on device strategy as well as adverse events in the first 12 months following implantation.[46] Of the 1420 VAD implantations, 37 (3%) were in patients less than 19 years of age. As this data accrual expands, valuable information will be gained to help HF specialists optimize timing and device selection for their growing patient population.

The use of these devices has offered a great opportunity to advanced pediatric HF patients. With the rapid growth in the technology of VADs and smaller size of devices available, the use of this approach will only continue to expand in children and adolescents. The role of VADs in children will most likely change over time. There is increasing interest in using these devices for destination therapy as an alternative to transplant as durability improves and smaller devices are being produced.[20] The concept of outpatient VAD management is increasingly discussed, both in patients who are being bridged to recovery or transplant as well as those with destination devices.[47] A robust effort involving a multidisciplinary approach is required for successful outpatient management but is being increasingly done in adult and pediatric patients. And, as patient selection and better medical management improve, lower costs will likely occur allowing for more widespread use. As devices are used for longer periods, cardiac surveillance will improve. Favorable effects of VAD support in the form of reverse or favorable remodeling can be seen with both short-term and long-term mechanical unloading.[48] As surveillance technologies and surrogate markers of myocardial recovery expand, increased numbers of successful explantations will likely occur.[49,50] This may lead to increased longevity of native hearts and avoid the need, at least temporarily, for cardiac transplantation.

REFERENCES

1. Heart Failure Society Of America. Evaluation and management of patients with acute decompensated heart failure. J Card Fail 2006;12:e86–103.
2. Fiser WP, Yetman AT, Gunselman RJ, et al. Pediatric arteriovenous extracorporeal membrane oxygenation (ECMO) as a bridge to cardiac transplantation. J Heart Lung Transplant 2003;22:770–7.
3. Hopper AO, Pageau J, Job L, et al. Extracorporeal membrane oxygenation for perioperative support in neonatal and pediatric cardiac transplantation. Artif Organs 1999;23:1006–9.
4. Gajarski RJ, Mosca RS, Ohye RG, et al. Use of extracorporeal life support as a bridge to pediatric cardiac transplantation. J Heart Lung Transplant 2003;22:28–34.
5. Stiller B, Hetzer R, Weng Y, et al. Heart transplantation in children after mechanical circulatory support with pulsatile pneumatic assist device. J Heart Lung Transplant 2003;22:1201–8.
6. Ishino K, Loebe M, Uhlemann F, et al. Circulatory support with paracorporeal pneumatic ventricular assist device (VAD) in infants and children. Eur J Cardiothorac Surg 1997;11:965–72.
7. Sidiropoulos A, Hotz H, Konertz W. Pediatric circulatory support. J Heart Lung Transplant 1998;17:1172–6.
8. Hetzer R, Loebe M, Potapov EV, et al. Circulatory support with pneumatic paracorporeal ventricular assist device in infants and children. Ann Thorac Surg 1998;66:1498–506.
9. Blume ED, Naftel DC, Bastardi HJ, et al. Outcomes of children bridged to heart transplantation with ventricular assist devices: a multi-institutional study. Circulation 2006;113:2313–9.
10. Morales DL, Braud BE, Price JF, et al. Use of mechanical circulatory support in pediatric patients with acute cardiac graft rejection. ASAIO J 2007;53:701–5.
11. del Nido PJ, Dalton HJ, Thompson AE, et al. Extracorporeal membrane oxygenator rescue in children during cardiac arrest after cardiac surgery. Circulation 1992;86:II300–4.
12. Duncan BW, Hraska V, Jonas RA, et al. Mechanical circulatory support in children with cardiac disease. J Thorac Cardiovasc Surg 1999;117:529–42.
13. Duncan BW, Ibrahim AE, Hraska V, et al. Use of rapid-deployment extracorporeal membrane oxygenation for the resuscitation of pediatric patients with heart disease after cardiac arrest. J Thorac Cardiovasc Surg 1998;116:305–11.
14. Jacobs JP, Ojito JW, McConaghey TW, et al. Rapid cardiopulmonary support for children with complex congenital heart disease. Ann Thorac Surg 2000;70:742–9 [discussion: 749–50].
15. Kolovos NS, Schuerer DJ, Moler FW, et al. Extracorporal life support for pulmonary hemorrhage in children: a case series. Crit Care Med 2002;30:577–80.
16. Meyer DM, Jessen ME. Results of extracorporeal membrane oxygenation in children with sepsis. The Extracorporeal Life Support Organization. Ann Thorac Surg 1997;63:756–61.
17. Ashton RC Jr, Oz MC, Michler RE, et al. Left ventricular assist device options in pediatric patients. ASAIO J 1995;41:M277–80.
18. DiGiorgi PL, Rao V, Naka Y, et al. Which patient, which pump? J Heart Lung Transplant 2003;22:221–35.
19. Helman DN, Addonizio LJ, Morales DL, et al. Implantable left ventricular assist devices can successfully bridge adolescent patients to transplant. J Heart Lung Transplant 2000;19:121–6.
20. Rose EA, Moskowitz AJ, Packer M, et al. The REMATCH trial: rationale, design, and end points. Randomized Evaluation of Mechanical Assistance for the Treatment of Congestive Heart Failure. Ann Thorac Surg 1999;67:723–30.
21. Lietz K, Long JW, Kfoury AG, et al. Outcomes of left ventricular assist device implantation as destination therapy in the post-REMATCH era: implications for patient selection. Circulation 2007;116:497–505.
22. Price JF, Mott AR, Dickerson HA, et al. Worsening renal function in children hospitalized with decompensated heart failure: evidence for a pediatric cardiorenal syndrome? Pediatr Crit Care Med 2008;9:279–84.
23. Wieselthaler GM, Schima H, Dworschak M, et al. First experiences with outpatient care of patients with implanted axial flow pumps. Artif Organs 2001;25:331–5.
24. Pitsis AA, Visouli AN, Burkhoff D, et al. Feasibility study of a temporary percutaneous left ventricular

assist device in cardiac surgery. Ann Thorac Surg 2007;84:1993–9.

25. Yoshikai M, Hamada M, Takarabe K, et al. Clinical use of centrifugal pumps and the roller pump in open heart surgery: a comparative evaluation. Artif Organs 1996;20:704–6.

26. Morgan IS, Codispoti M, Sanger K, et al. Superiority of centrifugal pump over roller pump in paediatric cardiac surgery: prospective randomised trial. Eur J Cardiothorac Surg 1998;13:526–32.

27. Thuys CA, Mullaly RJ, Horton SB, et al. Centrifugal ventricular assist in children under 6 kg. Eur J Cardiothorac Surg 1998;13:130–4.

28. Bennett M, Horton S, Thuys C, et al. Pump-induced haemolysis: a comparison of short-term ventricular assist devices. Perfusion 2004;19:107–11.

29. Reinhartz O, Stiller B, Eilers R, et al. Current clinical status of pulsatile pediatric circulatory support. ASAIO J 2002;48:455–9.

30. Miller LW, Pagani FD, Russell SD, et al. Use of a continuous-flow device in patients awaiting heart transplantation. N Engl J Med 2007;357:885–96.

31. Potapov EV, Loebe M, Nasseri BA, et al. Pulsatile flow in patients with a novel nonpulsatile implantable ventricular assist device. Circulation 2000;102:III183–7.

32. Griffith K, Jenkins E, Pagani FD. First American experience with the Terumo DuraHeart left ventricular assist system. Perfusion 2009;24:83–9.

33. Pinkney KA, Minich LL, Tani LY, et al. Current results with intra-aortic balloon pumping in infants and children. Ann Thorac Surg 2002;73:887–91.

34. Akomea-Agyin C, Kejriwal NK, Franks R, et al. Intra-aortic balloon pumping in children. Ann Thorac Surg 1999;67:1415–20.

35. Sarkar K, Kini AS. Percutaneous left ventricular support devices. Cardiol Clin 2010;28:169–84.

36. Sjauw KD, Konorza T, Erbel R, et al. Supported high-risk percutaneous coronary intervention with the Impella 2.5 device the Europella registry. J Am Coll Cardiol 2009;54:2430–4.

37. Sugiki H, Nakashima K, Vermes E, et al. Temporary right ventricular support with Impella Recover RD axial flow pump. Asian Cardiovasc Thorac Ann 2009;17:395–400.

38. Andrade JG, Al-Saloos H, Jeewa A, et al. Facilitated cardiac recovery in fulminant myocarditis: pediatric use of the Impella LP 5.0 pump. J Heart Lung Transplant 2010;29:96–7.

39. Gregoric ID, Bruckner BA, Jacob L, et al. Techniques and complications of TandemHeart ventricular assist

device insertion during cardiac procedures. ASAIO J 2009;55:251–4.

40. Greenberg B, Czerska B, Delgado RM, et al. Effects of continuous aortic flow augmentation in patients with exacerbation of heart failure inadequately responsive to medical therapy: results of the Multicenter Trial of the Orqis Medical Cancion System for the Enhanced Treatment of Heart Failure Unresponsive to Medical Therapy (MOMENTUM). Circulation 2008;118:1241–9.

41. Cooley DA, Liotta D, Hallman GL, et al. Orthotopic cardiac prosthesis for two-staged cardiac replacement. Am J Cardiol 1969;24:723–30.

42. Dowling RD, Gray LA Jr, Etoch SW, et al. Initial experience with the AbioCor implantable replacement heart system. J Thorac Cardiovasc Surg 2004;127:131–41.

43. Copeland JG, Smith RG, Arabia FA, et al. Cardiac replacement with a total artificial heart as a bridge to transplantation. N Engl J Med 2004;351:859–67.

44. Fukamachi K, Horvath DJ, Massiello AL, et al. An innovative, sensorless, pulsatile, continuous-flow total artificial heart: device design and initial in vitro study. J Heart Lung Transplant 2010;29:13–20.

45. Kirklin JK, Naftel DC, Stevenson LW, et al. INTERMACS database for durable devices for circulatory support: first annual report. J Heart Lung Transplant 2008;27:1065–72.

46. Kirklin JK, Naftel DC, Kormos RL, et al. Second INTERMACS annual report: more than 1000 primary left ventricular assist device implants. J Heart Lung Transplant 2010;29:1–10.

47. Wilson SR, Givertz MM, Stewart GC, et al. Ventricular assist devices the challenges of outpatient management. J Am Coll Cardiol 2009;54:1647–59.

48. Mohaptara B, Vick GW, Fraser CD Jr, et al. Short-term mechanical unloading and reverse remodeling of failing hearts in children. J Heart Lung Transplant 2010;29:98–104.

49. Raman SV, Sahu A, Merchant AZ, et al. Noninvasive assessment of left ventricular assist devices with cardiovascular computed tomography and impact on management. J Heart Lung Transplant 2010;29:79–85.

50. Mountis MM, Starling RC. Management of left ventricular assist devices after surgery: bridge, destination, and recovery. Curr Opin Cardiol 2009;24:252–6.

Heart Transplantation for Heart Failure in Children

Elfriede Pahl, MD[a],*, Anne I. Dipchand, MD[b],
Michael Burch, MD, FRCP, FRCPCH[c]

KEYWORDS
- Heart transplantation • Pediatrics • Heart failure
- Indications

Heart transplantation has become standard therapy for children with end-stage heart failure, with excellent short-term results and 1-year survival greater than 90%, with the exception of patients with complex congenital heart disease.[1–3] Late survival remains limited because of graft rejection, coronary allograft vasculopathy, infectious complications, and posttransplant lymphoproliferative disorders.[1,4–8] Appropriate timing of referral for heart transplantation must therefore be balanced with the patient's quality of life, alternative options for treatment, and a realistic estimation of the patient's potential survival without heart transplantation. Because of increasing waiting times in recent years and a limited donor pool, early referral and consultation with a transplant center are always appropriate because 17% to 25% of listed pediatric patients die on the transplant waiting list.[1,9]

INDICATIONS

In absolute numbers, dilated cardiomyopathy (DCM) with end-stage heart failure is the predominant diagnosis leading to heart transplantation in the 1- to 10-year age group, as well as in adolescents (**Fig. 1**).[1,10] In the infant population less than 1 year of age, the indication for transplant tends to be structural congenital heart disease, often not in the setting of heart failure. The proportion of infant recipients with cardiomyopathy and

end-stage heart failure has almost doubled in recent years (16% to 30%) (**Fig. 2**). This increase likely reflects less use of heart transplantation for neonates with hypoplastic left heart syndrome.[10]

Cardiomyopathies

Cardiomyopathies in the pediatric population are varied and the different types have different clinical courses, responses to treatment, and outcomes, as detailed throughout this issue. However, there is significant morbidity and mortality, with 40% to 45% of affected children undergoing heart transplantation or dying within 5 years of diagnosis.[11–13] Indications for listing for transplantation remain challenging and medical practice varies by institution and physician.

In a recent analysis of the Pediatric Heart Transplant Study (PHTS) database, survival after listing in 1320 patients with pediatric cardiomyopathy was reviewed, with the goal of defining risk factors or adverse outcomes both before and after transplant and to provide evidence with which to base decisions about listing in this diverse patient population.[14] Patients with DCM represented 83%, whereas patients with restrictive and hypertrophic cardiomyopathy (HCM) made up 11% and 6%, respectively. Patients with cardiomyopathy were high acuity, with 72% United Network for Organ Sharing (UNOS) status 1, 24% mechanically ventilated, and 14% on mechanical ventricular assist

a Department of Pediatrics, Children's Memorial Hospital, Northwestern Feinberg School of Medicine, 2300 Children's Pl, Cardiology Box 21, Chicago, IL 60614, USA
b Division of Cardiology, Labatt Family Heart Centre, Hospital for Sick Children, 555 University Avenue, Toronto, Ontario, Canada
c Department of Cardiology, Great Ormond Street Hospital, London, UK
* Corresponding author.
E-mail address: epahl@childrensmemorial.org

Heart Failure Clin 6 (2010) 575–589
doi:10.1016/j.hfc.2010.05.010

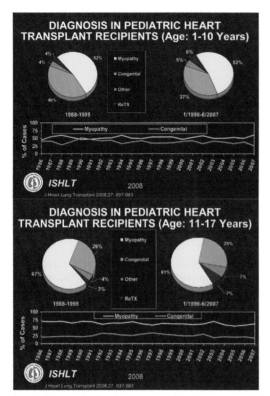

Fig. 1. Diagnosis for heart transplant, age 1 to 10 years and 10 to 17 years. (*From* Kirk R, Edwards LB, Aurora P, et al. Registry of the International Society For Heart And Lung Transplantation: Eleventh Official Pediatric Heart Transplantation Report-2008. J Heart Lung Transplantation 2008;27:970–7. Available at: www.ishlt.org.)

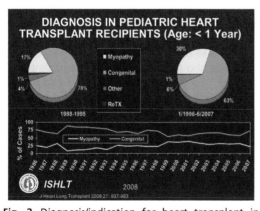

Fig. 2. Diagnosis/indication for heart transplant in infants less than 1 year of age. Comparison of early versus recent era. (*From* Kirk R, Edwards LB, Aurora P, et al. Registry of the International Society For Heart And Lung Transplantation: Eleventh Official Pediatric Heart Transplantation Report-2008. J Heart Lung Transplantation 2008;27:970–7. Available at: www. ishlt.org.)

device (VAD) support. Despite these factors, the waitlist mortality of 17% was lower than that of the noncardiomyopathy population (32%). Overall, looking at 10-year survival after listing, patients with cardiomyopathy did better using a clinical strategy of listing for transplantation compared with the noncardiomyopathy cohort (66% vs 53%). This finding supports data from the Pediatric Cardiomyopathy Registry (PCMR) and other single-center reports of the important role of heart transplantation in outcomes, when the rate of survival is greater than the rate of freedom from transplantation, and improvements seem related to transplantation itself rather than to improvements in heart failure therapy.[11,15,16]

DCM

Within the PHTS registry, amongst the 1320 patients with cardiomyopathy, 1098 had a dilated phenotype.[17] Ten-year survival after listing was 72% compared with a 64% survival at 5 years as reported for DCM.[17–20]

Patients with DCM are appropriate candidates for heart transplantation if reversible causes such as metabolic disorders (eg, carnitine deficiency or mitochondrial disorders), primary arrhythmias, anomalous origin of the left coronary artery from the pulmonary artery, and myocarditis have all been excluded. Two of 3 children with DCM have no known cause, and up to 40% progress to heart transplantation or death by 5 years after diagnosis.[11] Furthermore, patients with skeletal muscular dystrophy and certain mitochondrial disorders usually have the phenotype of DCM, and in select cases, these patients may be considered for heart transplantation. Data from the PHTS registry show that the cause of DCM was identified only 20% of the time in listed patients, and was not an independent risk factor for waitlist or posttransplant mortality.[17]

Listing practices vary for patients with DCM. Patient characteristics are outlined in **Table 1**, with the majority being high status and on inotropes, and 15% requiring mechanical support. Despite this, waitlist mortality was low at 11%, and reason for death while waiting was most commonly heart failure (45%). Factors significant for waitlist mortality included history of ventilation (relative risk [RR] 3.02; $P<.001$), extracorporeal membrane oxygenation (ECMO) (RR 2.17; $P = .001$), or arrhythmias (RR 1.53; $P = .03$). Cause, race, gender, age, size, blood group, UNOS status, inotropic or VAD support, surgical history, cardiac index, and pulmonary vascular resistance (PVR) at listing were not associated with waitlist mortality. Average wait time was 9.6 months, with an increase in high-status patients from

Table 1
Characteristics of 1098 patients with DCM

Characteristics	Listed for Transplant		Received Transplant	
	Total[a]	No. (%) or Mean ± SE	Total[a]	No. (%) or Mean ± SE
Demographics				
Male	1095	555 (51)	815	416 (51)
White	1089	698 (64)	811	517 (64)
Age, years	1098	7.3 ± 0.189	817	8.1 ± 0.217
Status				
Status 1	1064	814 (77)	786	669 (85)
Inotropes	1098	720 (66)	817	552 (68)
Ventilator	1098	305 (28)	817	164 (20)
ECMO	1098	92 (8)	817	64 (8)
VAD	1098	74 (7)	817	107 (13)
Condition at listing				
Arrhythmia	1098	250 (23)		
Failure to thrive	1098	131 (12)		
Renal insufficiency	1098	38 (3)		
Asthma	1098	33 (3)		
CVA	1098	22 (2)		
Diabetes	1098	5 (<1)		
Cause of DCM				
Idiopathic		888 (80.9)		
Myocarditis[b]		133 (12.1)		
Adriamycin toxicity		34 (3.1)		
Postpartum		3 (3.6)		
Other		40 (3.6)		

Abbreviations: CVA, cerebrovascular accident; SE, standard error.
[a] Number of patients with data available.
[b] Acute myocarditis versus DCM at any time after an episode of myocarditis were unable to be separated within the database and both patient types contribute to this group of patients.
From Kirk R, Naftel D, Hoffman TM, et al. Outcome of pediatric patients with dilated cardiomyopathy listed for transplant: a multi-institutional study. J Heart Lung Trans 2009;28:1322–8; with permission.

77% to 85% and an increase in VAD usage of 7% to 13% during that period. A large proportion of lower-acuity (UNOS status 2) patients were alive and waiting at 1 year (31%) and 2 years (22%) after transplant, which again raises the question as to whether relatively stable patients should undergo heart transplantation, rather than be followed conservatively. This subject has been debated elsewhere, with the conclusion that heart transplantation still conferred a survival benefit, even for lowest-status patients.[21]

In timing and indications for listing, in general, patients with DCM are listed if they cannot be weaned from inotropic support or mechanical support. Outpatients with frequent heart failure admissions, poor quality of life (ie, intractable heart failure and inability to attend school), severe growth failure requiring and/or despite enteral tube supplemental feeding may all benefit from being listed for heart transplantation. Patients with increased PVR, despite a trial of optimal medical therapy with diuretics, inotropes, and afterload reduction, may be listed for heart transplantation within the considerations noted later.

Restrictive cardiomyopathy

As discussed elsewhere in this issue, restrictive cardiomyopathy is a rare disease accounting for 2% to 5% of children with cardiomyopathy.[12] It comprises the second most common type of cardiomyopathy for which patients are referred for transplant.[14] This situation likely relates to the poor reported actuarial survival for this phenotype of less than 50% at 2 years, the high risk of sudden death, and the practice in some centers of listing at the time of diagnosis.[22–24] These patients often present late with symptoms of syncope or aborted sudden death, symptoms of right heart failure, and increased PVR at the time of diagnosis.

Zangwill and colleagues[25] reviewed the largest cohort of children with restrictive cardiomyopathy listed for heart transplant (n = 145). The mean age at listing was 8.1 ± 0.4 years; only 14 patients were less than 1 year of age. Sixty-one (44%) patients were listed as UNOS status 1, 48 (33%) required inotropic support, and 14 (10%) patients were ventilator dependent. Seven (5%) required mechanical support, with 6 on ECMO and 1 patient supported on a VAD at listing. As a treatment strategy in this cohort, 10-year survival after listing was 63%. Waitlist mortality for restrictive cardiomyopathy was 10%; however, in contrast to children with DCM, the most common causes of death were neurologic (27%) and sudden cardiac death (20%) as opposed to heart failure (13%). Patients who were UNOS 1 had a significantly increased risk of death while waiting (**Fig. 3**). In multivariable analysis, the only significant factors for waitlist mortality included younger age at listing (RR 1.5; P = .002 for 1-year-old vs 10-year-old patient at listing) and use of ECMO or VAD at listing (RR 11.7, P<.001). Of note was

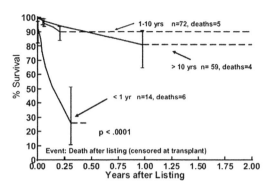

Fig. 4. Survival stratified by age-restrictive cardiomyopathy. PHTS: January 1993 to December 2006. Cardiomyopathy diagnosis: listed patients. Restrictive patients by age at listing, n = 145. Survival of patients with restrictive cardiomyopathy is shown by age at listing. (*From* Zangwill SD, Naftel D, L'Ecuyer T, et al. Outcomes of children with restrictive cardiomyopathy listed for heart transplant: a multi-institutional study. J Heart Lung Transplant 2009;28(12):1335–40.)

the effect of age on waitlist mortality, wherein infants less than 1 year of age were significantly more likely to die waiting than older patients (**Fig. 4**). Age at listing was not a significant factor for death after transplant, indicating that the effect of age on death occurs only during the waiting period.

In general, the patients in this cohort were less acutely unwell than the dilated cohort, yet overall survival if the patient received a transplant was better than the natural history of the disease. Risk factors for death while waiting reflected a higher-status or acutely unwell patient. Therefore, this patient population seems better served with early referral and listing before they deteriorate and meet high-status criteria. With regards to the infant group, one could hypothesize either a greater proportion of genetic-metabolic disorders or that age could be a surrogate for a more aggressive and/or malignant form of the disease with an earlier presentation.

Of note is the concern regarding increased pulmonary pressures and/or PVR in this patient population and potential effect on posttransplant survival. There is no consensus on routine cardiac catheterization and measurement of pulmonary hemodynamics in the pretransplant period. However, this strategy is practiced in some centers with guarded optimism when listing patients with a PVR of greater than 4 Wood units.

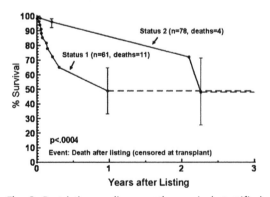

Fig. 3. Restrictive cardiomyopathy survival stratified by listing status 1 versus 2. PHTS: January 1993 to December 2006. Restrictive: listed patients, n = 145. Waitlist mortality for restrictive cardiomyopathy patients is shown by status at listing. Status 1 patients include all infants aged less than 6 months. There were 6 patients with missing data for status at listing. (*From* Zangwill SD, Naftel D, L'Ecuyer T, et al. Outcomes of children with restrictive cardiomyopathy listed for heart transplant: a multi-institutional study. J Heart Lung Transplant 2009;28(12):1335–40.)

HCM

Patients with HCM are rarely referred for transplantation, even although this is one of the more common types of cardiomyopathy, because these children rarely have symptoms of heart failure.[26,27] However, there are exceptions. A multicenter report by Gajarski and colleagues[26] from the PHTS identified 77 patients with HCM who were listed for heart transplantation (male 61%, white 79%). The mean age at listing was 7.6 years. At listing, 59% were UNOS status 1, 30% were on inotropic support, 27% were ventilated, and 8% were on ECMO. Arrhythmia had occurred in 27% and 14% had failure to thrive. Sixty-five percent underwent heart transplantation within 1 year. Overall, 25 patients died after listing; of these, 11 patients died while waiting and 14 died after heart transplantation. The investigators found poorest survival in infants who were less than 1 year of age at listing (**Fig. 5**). Whether infants less than 1 year of age should be offered heart transplantation needs to be individualized, given their poor outcomes compared with infants with DCM or congenital heart disease undergoing transplantation.

In the older age groups, other higher-risk patients with HCM, including patients who have ischemic symptoms from profound diastolic dysfunction that cannot be managed medically and are not surgical candidates, or who have already had surgical myomectomy, may also be considered for transplant. Rarely, there are instances of HCM progressing to severe systolic dysfunction, but this does not usually occur in the first 2 decades of life. Older patients requiring heart transplantation with HCM generally fare well.

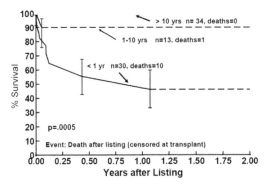

Fig. 5. Survival after listing by age in patients with HCM (censored at transplant). PHTS: January 1993 to December 2006. Cardiomyopathy diagnosis: listed patients. Hypertrophic patients by age at listing, n = 77. Survival curve of patients with HCM listed for heart transplant based on age as a function of time after listing. Compared with older age groups, infants had the highest mortality awaiting transplant, with most deaths occurring in the first 3 months after listing. (*From* Gajarski R, Naftel DC, Pahl E, et al. Outcomes of pediatric patients with hypertrophic cardiomyopathy listed for transplant. J Heart Lung Transplant 2009;28(12):1329–34.)

Anthracycline-induced cardiomyopathy

Although effective antineoplastic agents, anthracyclines are limited by their well-recognized and pervasive cardiotoxic effects. The incidence of late progressive cardiovascular disease in long-term survivors of cancer is established and may contribute to heart failure and death. Anthracycline cardiomyopathy leading to heart transplantation has been well described, even in pediatric patients, with good survival and low risk of cancer recurrence.[28,29] Pediatric cardiologists must work closely with oncologists to determine risk of cancer recurrence when deciding timing of listing, because a 5-year cancer-free period may be unrealistic and unnecessary in pediatric cancers.

Myocarditis

One of the most common reasons for referral for heart transplant is primary pump failure, as a result of profound acute systolic dysfunction. Primary pump failure may occur in the setting of acute myocarditis; however, most of these patients make a complete recovery if supported with inotropes, ventilation, and occasionally mechanical support; only a few undergo transplantation.[30,31] Lee and colleagues[30] reported outcomes on 36 pediatric cases of biopsy-proven myocarditis from 1984 to 1998, with 86% and 79% freedom from death/transplantation at 1 month and 2 years, respectively. However, there were 5 deaths within 72 hours of admission, as well as 1 late death at 1.9 years. A recent multicenter report from the PCMR found the incidence of death/transplant rate was 24% for 119 patients with biopsy-proven myocarditis compared with 47% in patients with idiopathic DCM, and echo left ventricular recovery at 2 years was significantly higher in the myocarditis group compared with patients with DCM.[31] Because of the risk of death from severe myocarditis, and prolonged waiting times in patients who are listed, a transplant center may consider listing if a patient with myocarditis requires mechanical support and/or after a prolonged period on support without signs of recovery of ventricular function. Patients with neonatal myocarditis from enterovirus may have a particularly fulminant course,[32] and those infrequent cases with giant cell myocarditis, although rare in children, are less likely to recover and should have early consideration for heart transplantation.[33]

The most severe cases of myocarditis may be supported by ECMO, as described in a multicenter registry report of 116 ECMO centers.[34] Survival outcomes for pediatric patients supported with ECMO for severe myocarditis identified 260 runs of ECMO for 255 patients, with survival to hospital discharge of 61%; only 7 patients (3%) underwent heart transplantation.

Congenital Heart Disease with Heart Failure

The second major category of patients who may be candidates for transplant are those with complex congenital heart disease with no other surgical options and refractory heart failure. This category includes neonates with complex heart disease including but not limited to (1) patients with hypoplastic left ventricle complex who are not candidates for Norwood-type palliation because of severe atrioventicular valve regurgitation or other technical considerations, (2) patients with severe truncus arteriosus who are not candidates for primary repair, (3) patients with pulmonary atresia with coronary sinusoids, and (4) patients with single ventricle physiology and severe atrioventricular valve regurgitation including complex heterotaxy syndromes.

Furthermore, increasing numbers of teenagers and young adults with systemic right ventricles from congenitally corrected transposition, or patients with simple transposition palliated with an atrial baffle procedure (ie, Mustard or Senning), develop congestive heart failure with atrial arrhythmias, risk of sudden death, and progressive multiorgan failure that may include significant hepatic and renal dysfunction, needing referral for heart transplantation.[2,3] In a multicenter report by Lamour and colleagues[2] from the PHTS, patients undergoing transplantation for congenital heart disease had good late survival after the initial 3-month period, with increased risk factors for perioperative mortality occurring in older age at transplant as well as in older donors and longer ischemic times. In addition, survival in patients who had undergone a Fontan procedure was lower (77% and 70% at 1 and 5 years) versus congenital patients who had not undergone a Fontan procedure (88% and 81%) at 1 and 5 years, respectively.

Bernstein and colleagues[35] reported a multicenter experience with heart transplantation in patients with single ventricle/failed Fontan procedure. The timing of listing of patients with protein-losing enteropathy (PLE) as well as plastic bronchitis[36] should be considered for those patients who fail medical therapy even if ventricular systolic function seems adequate, because these patients are at high risk for mortality during the next few years.[37] PLE has been treated with limited success with multimodal therapy; however, in patients who did not respond to medical therapy, PLE generally improved within weeks after heart transplantation, although this subset of patients were at higher risk for postoperative infections because of their immunodeficiencies.[35]

Heart transplantation may be necessary for patients with acute postoperative heart failure who are unable to be weaned from bypass surgery. These patients may be initially temporized with ECMO support[38]; however, if it becomes clear that the myocardium shows no signs of recovery, then heart transplantation should be considered if the patient meets candidacy requirements as outlined later. These patients may then be bridged to better long-term support with a VAD.[39]

ISCHEMIC HEART DISEASE

Although rare, another category of children for whom transplant should be considered is those with ischemic heart disease and resultant decreased myocardial function related to myocardial ischemia and infarction. This is a broad category and may include the rare patient with anomalous origin of the left coronary artery from the pulmonary artery who does not recover after reimplantation of the left coronary artery. Other examples are perioperative injury to a coronary artery when there is resultant severe and irrecoverable left ventricular dysfunction, for example after arterial switch repair for transposition of the great arteries or after a Ross operation. Indications for heart transplantation in patients with a history of Kawasaki disease were reported in a small multicenter series and included severe myocardial dysfunction, severe ventricular arrhythmias including cardiac arrest, and severe distal occlusive coronary artery disease.[40]

PRETRANSPLANT ASSESSMENT

Once referred, all patients should undergo a pretransplant assessment to identify indications for transplantation, identify potentially reversible causes of end-stage heart failure and optimize management, and identify contraindications that may preclude candidacy for organ transplantation. **Box 1** outlines the key components of a pretransplant assessment. Evaluation by an interdisciplinary team including social work, psychiatry, physiotherapy, occupational therapy, adolescent medicine, and key medical services including nephrology and anesthesia are critical to the transplantation process. Psychosocial assessment is vital, especially in the adolescent population, given the effect of nonadherence and risk-taking behaviors on graft and patient survival.[41,42]

Box 1
Pretransplant assessment testing

Echocardiogram

Cardiac catheterization (hemodynamics, anatomy)

Magnetic resonance imaging/magnetic resonance angiography or computed tomography angiography (anatomy)

Exercise test

Vascular ultrasound

Blood group

HLA antibody testing

Chemistry

- Renal function
- Liver function
- Lipid profile
- Immunoglobulins

Hematology

Infectious serologies

Because cardiomyopathies make up most of the diagnoses in patients with heart failure with an anatomically normal heart, a thorough workup for cause should be undertaken because certain genetic or metabolic conditions may be either amenable to treatment or, more likely, affect prognosis and eligibility for heart transplantation. Patients should be managed as per current state-of-the-art recommendations for the management of heart failure, as outlined elsewhere in this issue. Transplantation should be considered when patients are deteriorating despite optimal medical and supportive management. Functional class and heart failure stage should be assessed initially and in response to medical therapy, as outlined later. A full discussion of contraindications to pediatric heart transplantation is beyond the scope of this article but may be found elsewhere.[43]

Full Cardiac Assessment

If a patient is referred from a different center to the transplant center, there is often a need for a full cardiac evaluation, which may include electrocardiography, echocardiography, Holter monitoring, graded exercise testing, stress testing, cardiac catheterization, and other forms of cardiac imaging, including computed tomography or magnetic resonance imaging. Any potential alternative therapies should be explored, with further optimization of medical management and/or interventional or surgical options in lieu of heart transplantation.

Heart Failure Classification

One of the biggest challenges with congestive heart failure in childhood is the ability to objectively grade the degree of severity. This challenge is further compounded by the broad spectrum of age and development within the pediatric age range. Therefore, literature and guidelines regarding timing of listing vary with individual practice and/or lack of definition of objective and reproducible criteria for listing (**Box 2**). Several scoring systems have been proposed for grading heart failure in children. The most widely used is the Ross classification.[44] Another system has a 12-point scale based on quantity and duration of feeding, respiratory rate and pattern, heart rate, peripheral perfusion, presence of a diastolic filling sound, and degree of hepatomegaly.[45] With the New York University Pediatric Heart Failure Index a total score from 0 to 30 is obtained by adding together points based on physiologic indicators and the patient's specific medical regimen.[46] Overt heart failure symptoms occur late in the disease process, indicating a failure of compensatory mechanisms. Functional class

---

Box 2
Indications for heart transplantation/ evaluation and listing

- Intractable heart failure –

  inotrope dependence

  recurrent hospitalization for intravenous medications

- Severe failure to thrive because of congestive heart failure
- High pulmonary vascular resistance
- Recurrent ventricular tachycardia/ventricular fibrillation
- Hypertrophic cardiomyopathy

  severe ischemia, unresponsive to medical therapy

  severe diastolic dysfunction/ventilator dependence

- Kawasaki disease with severe ischemia
- Pulmonary atresia with coronary sinusoids
- Fontan-failed ± protein-losing enteropathy
- Severe myocarditis /heart failure, unable to wean from support
- Postcardiotomy pump failure, unable to wean from support

can be affected by adjustments in medical management and should not be the sole requirement for listing.

Both the New York Heart Association (NYHA) and Ross heart failure scales concentrate on current symptoms and do not discriminate well between early versus chronic or stable versus decompensated heart failure. Regardless of the specific diagnosis, a preliminary evaluation by the referring cardiologist generally includes a detailed history of symptoms, with an attempt to classify Ross symptoms[45] or NYHA class in older children and whether there has been a sudden or gradual change in clinical status. Growth and development, in particular a drop in growth percentiles, are useful information vis à vis severity of heart failure in the pediatric population. In particular, significant failure to gain adequate weight may be an indication for consideration for transplantation, especially in an infant, if optimal enteral feeds and heart failure therapy have been implemented.

Cardiopulmonary Exercise Testing

Formal cardiopulmonary testing provides an objective assessment of the degree of limitation that can be followed in a serial manner, is correlated with survival, and allows consistency across transplant programs if patients are old enough and cooperative enough to participate. Trends or changes in formal cardiopulmonary exercise testing are routinely assessed at adult centers, with a peak oxygen consumption less than 14 mL/min/m^2 correlating with poor survival.[47] Although some controversy exists about the degree of impairment in exercise required to justify transplantation, in general, adult patients with peak oxygen consumption (Vo_2) less than 10 mL/kg/min should be listed for transplant, and those with a Vo_2 greater than 18 mL/kg/min experience 1-year survival of more than 95% and should be followed expectantly.[48] Management of patients with a peak Vo_2 between 10 and 18 mL/kg/min remains controversial. In addition, a blunted systolic blood pressure response to exercise, and/or chronotropic incompetence, when associated with a peak Vo_2 less than 15 mL/kg/min or a peak Vo_2 less than 50% of predicted help redefine the prognostic value of intermediate Vo_2 values in adults.[48,49]

There are no objective numbers for exercise parameters that are generally accepted in the pediatric population, and percent predicted values have to be taken into consideration especially in younger patients. Published adult recommendations can only be extrapolated at this point. Pahl

and colleagues[50] recently reported serial exercise treadmill testing in a stable pediatric heart failure population, who were mostly NYHA class 1 and 2. This review included exercise tests in 56 patients from 1993 to 2007. The investigators correlated stress tests with a cardiac event, which was defined as death, listing for heart transplant, or hospitalization for heart failure. Receiver operating characteristic analysis was performed for lowest Vo_2max and endurance time per patient to predict a cardiac event. A peak Vo_2 of 21 and/or endurance less than 6.75 minutes were critical values to risk stratify children with heart failure who had a cardiac event. Patients with congenital heart disease had significantly lower Vo_2max and endurance times than those with DCM.

Interpretation of cardiopulmonary testing in patients with structural heart disease is more complicated. Baseline normal Vo_2 values for patients with different types of palliated congenital heart disease are not fully delineated, especially if one also considers age, size, and gender. Patients with single ventricle or cyanosis have even lower values. Therefore, the role of cardiopulmonary testing at present is to compare serial tests in the same patient over time for objective evidence of clinical deterioration in functional status, and to help guide timing of follow-up intervals.

PVR

There is a role for pulmonary vasoreactivity testing as part of the pretransplant assessment. Increased PVR is an independent risk factor for mortality both early and late after heart transplantation.[51,52] There is a continuum of increasing risk as PVR rises, and the actual degree of pulmonary hypertension precluding heart transplantation varies by multiple factors including age, diagnosis, and center experience. However, the reactivity of the vascular bed rather than the absolute measure of PVR correlates with outcome.[52–54] Addonizio and colleagues[54] looked at PVR Index (PVRI) values in 82 patients ranging in age from 4 to 61 years; no patient with a PVRI of less than 6 units developed right ventricular (RV) failure, and 28 of 33 patients with a PVRI greater than 6 and 10 of 12 patients with a PVRI greater than 9 were successfully transplanted, although at a higher risk of RV failure (40%) and mortality (15%). Assessment of PVR and/or vasoreactivity with a diagnosis of any form of single ventricle anatomy, some complex congenital heart diseases with variable sources of pulmonary blood flow, or restrictive cardiomyopathy may be challenging or not possible.

HLA Sensitization

Panel-reactive antibody (PRA) testing during the pretransplant assessment identifies the presence of anti-HLA antibodies, which may increase the risk of antibody-mediated rejection after transplantation. High PRA titers (>10%) are associated with an increased incidence of rejection and reduced survival after heart transplantation.[55] Common sensitizing events in the pediatric heart failure population include repair of congenital heart disease using homograft material,[56] and the increasing use of VADs.[57] Although cross-matching for HLA antibodies is time consuming and not applicable across longer distances, virtual cross-matching is possible. This process involves tissue-typing laboratories assessing the HLA status of the potential donor and considering the recipient's HLA antibodies. The antibodies can be specified and quantified using the Luminex system. This process is widely practiced but does mean many donors are declined because of HLA type and success depends on a wide donor pool. Data from Pittsburgh[58] have shown that if a policy of requiring a negative, prospective cross-match (real or virtual) for highly sensitized children is adopted there are longer waiting list times and a higher mortality after listing. There are increasing reports of successful transplantation in highly sensitized patients and/or across a positive cross-match.[59] The optimal immuno-suppression strategy and long-term outcomes including the incidence of allograft vasculopathy remain to be determined.

ABO-incompatible heart transplantation

Infants continued to experience a high waitlist mortality in 2009 despite the first report of short-term success with intentional ABO-incompatible heart transplantation in,[60] and a clear effect on, institutional waitlist mortality.[61,62] Dipchand and colleagues[63] have recently reported equivalent clinical outcomes for ABO-incompatible and ABO-compatible infant heart transplant recipients with a sustained and significantly lower waitlist mortality for both groups. This practice is becoming more widespread in Europe as well. In the United States, ABO-incompatible transplantation is limited such that the amount of antibody quantified by isohemagglutination must be 1 in 4 or less and recipients must be category 1A, and less than a certain age. In Canada and the United Kingdom blood group mismatches are used with wider titers and are offered to all categories of patients on the list. The latter practice may explain the improved results in Canada and the United Kingdom with this type of transplant. Because of these results, and prolonged waiting times particularly in young infants with donor scarcity, all appropriate pediatric patients should be given the opportunity to be listed for heart transplantation from the first available donor of appropriate size, without regard to donor blood type, if they have absent or low levels of donor-directed antibodies.[63]

The upper age limit at which ABO-incompatible heart transplantation is contraindicated remains controversial and unanswered. The oldest reported patients in the literature are 40 months and 5 years old.[64,65] However, age itself is clearly not the primary risk indicator, and serves only as a surrogate marker for an individual's ability to produce isohemagglutinins. The absolute titer above which transplantation is a contraindication also remains unclear, with successful reports in the literature with isohemagglutinin titers as high as 1:128.[63]

Contraindications

Are there children who are not eligible for heart transplant? There are few absolute contraindications and most are now considered relative. A high PVR remains an absolute contraindication, but children with moderate increase of resistance have received transplants, although at higher risk. The use of a Berlin Heart to reduce resistance before transplant has also been successful. The presence of active sepsis may contraindicate transplant, yet many centers have experience of transplant for patients on ECMO on antibiotics. Infectious diseases often cause concern with future immunosuppression. Yet even patients positive for the human immunodeficiency virus have undergone transplantation.[66] The risks are clearly greater in patients with full-blown AIDS with low T-cell counts. Other patients with chronic infectious diseases such as hepatitis B/C and Chagas disease have also received transplants.[67,68] However, most centers are cautious in their selection and consult their infectious disease colleagues for advice in these unusual settings.

Anatomic considerations are also rarely contraindications to transplant, with pediatric heart surgeons capable of correcting even the most complex venous and arterial anomalies. However, small pulmonary artery size/distortion is a recognized risk factor for successful transplantation.[3] In addition, renal or liver disease is not an absolute contraindication but contributes to morbidity. Combined liver and renal transplant has been performed with heart transplantation, and in particular is more common in adult congenital patients with

> **Box 3**
> **Canadian listing status for cardiac transplantation: pediatric**
>
> When patients have been listed for transplantation, they are assigned a listing status according to their disease stability and the likelihood of survival without transplantation. The following status criteria have been developed by the Canadian Cardiac Transplant Network for listing of cardiac transplant recipients across the country. The criteria below are to be applied to patients for whom a decision has already been made about the appropriateness of heart transplantation. It is not meant to represent criteria for listing. All patients must be proved neurologically eligible for listing.
>
> *General Principles for the Pediatric Age Group (fetal to 18 years):*
>
> 1. The option for listing across compatible blood groups (ie, ABO-incompatible heart transplantation) should exist in any pediatric patient in whom it is clinically appropriate.[1] Eligibility for ABO-I listing is to be determined by a transplant physician or surgeon with the appropriate clinical expertise.
> 2. Organ allocation is made preferentially to postnatal patients regardless of status. There may be circumstances where an in utero[2] patient is deemed to have "life threatening CHD not amenable to medical or surgical temporizing therapy" and may be listed as a Status 4 at the discretion of the listing program. Allocation of a donor organ to an in utero patient ahead of any postnatal patient (regardless of listing status) requires mandatory discussion physician-to-physician. The program with the Status 4 patient should be notified as per the principles of organ sharing and initiate the discussion regarding the possibility of reallocation of the donor heart to the in utero candidate. In utero listing: prenatal testing should confirm that the fetus is viable and medically suitable to receive a transplant; the risk of associated complications becomes appropriately low at approximately 35 to 36 weeks' gestational age; waiting time recommences at the time of birth.
> 3. Hearts from donors less than 18 years of age are first considered for recipients less than 18 years of age (pursuant to size, blood type and clinical status). However, a suitable-sized pediatric donor may be better suited for a higher-status older recipient and consideration for reallocation should proceed as per the principles of organ sharing.
>
> *Status Criteria: Pediatric Cardiac Transplant*
>
> Status 4 (All status 4 patients should be discussed and approved as status 4 with all other centers supported by the regional Organ Procurement Organization before listing)
>
> 1. VAD in a patient weighing less than 8 kg
> 2. Mechanically ventilated on high-dose single or multiple inotropes ± mechanical support (eg, IABP, ECMO, Abiomed [Danvers, MA, USA] BV5000, or Biomedicus [Perfusion.com INC, Fort Myers, FL, USA]), excluding VADs
> 3. VAD malfunction or complication such as thromboembolism, systemic device-related infection, mechanical failure, or life-threatening arrhythmia
> 4. Patients should be recertified every 7 days as a status 4 by a qualified physician if still medically appropriate
>
> Status 4S
>
> 1. High PRA (>80%) or increased PRA (>20%) with 3 prior positive cross-matches (in the setting of negative virtual or actual donor/recipient specific cross-match).
>
> Status 3.5
>
> 1. Hospitalized patient with a VAD
> 2. Less than 6 months of age with congenital heart disease: prostaglandin dependent
> 3. High dose multiple inotropes in hospital and patients not candidates for VAD therapy or no VAD available
> 4. Acute refractory ventricular arrhythmias
>
> Status 3
>
> 1. VAD not meeting status 4 criteria including outpatient VAD
> 2. Less than 6 months of age with congenital heart disease
> 3. Cyanotic congenital heart disease with resting saturation less than 65%
> 4. Congenital heart disease: arterial shunt dependent (ie, Norwood)
> 5. Patients on inotropes in hospital, not meeting above criteria
> 6. Inpatient with CPAP/BIPAP support for HF management
> 7. Heart-lung recipient candidates

Status 2

1. At home with intermittent CPAP/BIPAP support for HF management
2. In hospital for management of heart disease/HF not meeting the above criteria
3. Growth failure: less than fifth percentile for weight and/or height or loss of 1.5 SD of expected growth (weight or height)
4. Cyanotic congenital heart disease with resting saturation 65% to 75% or prolonged desaturation to less than 60% with modest activity (ie, walking, feeding)
5. Fontan palliation with protein-losing enteropathy
6. Multiple organ transplant recipient candidates

Status 1

1. All other out-of-hospital patients
2. In utero (congenital heart disease or heart failure)

Abbreviations: BIPAP, bilevel positive airway pressure; CPAP, continuous positive airway pressure; HF, heart failure; PRA, panel-reactive antibody; SD, standard deviation; VAD, ventricular assist device.

long-standing hepatic insufficiency and cirrhosis, and in patients who are on dialysis at the time of listing for heart transplantation. Previous malignancy is not a contraindication, as noted earlier, but the length of time that a patient has been in remission before transplant varies between countries and among centers; careful consultation with an oncologist is crucial to make an appropriate decision. Adverse social circumstances may be overcome with strong support.[69] Learning difficulties, cerebral damage, and chromosomal abnormalities are also relative rather than absolute contraindications, with many centers offering transplantation. For many of these conditions the decision-making process needs to be multidisciplinary and individualized for the child and family.

THE CHILD ON THE WAITING LIST FOR HEART TRANSPLANTATION

When to list a child for heart transplantation? How to prioritize children on the list? Who is not a candidate for a heart transplant? These problems face pediatric transplant teams throughout the developed world. However, there is no simple answer. Experience and clinical judgment matter more than reliance on numbers. Waiting list mortality is multifactorial, reflecting donor availability, acuity of the waiting recipient (status), diagnosis, and blood type. Influencing donor availability is difficult, but knowledge of waiting list mortality data can often play a role in decision making around appropriate timing for listing a patient for transplant. However, in adolescents with DCM for whom reliable exercise test data are available, the numerical values from adult criteria can be helpful, as discussed earlier. Even so, data can be different in patients on β-blockers and absolute cutoffs are difficult. As discussed earlier,

metabolic exercise testing is rarely the primary data source for decision making on listing for transplant in younger children and those with congenital heart disease. In adolescents with congenital heart disease a V_E/V_{CO_2} seems more useful than simple oxygen consumption.[70] Impaired function on echocardiography is a poor discriminator of prognosis. A similarly low ejection/shortening fraction can be seen in children with no symptoms and those with NYHA 4/Ross 4. This situation creates problems in pediatrics, where there can be pressure to list for transplant because of poor function on echocardiography. However, because of the limitations of exercise testing in the young, there has been a search for alternative prognostic markers. As in adults, natriuretic peptide can be helpful in defining prognosis and seems to correlate well with symptoms, more than echocardiography.[71,72] Natriuretic peptides have the advantage of being useful across all age groups, although the data available concentrate more on children with myocardial rather than congenital heart disease, in which peptide levels may vary. Weight gain and growth are important markers in pediatric cardiology. An infant or young child who fails to thrive with heart failure despite optimal medical therapy and supplemented nutrition is generally considered to have a poor prognosis.

Pretransplant diagnosis also affects posttransplant survival. For patients with congenital heart disease, there is a significantly higher early mortality compared with patients transplanted for cardiomyopathy.[17] Guidelines are increasingly being developed specifically applicable to the pediatric and adult congenital population, striving to identify patients who are at the greatest risk of dying and who derive the greatest benefit from heart transplantation. However, even these guidelines are controversial. Two published consensus reports on listing pediatric patients for heart transplantation exist but are predominantly based on expert opinion as opposed to multi-center clinical trials.[73,74]

As noted earlier, timing of listing with a diagnosis of restrictive cardiomyopathy remains controversial. However, the most recent consensus listing guidelines recommend listing at or shortly after the time of diagnosis because of the limited available medical interventions and the concern about the development of a nonreactive pulmonary vascular bed.[74] The emergence of safer long-term mechanical support with the Berlin Heart has allowed an alternative approach of decompressing left atrial pressure and allowing PVR to decrease over weeks or even months before transplant.[75]

The term waiting list is a misleading term for transplantation. Not all donor organs are suitable for all recipients. Size, blood group, and HLA typing of donors are considered when allocating organs. Once a child is on the list for transplantation it is prudent to ensure those at greatest risk of death are given priority. How this is done and what criteria are used varies around the world. In larger countries there is geographic priority for local recipients.

The United States are divided into 11 regions, which are managed by a federally designated organ-procurement organization, the UNOS,[76] which is a national body. The UNOS system also allows prioritization of the most ill patients. Organs are allocated first to the local region and then referred to a nearby area. This system reduces ischemic time of the donor organ. The highest-priority pediatric patients are categorized as type 1A and are in hospital on inotropes or a mechanical assist and are often ventilated. The next priority group is category 1B patients. These children are on lower-dose intravenous medications either in hospital or at home. As in Europe, there are virtually no cases of children with mechanical support being discharged home, unlike in adults.

In 1999, the pediatric heart allocation system was revised in the United States. Almond and colleagues[9] recently reported on the effect of the change in waiting list mortality since 1999, to determine whether the revised allocation system has affected survival. In the United States, equal 1A status is assigned to patients who are on ECMO, ventilator support, or merely on inotropes. This study found that patients on ECMO had a 12-fold higher mortality, and that the highest risk of dying while waiting was for patients who were on ECMO, ventilated, on dialysis support, and of non-White race. A more optimal organ allocation system may be indicated for pediatric heart donors and recipients.

In the United Kingdom, there is an urgent transplant list for the most ill patients. Those who are in hospital on inotropes can be listed urgently. In pediatrics, there are few patients on mechanical support at home. The final group of patients (1B) are those who are stable at home. This system is mirrored in most countries, with slight variations. For example in Germany and the European transplant community an urgency-based heart allocation algorithm was adopted in August 2000. The UK transplant service adopted an urgent allocation system in 1999. In both regions, the results of transplant for the sickest patients have improved, with fewer deaths on the waiting list. In the United Kingdom all children on Berlin Heart assist remain in hospital at present and are urgently listed. Also in the United Kingdom the severe shortage of organs for infants and children weighing less than 15 kg has limited urgent listing in this group to those on positive pressure ventilation or mechanical assist.

The outcomes for children on the waiting list who are bridged to transplant with mechanical support are good. A review of the UNOS data by Davies and colleagues[77] showed comparable outcomes after transplant in children on mechanical support with children not on mechanical support. However, this study also showed that early survival among those undergoing ECMO and infants on mechanical support was poor.

From the Canadian perspective, the listing algorithm and status levels are more detailed in an attempt to address the fundamental issue of ensuring the sickest recipient is the first to be allocated an organ. **Box 3** outlines the most recent iteration of the Canadian pediatric listing algorithm from October 2009, which separates short-term mechanical support and mechanical support with complications from only intravenous inotropes and mechanical ventilation.

As discussed earlier, patients sensitized to HLA types are a considerable problem in the listing process. At present, there is no prioritization for these sensitized patients within the UNOS system, although it does exist in the Canadian system. In the United Kingdom a proposal has been made to include these patients in the priority scheme, at a second level behind those conventionally urgently listed. The risk of sudden death on the transplant list is a concern. Sudden death in children seems less common than in adults, and data from the PHTS group[78] show that only 1.3% of pediatric patients listed in the United States died suddenly or from an arrhythmia.

The presence of congenital heart disease and UNOS status were not associated with an increased risk of sudden death. This study did not support the uniform use of implantable cardiac defibrillators in children on the transplant list.

SUMMARY

Heart transplantation extends the life expectancy and quality of life in children with end-stage heart failure. The indications and contraindications for heart transplantation are variable, and must be individualized for patients and their family. The evaluation process is extensive and multidisciplinary. Patients should be referred early with consultation to a heart failure/transplantation center to optimize the appropriate timing for listing, because waiting times can be prolonged, and mortality on the waiting list is significant. Outcomes after heart transplantation continue to improve, even for the most complex patients, and even patients with significant medical challenges can be stabilized and survive to a successful transplant.

REFERENCES

1. Kirk R, Edwards LB, Aurora P, et al. Registry of The International Society for Heart and Lung Transplantation: eleventh official pediatric heart transplantation report-2008. J Heart Lung Transplant 2008;27: 970–7.
2. Lamour JM, Kanter KR, Naftel DC, et al. Cardiac Transplant Registry Database. Pediatric Heart Transplant Study. The effect of age, diagnosis, and previous surgery in children and adults undergoing heart transplantation for congenital heart disease. J Am Coll Cardiol 2009;54:160–5.
3. Chen JM, Davies RR, Mital SR, et al. Trends and outcomes in transplantation for complex congenital heart disease: 1984 to 2004. Ann Thorac Surg 2004;78(4):1352–61 [discussion: 1352–61]. Review.
4. Webber SA, Naftel DC, Parker J, et al. Late rejection episodes more than 1 year after pediatric heart transplantation: risk factors and outcomes. J Heart Lung Transplant 2003;22(8):869–75.
5. Pahl E, Naftel DC, Canter CE, et al. Death after rejection with severe hemodynamic compromise in pediatric heart transplant recipients: a multi-institutional study. J Heart Lung Transplant 2001;20:279–87.
6. Schowengerdt KO, Naftel DC, Seib PM, et al. Infection after pediatric heart transplantation: results of a multiinstitutional study. J Heart Lung Transplant 1997;12:1207–16.
7. Webber SA, Naftel DC, Fricker FJ, et al. Lymphoproliferative disorders after paediatric heart transplantation: a multi-institutional study. Lancet 2006;367(9506):233–9.
8. Pahl E, Naftel DC, Kuhn MA, et al. The impact and outcome of transplant coronary artery disease in a pediatric population: a 9-year multi-institutional study. J Heart Lung Transplant 2005;24:645–51.
9. Almond CS, Thiagarajan RR, Piercey GE, et al. Waiting list mortality among children listed for heart transplantation in the United States. Circulation 2009;119(5):717–27.
10. International Society of Heart and Lung Transplantation. Available at: http://www.ishlt.org/registries/slides.asp2008. Accessed July 2, 2010.
11. Towbin JA, Lowe AM, Colan SD, et al. Incidence, causes, and outcomes of dilated cardiomyopathy in children. JAMA 2006;296:1867–76.
12. Lipshultz S, Sleeper L, Towbin J, et al. The incidence of pediatric cardiomyopathy in two regions of the United States. N Engl J Med 2003;348:1647–55.
13. Cox GF, Sleeper LA, Lowe AM, et al. Variables associated with a known etiology of cardiomyopathy in children: a retrospective analysis of the Pediatric Cardiomyopathy Registry (PCMR) from 1990–1995. Circulation 2001;104(Suppl II):588.
14. Dipchand AI, Naftel DC, Feingold B, et al. Outcomes of children with cardiomyopathy listed for transplant: a multi-institutional study. J Heart Lung Transplant 2009;28(12):1312–21.
15. Tsirka AE, Trinkaus K, Chen SC, et al. Improved outcomes of pediatric dilated cardiomyopathy with utilization of heart transplantation. J Am Coll Cardiol 2004;44:391–7.
16. Abraham JR, Redington AN, Dipchand AI, et al. Effect of medical therapy and transplantation on the natural history of pediatric dilated cardiomyopathy: a 25 year retrospective study [abstract]. Circulation 2006;114(Suppl II):451.
17. Kirk R, Naftel D, Hoffman TM, et al. Outcome of pediatric patients with dilated cardiomyopathy listed for transplant: a multi-institutional study. J Heart Lung Transplant 2009;28(12):1322–8.
18. Akagi T, Benson LN, Lightfoot NE, et al. Natural history of dilated cardiomyopathy in children. Am Heart J 1991;121:1502–6.
19. Burch M, Siddiqi SA, Celermajer DS, et al. Dilated cardiomyopathy in children: determinants of outcome. Br Heart J 1994;7:246–50.
20. Arola A, Tuominen J, Ruuskanen O, et al. Idiopathic dilated cardiomyopathy in children: prognostic indicators and outcome. Pediatrics 1998;101:369–76.
21. Kirklin J, Naftel D, Caldwell RL, et al. Should status II patients be removed from the pediatric heart transplant waiting list? A multi-institutional study. J Heart Lung Transplant 2006;25:271–5.
22. Chen S, Balfour IC, Jureidini S. Clinical spectrum of restrictive cardiomyopathy in children. J Heart Lung Transplant 2001;20:90–2.

23. Weller RJ, Weintraub R, Addonizio LJ, et al. Outcome of restrictive cardiomyopathy in children. Am J Cardiol 2002;90:501–6.

24. Rivenes SM, Kearney DL, Smith E, et al. Sudden death and cardiovascular collapse in children with restrictive cardiomyopathy. Circulation 2000;102(8): 876–82.

25. Zangwill SD, Naftel D, L'Ecuyer T, et al. Outcomes of children with restrictive cardiomyopathy listed for heart transplant: a multi-institutional study. J Heart Lung Transplant 2009;28(12):1335–40.

26. Gajarski R, Naftel D, Pahl E, et al. Outcomes of pediatric patients with hypertrophic cardiomyopathy. J Heart Lung Transplant 2009;28(12):1329–34.

27. Colan SD, Lipshultz SE, Lowe AM, et al. Epidemiology and cause-specific outcome of hypertrophic cardiomyopathy in children. Circulation 2007;115: 773–81.

28. Ward KM, Binns H, Chin C, et al. Pediatric heart transplantation for anthracycline cardiomyopathy: cancer recurrence is rare. J Heart Lung Transplant 2004;23:1040–5.

29. Morgan E, Pahl E. Early heart transplant in a child with advanced lymphoma. Pediatr Transplant 2002; 6:509–12.

30. Lee KJ, McCrindle BW, Bohn DJ, et al. Clinical outcomes of acute myocarditis in childhood. Heart 1999;82:226–33.

31. Foerster S, Canter C, Carey A, et al. A comparative analysis of outcomes for pediatric patients with biopsy-proven myocarditis, clinically-diagnosed myocarditis and idiopathic dilated cardiomyopathy. Circulation 2007;1007(Suppl II):565.

32. Verma NA, Zheng XT, Harris MU, et al. Outbreak of life-threatening coxsackievirus B1 myocarditis in neonates. Clin Infect Dis 2009;49(5):759–63.

33. Cooper LT. Giant cell myocarditis in children. Prog Pediatr Cardiol 2007;24(1):47–9.

34. Rajagopal SK, Almond CS, Laussen PC, et al. Extracorporeal membrane oxygenation for the support of infants, children, and young adults with acute myocarditis: a review of the Extracorporeal Life Support Organization Registry. Crit Care Med 2010;38(2):382–7.

35. Bernstein D, Naftel D, Chin C, et al. Outcome of listing for cardiac transplantation for failed Fontan: a multi-institutional study. Circulation 2006;114(4):273–80.

36. Costello JM, Steinhorn D, McColley S, et al. Treatment of plastic bronchitis in a Fontan patient with tissue plasminogen activator: a case report and review of the literature. Pediatrics 2002;109(4):e64.

37. Griffiths ER, Kaza AK, Wyler von Ballmoos MC, et al. Evaluating failing Fontans for heart transplantation: predictors of death. Ann Thorac Surg 2009;88(2): 558–63.

38. del Nido PJ, Armitage JM, Fricker FJ, et al. Extracorporeal membrane oxygenation support as a bridge to pediatric heart transplantation. Circulation 1994; 90(5 Pt 2):II66–9.

39. Blume ED, Naftel DC, Bastardi HJ, et al. Outcomes of children bridged to heart transplantation with ventricular assist devices: a multi-institutional study. Circulation 2006;113(19):2313–9.

40. Checchia PA, Pahl E, Shaddy RE, et al. Cardiac transplantation for Kawasaki disease. Pediatrics 1997;100(4):695–9.

41. Wray J, Radley-Smith R. Longitudinal assessment of psychological functioning in children after heart or heart-lung transplantation. J Heart Lung Transplant 2006;25(3):345–52.

42. Ringewald JM, Gidding SS, Crawford SE, et al. Nonadherence is associated with late rejection in pediatric heart transplant recipients. J Pediatr 2001; 139:75–8.

43. Canter CE, Kirklin JK. ISHLT monograph series. Pediatric heart transplantation, vol. 2. Philadelphia (PA): Elsevier; 2007.

44. Ross RD, Daniels SR, Schwartz DC, et al. Plasma norepinephrine levels in infants and children with congestive heart failure. Am J Cardiol 1987;59: 911–4.

45. Ross RD, Bollinger RO, Pinsky WW. Grading the severity of congestive heart failure in infants. Pediatr Cardiol 1992;13:72–5.

46. Connolly D, Rutkowski M, Auslender M, et al. The New York University Pediatric Heart Failure Index: a new method of quantifying chronic heart failure severity in children. J Pediatr 2001;138:644–8.

47. Mancini DM, Eisen H, Kussmaul W, et al. Value of peak exercise O_2 for optimal cardiac transplantation in ambulatory patients with heart failure. Circulation 1991;83:778–86.

48. Miller LW. Listing criteria for cardiac transplantation: results of an American Society of Transplant Physicians-National Institutes of Health Conference. Transplantation 1998;66:947–51.

49. Pardaens K, Van Cleemput J, Vanhaecke J, et al. Peak oxygen uptake better predicts outcome than submaximal respiratory data in heart transplant candidates. Circulation 2000;101:1152–7.

50. Pahl E, Devries J, Ward K, et al. Exercise stress tests in children with heart failure: peak oxygen consumption and endurance correlate with adverse cardiac events. J Heart Lung Transplant 2009;28:S235.

51. Espinoza C, Manito N, Roca J, et al. Reversibility of pulmonary hypertension in patients evaluated for orthotopic heart transplantation: importance in the postoperative morbidity and mortality. Transplant Proc 1999;31:2503–4.

52. Gajarski RJ, Towbin JA, Bricker JT, et al. Intermediate follow-up of pediatric heart transplant recipients with elevated pulmonary vascular resistance index. J Am Coll Cardiol 1994;23:1682–7.

53. Zales VR, Pahl E, Backer CL, et al. Pharmacologic reduction of pretransplantation pulmonary vascular resistance predicts outcome after pediatric cardiac transplantation. J Heart Lung Transplant 1993;12(6 pt 1):965–72.

54. Addonizio LJ, Gersony WM, Robbins RC, et al. Elevated pulmonary vascular resistance and cardiac transplantation. Circulation 1987;76(5 pt 2):V52–5.

55. Kobashigawa JA, Sabad A, Drinkwater D, et al. Pre-transplant panel reactive-antibody screens. Are they truly a marker for poor outcome after cardiac transplantation? Circulation 1996;94:II294–297.

56. Breinholt JP 3rd, Hawkins JA, Lambert LM, et al. A prospective analysis of the immunogenicity of cryopreserved nonvalved allografts used in pediatric heart surgery. Circulation 2000;102(19 Suppl 3):III179–82.

57. Pagani FD, Dyke DB, Wright S, et al. Development of anti-major histocompatibility complex class I or II antibodies following left ventricular assist device implantation: effects on subsequent allograft rejection and survival. J Heart Lung Transplant 2001;20:646–53.

58. Feingold B, Bowman P, Zeevi A, et al. Survival in allosensitized children after listing for cardiac transplantation. J Heart Lung Transplant 2007;26(6):565–71.

59. Pollock-BarZiv SM, den Hollander N, Ngan B, et al. Pediatric heart transplantation in human leukocyte antigen sensitized patients: evolving management and assessment of intermediate-term outcomes in a high-risk population. Circulation 2007;116:172–8.

60. West LJ, Pollock-Barziv SM, Dipchand AI, et al. ABO-incompatible heart transplantation in infants. N Engl J Med 2001;344(11):793–800.

61. West LJ, Karamlou T, Dipchand AI, et al. Impact on outcomes after listing and transplantation, of a strategy to accept ABO blood group-incompatible donor hearts for neonates and infants. J Thorac Cardiovasc Surg 2006;131(2):455–61.

62. Goldman AP, Cassidy J, de Leval M, et al. The waiting game: bridging to paediatric heart transplantation. Lancet 2003;362(9400):1967–70.

63. Dipchand AI, Pollock BarZiv SM, Manlhiot C, et al. Equivalent outcomes for pediatric heart transplantation recipients: ABO-blood group incompatible versus ABO-compatible. Am J Transplant 2009;9:1–9.

64. Roche SL, Burch M, O'Sullivan J, et al. Multicenter experience of ABO-incompatible pediatric cardiac transplantation. Am J Transplant 2008;8(1):208–15.

65. Bucin D, Johansson S, Malm T, et al. Heart transplantation across the antibodies against HLA and ABO. Transpl Int 2006;19(3):239–44.

66. Uriel N, Jorde UP, Cotarlan V, et al. Heart transplantation in human immunodeficiency virus-positive patients. J Heart Lung Transplant 2009;28(7):667–9.

67. Dimopoulos K, Okonko DO, Diller GP, et al. Abnormal ventilatory response to exercise in adults with congenital heart disease relates to cyanosis and predicts survival. Circulation 2006;113(24):2796–802.

68. Bern C, Montgomery SP, Herwaldt BL, et al. Evaluation and treatment of Chagas disease in the United States: a systematic review. JAMA 2007;298(18):2171–81.

69. Gasink LB, Blumberg EA, Localio AR, et al. Hepatitis C virus seropositivity in organ donors and survival in heart transplant recipients. JAMA 2006;296(15):1843–50.

70. Brown KL, Ramaiah R, Fenton M, et al. Adverse family social circumstances and outcome in pediatric cardiac transplant recipients at a UK center. J Heart Lung Transplant 2009;28(12):1267–72.

71. Price JF, Thomas AK, Grenier M, et al. B-type natriuretic peptide predicts adverse cardiovascular events in pediatric outpatients with chronic left ventricular systolic dysfunction. Circulation 2006;114(10):1063–9.

72. Mangat J, Carter C, Riley G, et al. The clinical utility of brain natriuretic peptide in paediatric left ventricular failure. Eur J Heart Fail 2009;11(1):48–52.

73. Dipchand AI, Cecere R, Delgado D, et al. Canadian consensus on paediatric and adult congenital heart transplantation 2004. Can J Cardiol 2005;21(13):1145–8.

74. Canter CE, Shaddy RE, Bernstein D, et al. Indications for heart transplantation in pediatric heart disease. Circulation 2007;115(5):658–76.

75. Gandhi SK, Grady RM, Huddleston CB, et al. Beyond Berlin: heart transplantation in the "untransplantable". J Thorac Cardiovasc Surg 2008;136(2):529–31.

76. United Network for Organ Sharing. Available at: UNOS.org. Accessed July 2, 2010.

77. Davies RR, Russo MJ, Hong KN, et al. The use of mechanical circulatory support as a bridge to transplantation in pediatric patients: an analysis of the United Network for Organ Sharing database. J Thorac Cardiovasc Surg 2008;135(2):421–7.

78. Rhee EK, Canter CE, Basile S, et al. Sudden death prior to pediatric heart transplantation: would implantable defibrillators improve outcome? J Heart Lung Transplant 2007;26(5):447–52.

Novel Therapies in Childhood Heart Failure: Today and Tomorrow

Daniel J. Penny, MD, PhD, Giles Wesley Vick III, MD, PhD*

KEYWORDS

- Pediatric heart failure • Diagnostic technology
- Cardiomyopathies • Ventricular dysfunction

Heart failure is an important cause of morbidity and mortality in individuals of all ages. The constellation of characteristics associated with heart failure is well known. These characteristics include diminished tissue perfusion, peripheral vasoconstriction and edema, and pulmonary congestion, frequently but not always accompanied by diminished cardiac contractile action. The many-faceted nature of the clinical heart failure syndrome has historically frustrated attempts to develop an overarching explanative theory.[1] However, much useful information has been gained by basic and clinical investigation, even though a comprehensive understanding of heart failure has been elusive.

In any event, 3 verities do seem clear. (1) Heart failure is a growing problem, in both adult and pediatric populations.[2,3] (2) Standard medical therapy, as of 2010, can have positive effects, but these are usually limited and progressively diminish with time in most patients.[4] (3) If we want curative or near-curative therapy that will return patients to a normal state of health at a feasible cost, we need to develop much better diagnostic and therapeutic technologies.[5,6]

This review does not deal with pediatric heart failure secondary to volume or pressure overload. In most cases, effective corrective or palliative therapy for these types of pediatric heart failure is already available in the form of surgery or interventional catheterization.[7,8] Rather, the authors address the vexing group of heart failure etiologies that include cardiomyopathies and other ventricular dysfunctions of various types, for which current therapy is only modestly effective. There are certainly many unique aspects to heart failure in patients with pediatric and congenital heart disease.[9–11] However, many of the innovative approaches that are being developed for the care of adults with heart failure will be applicable to heart failure in childhood.[7,8]

BIOLOGIC COMPLEXITY OF HEART FAILURE

The authors are of the opinion that developing the radically new technologies required to completely cure the most common types of heart failure will require us to acknowledge and embrace the vast biologic complexity of these types of heart failure.[12] The study of heart failure is, as is the study of biology in general,[13] at its core a study of information (**Fig. 1**). A great deal of scientific progress has resulted from reductionist approaches to analyzing biologic information, and these approaches continue to be useful and to be needed. However, mechanistic understanding acquired at the molecular level must be integrated at the level of the organ and organism if it is to have clinical utility.[14,15]

The amount of information encoded in just the individual genetic and epigenetic components of animals and humans is massive. However, the

Section of Pediatric Cardiology, Department of Pediatrics, Baylor College of Medicine, Texas Children's Hospital, 6621 Fannin Street, Houston, TX 77030, USA
* Corresponding author.
E-mail address: gvick@bcm.tmc.edu

Heart Failure Clin 6 (2010) 591–621
doi:10.1016/j.hfc.2010.06.003

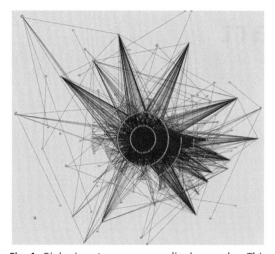

Fig. 1. Biologic systems are exceedingly complex. This figure, constructed with the aid of the Cytoscape computer software program from data generated by Stelzl and colleagues is a reconstruction of the human protein-protein interaction network. This static figure, complicated as it is, greatly underestimates the complexity of the actual biologic networks, which are in constant flux and which have many rapidly changing quantitative relationships between components. (*Data from* Stelzl U, Worm U, Lalowski M, et al. A human protein-protein interaction network: a resource for annotating the proteome. Cell 2005;122(6):957–68.)

most important aspects of animal and human complexity lie in the pervasive interconnectedness of these components, including widespread epistatic and pleiotropic mechanisms and a multitude of other interactions, the large time-dependent flux of these components, and the daunting fact that no 2 animals or humans are precisely identical, not even monozygotic human twins or inbred mice strains.[16–18] Two organisms may share the same genetic information but they never contain exactly corresponding epigenomes.

Furthermore, biologic component parts acting together have complicated emergent properties that are not shared by any of the components individually. For instance, both myofibrils and mitochondria are important constituents of individual cardiac cells. However, neither myofibrils nor mitochondria by themselves are capable of pumping blood. Generating a cardiac output is an emergent property possessed only by the intact heart and is produced by extraordinarily intricate interaction between the many trillions of individual elements of the heart. The necessity of characterizing the emergent physiologic parameters affected by heart failure adds many additional layers to the informational complexity of the disorder.

SYSTEMS BIOLOGY

The developing science of systems biology offers promising approaches to help clinicians and researchers practically deal with the tsunami of biologic information that threatens to overwhelm them.[19–22] It is important to recognize that "brute force" application of standard computational and statistical methods has limited applicability for the modeling of biologic systems, because these methods become rapidly overwhelmed by large numbers of input variables and immense amounts of data. This "curse of dimensionality" causes computational overhead to grow so rapidly that feasible limits of data processing are quickly exceeded in the absence of substantial simplifying algorithmic assumptions.[23] For example, moderately detailed quantum mechanical modeling of the folding of even one protein requires months of processing time on an advanced supercomputer.[24]

The most important such simplification is recognition that biologic systems are modular,[25–27] being composed of a limited number of major subsystems or "final common pathways" (**Fig. 2**).[28,29] Heart failure cannot occur without considerable malfunction in at least one major subsystem or final common pathway. This "final common pathway" hypothesis provides a straightforward way to perform biologically relevant dimensionality reduction for investigational purposes, and facilitates a reasonable strategy to guide diagnosis and therapy.

The second important simplification is that biologic processes have a networked organizational structure that can be described in an effective manner by network theory, a branch of mathematical topology.[30–32] Networks are made up of nodes, and the connections between nodes that are termed edges. The edge or connection between 2 nodes delineates how the nodes are related. If directional information is associated with an edge, the edge is said to be directed. If not, the edge is undirected. The nodes in biologic systems can represent various molecular entities such as genes, proteins, promoters, introns, or metabolites. A node can also represent the aggregate behavior of multiple such entities combined into a single module. In most cases each individual node will exhibit a characteristic complex functionality. The cellular nature of biologic systems dramatically increases both their intrinsic network density and their overall robustness.

It is important to recognize that there are not "privileged" levels of information or causality in biologic networks.[14] In our electronic computer systems, the "program" that governs the machine

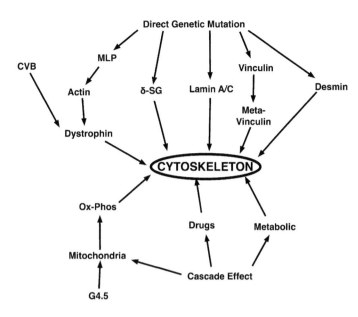

Fig. 2. Biologic systems are modular with final common pathways for dysfunction. Multiple effects can cause dysfunction of the cytoskeletal modules of the cardiomyocyte. Direct genetic mutations as well as Coxsackie B (CVB) viral infection can lead to failure of the cytoskeleton to function properly. In addition, event cascades precipitated by binding partner disruption, acquired disruption from medications, metabolic derangements, or inefficient mitochondrial energy production can render the cardiac cytoskeleton unable to perform its tasks. CVB, Coxsackievirus B; Ox-Phos, oxidative phosphorylation; MLP, muscle LIM protein; Lamin A/C, protein belonging to the lamin family of proteins that is encoded in humans by the LMNA gene; δ-SG, δ-sarcoglycan; G4.5, Tafazzin, a protein highly expressed in skeletal and cardiac muscle. (*Modified from* Towbin JA, Bowles NE. Molecular genetics of left ventricular dysfunction, Curr Mol Med 2001;1(1):81–90; with permission.)

is typically discrete, readily identifiable, and separate from the data stored in the computer and from the processes controlled by the program. No such separation is present in biologic systems. Digital information may indeed flow from the DNA to RNA to protein synthesis and eventually cause modification of macroscopic analog characteristics such as cardiac output or blood pressure (**Fig. 3**A). However, feedback from the effect of these macroscopic analog parameters will then modify the expression of the DNA. Information and conditional directives are constantly flowing back and forth between macroscopic structures and variable levels of the microscopic structure of biologic systems, and also within these structures and levels (**Fig. 3**B).

BIOLOGIC NETWORKS

Watts and Strogatz demonstrated in 1998 that the neural network of the nematode *Caenorhabditis elegans* could be modeled by a class of network graphs that contained highly clustered subnodes, in which most nodes were not neighbors, but in which most nodes could be reached from each other in a small number of steps.[33] Watts and Strogatz termed this class of networks "small-world networks". Many subsequent studies have demonstrated that a wide variety of biologic systems are best characterized as small-world networks. Barabasi and Albert discovered how small-world networks could be mathematically defined.[34,35]

Networks can potentially be connected in several ways. The nodes can be connected in a regular fashion or a random fashion. When connections are assigned regularly or randomly, the number of connections per node will have an approximately normal distribution, with a peak value that gives a characteristic network "scale". A third way that networks can be connected is with a large number of nodes of relatively low connectivity and a small number of highly connected nodes. In this type of network the number of nodes (*N*) with a given number of connections (*k*) usually diminishes in accordance with a power law

$$N(k) \sim k^{-g}$$

where *g* is usually between 2 and 3. The function *N(k)* is a so-called fat-tailed distribution that does not have a characteristic peak value. Networks whose organization follows this type of power law distribution thus do not have an identifiable peak value or "scale" and are termed "scale-free".

This scale-free organization is a consequence of 2 fundamental mechanisms that are related to the fundamental biologic nature of the nodes: preferential attachment and sequential growth. New nodes tend to be preferentially connected to nodes that are already highly connected, a manner of development often termed "the rich get richer". Recurrent networking patterns or motifs such as autoregulation and negative feedback are prevalent in living systems (**Fig. 4**).[36]

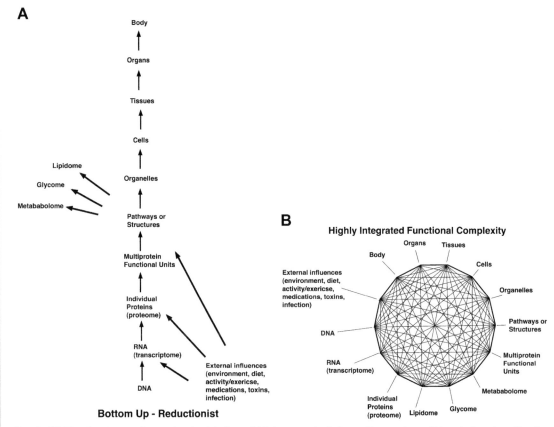

Fig. 3. (*A*) The "bottom-up" or reductionist view of biology posits information and conditional directives flowing from DNA to proteins and thence to higher levels of organization. Causation is believed to follow the "central dogma" described by Crick and to originate primarily in the DNA sequence, the "le programme génétique" of Monod. (*B*) Highly integrated functional complexity. An alternative model of biologic organisms as systems of vast and highly integrated functional complexity is finding increasing experimental support. In this model, causation is neither "bottom-up" nor "top-down" but is broadly distributed among the varying levels of the biologic system, with information and conditional directives flowing back and forth between macroscopic structures and variable levels of the microscopic structure of the systems, and also within these structures and levels. Note that the quantitative relationships between the components of these highly integrated systems are not fixed but are highly dynamic and variable. This model in no way diminishes the critical role of the DNA sequence in providing the essential "dictionary" of life. However, it emphasizes that the specific expression of this "dictionary" is dependent on the properties of the biologic system as a whole in addition to those of the "dictionary" itself. The model has similarities to the paradigm proposed by Noble[14] but is not identical.

There are important practical consequences to the scale-free organization of biologic networks. The networks tend to be robust to many types of stress.[37] This robustness can be accounted for in part by noting that a network allows the same output to be produced by multiple pathways. Consider how the Internet architecture (which is also scale-free) facilitates signal transmission between 2 points even if one connecting route is blocked. The pervasive presence of biologic networking can thus at least partially explain why complete knockout of presumably important genes may have minimal or no phenotypic effect. However, disabling highly connected network "hubs" and final common pathways can be profoundly disruptive to networks with scale-free topology. Such "nexus" nodes and final common pathways can be essential to the functioning of the organism. Their dysfunction may result in disease, and they may also be attractive therapeutic targets. Focus on these "nexus" nodes and final common pathways is an appealing strategy for biologically meaningful data dimensionality reduction.

Multiple possible separate pathways for the origin of given phenotypic states is a corollary of the networked control structure of living organisms. A phenotypic change could result as a consequence of inherited genetic information encoded in the DNA sequence. However, in

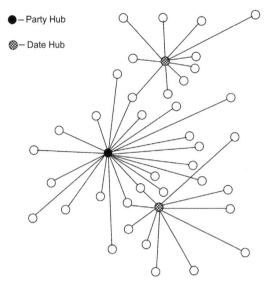

● — Party Hub

◉ — Date Hub

Fig. 4. Many biologic processes are organized into scale-free networks. Integrated processes at multiple different levels are networked together in the functioning of the normal and diseased heart. Most nodes in these networks have only a few connections, but a few nodes, the "hub" nodes, are highly interconnected. Biologic systems are typically robustly tolerant to dysfunction of outlying nodes, but can be severely affected by impairment of hubs. Hub nodes can be subdivided into 2 categories, "party hubs" and "date hubs." Party hubs have simultaneous interaction with most of their partners. Date hubs interact with different partners at different times and locations. Date hubs are generally the most critical to the maintenance of network topology.

many cases the phenotypic change could also result from inherited or acquired changes in the epigenome controlling DNA expression, including noncoding RNAs, histone modifications, chromatin configuration, DNA methylation states, and mRNA splicing as well as alterations in the rate of protein or mRNA degradation and in protein phosphorylation or glycosylation. Direct environmental influence such as infection, toxins, or stress could also produce the phenotypic change.

A good example of multiple pathways of phenotypic origin can be seen in the case of anomalies of the dystrophin molecule. The dystrophin molecule is a critical component of the myocardial cytoskeleton.[38] When dystrophin does not function appropriately, myocardial sarcolemmal disruption results, causing cardiomyopathy and heart failure.[39] It is well known that DNA mutations can cause formation of dysfunctional dystrophin. However, the enterovirus protease 2A can cleave dystrophin and also cause the molecule to malfunction.[40] Sarcolemmal dysfunction, cardiomyopathy, and heart failure are caused by both the

DNA mutation and the viral infection. The dystrophin molecule can also be damaged by the chronic mechanical stress of dilated cardiomyopathy.[41] It follows that cardiomyopathy, once initiated, can become a vicious cycle, with heart failure itself causing myocardial structural changes that produce more severe heart failure. Fortunately, recent experimental evidence suggests that the cycle can be interrupted and even reversed in selected cases by appropriately timed mechanical support.[42,43]

NONLINEAR NATURE OF BIOLOGIC NETWORKS

Biologic networks are dynamic in nature and highly nonlinear, as one might expect, because the underlying biologic systems themselves operate far from thermodynamic equilibrium.[36,44,45] Unfortunately, these properties complicate the study of biologic networks, because output of a nonlinear system does not bear a proportional relationship to the input, and because the global system behavior of a nonlinear system is not a simple summation of its constituent parts.[46,47]

Nonlinear biologic systems frequently exhibit what is termed "chaotic" behavior.[48] The usual popular understanding of chaos is a state of utter confusion or disorder. However, the mathematical and scientific definition of chaos differs from the vernacular. Chaotic systems, at least for mathematicians and scientists, are typically deterministic. That is, their behavior is definitely not random and is governed by the initial conditions of the system. Probably the most important property of chaotic systems is their extreme sensitivity to very small changes, often referred to as the "butterfly effect." A related property is the propensity of these systems to abruptly change from one pattern of response to another substantially different response pattern, called a "bifurcation." For example, the beat-to-beat alteration in QRS amplitude and axis sometimes seen in cardiac tamponade is a type of bifurcation response. Bifurcation responses in chaotic systems can on occasion be catastrophic, in that their initiation causes a sudden and total failure of the system from which it does not recover. Without outside intervention, chaotic systems undergoing catastrophic bifurcation responses will revert to thermodynamic equilibrium. Cardiac ventricular fibrillation is a good example of this phenomenon.

Because of the dynamical instability of chaotic systems, precise long-term prediction of their exact state is not possible. However, the overall behavior of deterministic chaotic systems can be ascertained. If we plot the development of a chaotic system over an extended time period a characteristic pattern will emerge. Such patterns are called "attractors". Attractors with complicated structures, as are typically found in biology, are called "strange attractors" and often have characteristics similar to a type of geometric construct known as "fractals". Fractals are irregular figures with noninteger or fractional dimensions. By contrast, the classic geometric forms of lines, circles, and spheres have 1, 2, and 3 dimensions, respectively. The detail apparent on inspection of fractals increases as one inspects them more closely. The wrinkly pattern of a fractal is qualitatively similar at variable levels of magnification, a property referred to as self-similarity. Fractal geometry is widely seen in nature. Coastlines, clouds, and lightning flashes are good examples. Many biologic structures, including the bronchial tree, the vascular system, the folds of the cerebral cortex, and the His-Purkinje network exhibit a fractal structure.

Several investigators have applied the mathematical techniques of nonlinear analysis to the study of heart rate variability. It is clear that cardiac rate patterns of normal subjects exhibit fluctuations on different time scales, that is, at different levels of temporal magnification, that are statistically self-similar. Poon and Merrill[49] studied healthy subjects and patients with severe congestive heart failure, and found that short-term variations of the cardiac beat-to-beat interval showed a consistently and strongly chaotic character in all normals. However, in congestive heart failure the chaotic fluctuations were replaced by low-frequency intermittent oscillations and a decrease in temporal variability (**Fig. 5**). Thus, the normally chaotic features of cardiac rhythm were substantially reduced in the abnormal hearts. More recently, Arzeno and colleagues have demonstrated that heart rate chaos analysis can be

effectively employed as a mortality predictor in mild to moderate heart failure.[50]

There are many additional aspects of the dynamic heart failure syndrome that could potentially be usefully characterized by nonlinear and network analysis, both at the macro level and in the molecular systems of the heart and other involved organs and structures. It is clear that much remains to be done in this field.

DIAGNOSIS AND THERAPY FOR HEART FAILURE AND CAUSALITY

The predominant paradigm in heart failure diagnosis and therapy has been predicated on simple linear cause and effect models of disease. Sometimes these models are very effectual. Many of the heart failure syndromes seen at the initial presentation of patients with congenital cardiovascular disease are actually characterized quite well by such an approach. For example, the poor peripheral perfusion and pulmonary edema frequently seen in untreated infants with severe coarctation of the aorta and large ventricular septal defect is directly attributable to structural anatomic anomalies in the circulation. Therapy that mends these defects in anatomy effectively and rapidly corrects the heart failure syndrome caused by them. Linear cause and effect models also for the most part characterize acquired cardiac valvular diseases well. These diseases are similarly effectively treated with mechanical therapeutic interventions by interventional catheterization or surgery. Linear cause and effect can explain acute viral myocarditis reasonably satisfactorily also. Although the potency of currently available antiviral therapy may be limited, the action of the patients' immune system often can eventually neutralize the viral infection. Supportive treatment, sometimes even including temporary mechanical ventricular

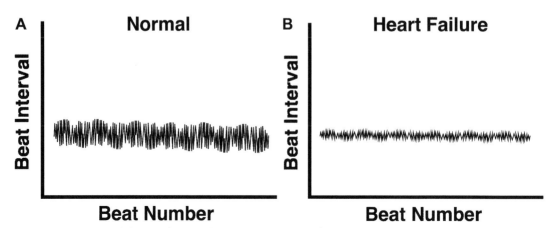

Fig. 5. Heart rate variability is substantially reduced with heart failure (*B*) in comparison with normal (*A*).

assistance while the immune system response is building, can frequently facilitate a complete recovery.

Even heart failure secondary to monogenetic cardiomyopathic disorders is in principle explicable by a simple linear cause and effect model, because a single identifiable proximate causation is known. However, in contradistinction to cardiac anatomic anomalies, our therapeutic technology does not yet allow us to correct genetic disorders directly, even when they are known. Because developed vertebrates are composed of trillions of cells, such correction in developed vertebrates would require trillions of precise molecular operations. Therefore, clinical diagnostic characterization and therapy for these disorders must currently deal with the manifold downstream manifestations of the primary defect. Because most patients are genetically different, and because all patients are epigenetically different, these downstream phenotypic manifestations will be different for different individuals, even if they share the same monogenetic defect.

Unfortunately, the most common types of heart failure now faced by cardiologists do not have simple structural etiologies. In most cases there is not even a known direct cause for the heart failure (see **Fig. 3**B). For example, the cellular and circulatory malfunctions in advanced heart failure are pervasive,[51–54] involving diverse derangements in such processes as: cellular calcium cycling and the proteins regulating this cycling; myosin isoform synthesis and functioning; cytoskeletal protein function; cardiac extracellular matrix homeostasis; mitochondrial energy production; catecholamine synthesis; adrenergic receptor production; free fatty acid synthesis; mitochondrial coupling of adenosine diphosphate phosphorylation to respiration; cardiolipin production; regulation of the mediators of cellular proliferation; the inflammatory response mechanisms; autophagy; and apoptosis. All of these subsystem processes are critical to normal cardiac functioning. When they are observed to be malfunctioning in concert, attributing causation is exceedingly problematic. Investigators are prone to champion the importance of one subsystem or another, but without a comprehensive explanatory model they are truly analogous to the blind men investigating the elephant. The elephant of advanced heart failure is far more than the sum of its parts and the emergent properties of the elephant cannot be adequately characterized by describing each individual part.

Although proximate causes always exist, the highly networked character of living organisms suggests that there will usually not be a unique proximate cause or even a unique set of proximate causes for the widespread derangements of heart failure (**Fig. 6**).[55,56] Indeed, it may never be possible to ascertain primary causation once heart failure becomes evident. Thus, we usually have a causality problem of diagnosis in addition to the problem of not having a single clear therapeutic option.

Because of the highly complex networked nature of biologic reality, it follows that diagnosis and therapy for most heart failure patients must also be complicated if such diagnosis and therapy is to be truly effective. Instead of a single diagnostic test that can characterize the severity of the heart failure on a linear scale, we must think of large diagnostic matrices that will incorporate information from multiple affected biologic modules or final common pathways. Instead of a therapeutic "magic bullet" that will cure with a single well-aimed intervention, we must acknowledge that the best we can hope for, at least in the near term, is a "magic shotgun" that will correct the heart failure syndrome via many separate positive actions at multiple sites (**Fig. 7**).[57–60]

NECESSITY OF IMPROVEMENT IN DIAGNOSTIC CHARACTERIZATION OF HEART FAILURE

In the authors' opinion, improvement in the therapy for heart failure can occur most rapidly only if there is concomitant progress in the diagnostic characterization of heart failure syndromes. As noted earlier, every patient is unique, and this uniqueness extends to every period in the life of the patient, so that the identical context never repeats. As Heraclitus of Ephesus stated: "you never step in the same river twice." A therapy that may be beneficial at one point in time may be ineffective or even deleterious at another point in the development of the patient and the illness because of changes in the pathophysiological milieu. This situation is clearly evident in heart failure when disease progression may necessitate withdrawal of β-blockers and angiotensin-converting enzyme inhibitors for symptomatic hypotension or progressive renal dysfunction.[1,4] It follows that it is necessary to define the state of the heart failure illness at each inflection point in its course. Thus, periodic and robust diagnostic feedback is a critical part of therapeutic efforts and is particularly important in the initiation of new therapies.

The history and physical examination continues to be the cornerstone of diagnosis in heart

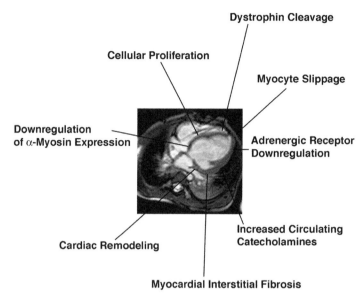

Fig. 6. Multiple processes are deranged in the heart failure phenotype. Once heart failure has advanced beyond the early stage, no single causation for the heart failure may be identifiable.

failure. The standard electrocardogram, chest radiograph, and echocardiogram are also routinely employed, as is standard functional and anatomic cardiac magnetic resonance imaging (MRI). Once the diagnosis of heart failure has been made, evaluation of hemodynamic and volume status on a continuing basis are important facets of follow-up medical care.

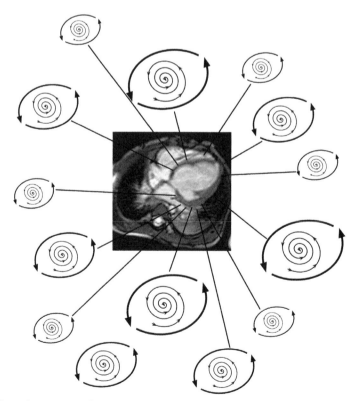

Fig. 7. A vast number of separate self-propagating deleterious positive feedback cycles (vicious cycles) provide the substrate for ventricular remodeling and the progression of heart failure.

Enhancements in remote and ambulatory monitoring technology have major potential to facilitate early identification of incipient heart failure exacerbation while it is still amenable to amelioration by modification of outpatient treatments.[61,62] Such early identification could substantially reduce the medical costs of heart failure, which are in large part secondary to acute and repeat hospital admissions.[63] Some of this remote and ambulatory monitoring technology, such as recording patient weight, is relatively mundane. However, recent advances in biosensor technology have produced very small implantable devices that do not require batteries and which can transmit central venous, arterial, and cardiac chamber pressure data wirelessly to external receivers.[64–66] Many other types of microsensors for biologically and clinically important parameters, such as metabolites, oxygen saturation, and impedance are possible, and in principle might be incorporated into multifunction implantable monitoring devices.[67] It is clear that we are on the verge of a new era in terms of clinical monitoring of heart failure. Even early systems for ambulatory and remote monitoring have shown considerable promise.[68,69] In the future, we will have the capability to replace single-point, invasive, and expensive in-hospital assessments with continuous outpatient monitoring in many scenarios.

A plethora of new diagnostic methods is now available to the clinician. It is important that physicians caring for patients with heart failure become acquainted with the strengths and weaknesses of these new techniques so that they can be appropriately utilized. A comprehensive treatment of the large number of new diagnostic techniques applicable to heart failure is well beyond the scope of this article. However, many of these techniques do share the common theme of being tools for molecular diagnosis. As we move toward more specific biologic therapy for heart failure, diagnosis is also moving toward improved specificity. Another common theme is that the newer modalities tend to address the modular nature of the underlying biology of heart failure. Excellent current examples of these themes are seen in the very active current research on biomarkers.[70–72] Important facets of the heart failure syndromes include neurohormonal activation, remodeling of the cardiac extracellular matrix, inflammation, myocyte stress and injury, and cardiac oxidative stress. It is now possible to evaluate the blood concentrations of various biochemical compounds that are components of each of these facets.

For instance, the precursor of brain natriuretic peptide (prepro-BNP) is produced by myocytes undergoing hemodynamic stress. It is then converted into the proBNP carboxy terminal peptide. proBNP is further processed by corin, a transmembrane serine protease, which produces NT-pro-BNP, an inactive 76-amino-acid amino terminal fragment and the biologically active 32-amino-acid carboxyl terminal fragment BNP.[73] BNP reduces the activity of the renin-angiotensin-aldosterone system. BNP also produces natriuresis, diuresis, and arterial vasodilation. Serum measurements of BNP and NT-pro-BNP have been found to be useful in the identification and management of heart failure. The myofibrillar protein troponin I is a marker for cardiac injury. Its elevation in serum has been shown to be a predictor of poor patient outcome.[74]

Patients with heart failure have abnormally elevated levels of plasma norephinephrine.[71] These patients have an activated renin-angiotensin-aldosterone system; they have elevated levels of big endothelin-1, secreted by vascular endothelial cells and a precursor of endothelin-1 itself, which stimulates vascular smooth muscle contraction and ventricular and blood vessel fibrosis, and potentiates circulating neurohormones. High serum concentrations of all of these neurohormonally related compounds are associated with poor prognosis.

As heart failure advances, there is a progressive ventricular remodeling process.[75] This process is associated with an imbalance between the matrix metalloproteinases that degrade fibrillar collagen and the tissue inhibitors of these enzymes. Plasma matrix metalloproteinase levels are elevated in patients with ventricular remodeling and dilation. Ventricular remodeling is also associated with an increase in cardiac collagen content. This increase in cardiac fibrosis can adversely affect ventricular function. Increased collagen synthesis is reflected in increased plasma procollagen levels. Cicoira and colleagues[76] measured plasma procollagen type III in patients with heart failure and found this parameter to be an independent predictor of poor outcome.

Extensive data suggest that increased oxidative stress is associated with pathologic changes in heart failure, and there appears to be correlation between the degree of oxidative stress and the severity of the heart failure.[77] Early studies indicated that inefficient mitochondrial metabolism and depleted antioxidant defenses could result in the production of toxic free radicals and consequent cellular damage and cell death. Later investigative efforts have demonstrated that the reactive oxygen species engendered by oxidative stress can have considerably more subtle effects by influencing intracellular signaling pathways that employ reactive oxygen species for signal transduction.

Direct measurement of reactive oxygen species in humans is problematic. Therefore, surrogate markers of oxidative stress have been employed. Such surrogate markers include plasma myeloperoxidase and malondialdehyde (indicators of leukocyte activation), oxidized lipoproteins, plasma and urine isoprostanes, and urinary biopyrrins (oxidative metabolites of bilirubin). Increased xanthine oxidase activity appears to be associated with increased levels of oxidative stress in heart failure. Because uric acid production is elevated in the presence of elevated xanthine oxidase, plasma uric acid may also prove to be a surrogate marker of oxidative stress.[71]

An intriguing body of work has identified a population of circulating endogenous endothelial progenitor cells. Multiple studies have found inverse correlations between the numbers of these cells and cardiovascular risk factors.[78–83] Patients with advanced heart failure have been noted to have substantially lower concentrations of these cells in their blood than age-matched controls.

Many other biomarkers have been demonstrated to give prognostic information in patients with heart failure. One exciting area of biomarker investigation is in molecular imaging.[84–87] Blood biomarkers are advantageous for many purposes because they are so readily obtained. However, blood biomarkers do not directly provide information about the heart. With modern imaging techniques it is possible to go beyond purely anatomic imaging to characterize tissue and directly visualize several biologic processes.

Viability scanning has come into widespread use in cardiology over the past several years, and may be considered to be a simple version of molecular and cellular imaging. Early myocardial viability studies were performed with positron emission tomography (PET) using the [18]fluorodeoxyglucose tracer. Single-photon emission computed tomography (SPECT) and stress echocardiography were also shown to be effective methods for distinguishing viable from nonviable myocardium. More recently, gadolinium contrast-enhanced MRI has been employed to evaluate myocardial viability. MRI has the advantages of not requiring radiation, of providing high resolution, and of not being dependent on acoustic windows. Many patients with heart failure have sustained myocardial damage and have replaced damaged regions of myocardium with fibrotic tissue. Knowledge of the presence and character of these regions is potentially clinically useful in patients with heart failure, because several studies suggest that their

existence and extent correlates with prognosis and susceptibility to arrhythmias.[88,89]

More sophisticated types of molecular imaging with PET, SPECT, and MRI are under active development. Targeted imaging agents for each of these imaging modalities have been devised, and several biologic processes of importance can now be visualized in vivo. For instance, myocardial apoptosis can be assessed.[90] The most commonly employed methods for apoptosis characterization by noninvasive imaging detect the molecule phosphatidylserine on the outer portion of the myocardial cell membrane. Normally, phosphatidylserine is sequestered on the inner myocardial plasma membrane. When myocardial cells are stressed, the phosphatidylserine is translocated to the outer surface of the membrane. Phosphatidylserine functions physiologically in that location as a marker for the macrophages that phagocytose apoptotic cells and remove them. Ligands that bind to phosphatidylserine with high affinity are available. The most widely used of these is the protein annexin V. Annexin V has been conjugated to positron emitters for PET, to radioisotopes for SPECT, to liposomes containing gadolinium for MRI, and to fluorescent markers for optical imaging.[91] Additional targets of molecular imaging that are being investigated in heart failure models include imaging of protease activity, inflammation, thrombosis, and angiogenesis. Many types of advanced nanomolecular tools such as quantum dots and molecular beacons are being employed by these studies.[92–94]

Imaging of myocardial metabolism has been possible for many years with PET. The development of small medical cyclotrons and the increasing clinical availability of PET should significantly increase the possibilities for clinical research with this valuable technique. Myocardial metabolism can also be evaluated with magnetic resonance spectroscopy (MRS).[95,96] Because of the technical limitations of low signal, cardiac MRS studies have been time consuming and difficult to perform. However, the development of large-bore high-field MRI systems and particularly the exciting implementation of hyperpolarization methods have made it possible to obtain greatly increased MRS signal from animals and patients. These methods may produce a renaissance in cardiac MRS.[97]

Noninvasive molecular imaging techniques are particularly important for the evaluation of genetic and cellular therapies for heart failure. It is essential to be able to track the incorporation and functioning of inserted genetic material. Groundbreaking experimental work led to the concept of "reporter genes."[98–101] Reporter genes are transgenes inserted into an organism. These genes usually produce a reporter protein that can be detected by an assay. The gene encoding the jellyfish green fluorescent protein is a commonly employed reporter gene. When this gene is expressed, the organism into which it is inserted will glow green under a blue light. If a therapeutic transgene is contained on the same gene insertion vector as the reporter, detection of the reporter is indicative that the therapeutic transgene has also been inserted in the target cell. A wide variety of reporter genes are now available. These genes have been adapted so that their expression is detectable by PET, SPECT, and MRI as well as by optical imaging methods. With reporter genes it is possible to noninvasively monitor gene therapy. Reporter gene methods also have important applicability for evaluating the efficacy of stem cell therapy.[94,102]

The patient genome can also be considered to be a biomarker.[103] A substantial portion of the variability in patient outcomes and responses to treatment in heart failure is unquestionably secondary to variations in patient DNA sequence characteristics. Until very recently, investigation of this genetic component of the heart failure syndrome was stymied because sequencing even sizable portions of a patient genome was economically unfeasible. Thus, family linkage studies and candidate gene approaches were previously the only practical methods to evaluate the genetic component of heart failure. These approaches, although technically demanding and tedious to perform with the limited tools available to early cardiac geneticists, were extraordinarily successful in identifying the genetic causes of the inherited cardiomyopathies, and have made accurate clinical diagnosis of these disorders straightforward in many cases.[104–107] The primary challenge now is to explain the genetic components of heart failure in patients that have phenotypic heart failure but do not fit into known genetic cardiomyopathic categories.

Pharmacogenomics, the use of genomic techniques to identify patients who might be vulnerable to drug toxicities or who might be optimal candidates for particular drug strategies, is an area of active investigation.[108] There are large variations among individuals in response to drug therapies. A substantial amount of this variation is secondary to genetic differences. Current medical guidelines make recommendations based on average response. Personalized medical recommendations based on pharmacogenomics could make medical therapy safer and more effective.[109]

The genes coding the β-adrenergic receptors are obvious candidates in this regard.[110] Indeed,

several studies now suggest that polymorphisms in the β1-adrenergic receptor gene and β2-adrenergic receptor gene can contribute to variability in response to β-blocker therapy. There are 2 common genetic polymorphisms for the β1-adrenergic receptor and 3 common genetic polymorphisms for the β2-adrenergic receptor. The Beta Blocker Evaluation of Survival Test (BEST) assessed the impact of the nonselective β-blocker bucindolol on patients with differing β1-adrenergic receptor (ADRB1) genotypes. A substantial reduction in hospitalization and improvement in survival was noted with bucindolol treatment in patients with the homozygous Arg389Arg genotype. By contrast, minimal effect of the therapy was seen in those patients homozygous or heterozygous for the Gly389 allele.[111,112] The G-protein receptor kinase 5 (GRK5) protein is an important regulator of cardiac β-adrenergic signaling. Polymorphisms in the gene encoding GRK-5 have also been found to affect the results of β-blocker therapy.[113,114]

A recent study by Cresci and colleagues has provided additional confirmation of the effects of β-adrenergic receptor polymorphisms on variability in response to therapy in heart failure patients.[115] A prospective cohort of 2460 patients (1749 Caucasian and 711 African American) was genotyped for the ADRB1 Arg389>Gly polymorphism and the GRK5 Gln41>Leu polymorphism. During the median 46-month follow-up period, there were 765 deaths. Both polymorphisms were noted to significantly affect response to β-blockers. The investigators concluded that differences in β-adrenergic receptor signaling pathway gene polymorphisms are the primary factors accounting for observed differences in β-blocker treatment effect between African Americans and Caucasians.

Investigational results suggest that there are many other genetic variations that contribute to variability in response to heart failure therapy, including polymorphisms in the genes coding for angiotensin-converting enzyme and aldosterone synthase. Cardiovascular pharmacogenomics is in its infancy, but these early studies portend considerable promise for the vision of personalized medicine.

Next-generation DNA sequencing methods have now reduced the price of sequencing cardiovascularly relevant subsets of the human genome to very reasonable levels.[116,117] There is a variety of these highly automated new techniques. It is difficult to predict at this time which one will become dominant. However, it is very clear that the actual cost of providing reliable DNA sequence data in genomic quantities will soon drop so low that the expense of obtaining a patient's entire

DNA sequence will be only a minor factor in deciding whether or not to actually collect the sequence data.

Thus the technical aspect of acquiring the necessary raw data for extensive evaluations of the genetic correlations with phenotype in patients with heart failure is becoming very straightforward. Unfortunately, the process of making meaningful clinical predictions based on this data is just beginning.[118] Early after completion of the Human Genome Project, there was substantial optimism that much of the genetic variability of human disease would be explicable on the basis of common genomic variants. It was quickly determined that the human genome has a haplotypic structure that makes possible accurate prediction of genetic variance at one locus from genetic variance at an adjacent locus.[119] It is thus feasible to assess for common variability throughout the genome by genotyping approximately 500,000 markers, typically single nucleotide polymorphisms (SNPs).[120] Multiple genome-wide association studies (GWASs) were made of common disease processes, based on SNP genotyping. The hope was that the genetic component of common diseases would be explicable on the basis of commonly inherited genotypes. Although the GWAS studies provided many useful insights, particularly regarding disease pathways,[121,122] these studies for the most part failed to explain more than a small fraction of the observed phenotypic variability.[123]

Overall, the large-scale GWAS studies to date have provided support for the alternative "rare-variant" hypothesis of genetic influence on phenotype.[124,125] This hypothesis postulates that the variability in genetic control of phenotype is primarily secondary to rare point mutations or structural variations (such as copy number variations) that have relatively large effects. Considering the vast amount of genetic sequence information that will shortly be readily available to researchers and clinicians, innovative bioinformatic strategies will be required to separate the needles of disease causing rare gene variants from the haystacks of rare variants that are essentially neutral in effect. However, great potential is also present because identification of causative rare variants may stimulate novel therapeutic strategies.

Dramatic improvement in multiplexed and high throughput assays now also makes it possible to obtain comprehensive assessments of the proteome, transcriptome, and metabolome of samples taken from patients with heart failure. Again, as with the next generation of genomic techniques, innovative bioinformatic approaches that go beyond inherently problematic associative analyses are needed if these data are to assist in providing mechanistic insights and to be useful clinically. The inherent danger with acquisition of large amounts of data from the new "omics" technology is that physicians and medical scientists will be enticed by the lure of opportunities for scientific "stamp-collecting" and not pursue the difficult task of distilling coherent understanding from the acquired information.[126] The goal is to move from characterization of diseases primarily by symptoms and a few functional parameters to a molecular systems pathologic characterization of disease states relative to healthy states, and to go further by delineating system response profiles to various treatments.

THE CURRENT STATE OF MEDICAL THERAPY, 2010

Medical therapy for heart failure has relied on a variety of small molecule compounds. Digoxin and diuretics have historically been utilized in patients with heart failure because they provide symptomatic relief. These medications continue to be used when symptoms warrant. However, neither digoxin nor diuretics have been shown to improve survival in patients with cardiac failure.[3,127]

The most successful small molecule approaches to heart failure to date have blocked neurohormonal signaling pathways activated by the decline in cardiac function. Although neurohormonal stimulation can have beneficial short-term effects when cardiac output transiently decreases, chronic stimulation of the sympathetic nervous system and chronically increased production of angiotensin II, endothelin, and natriuretic peptides is toxic.

Inhibitors of the renin-angiotensin-aldosterone system have been extensively studied in adult populations, and definitely improve survival and reduce symptoms in the studied groups. Similarly, β-blockers have been shown to improve symptoms and survival in large groups of adults with heart failure in comparison with controls having the same degree of illness. Unfortunately, the positive effects of these medicines statistically only serves to reduce the rate of heart failure progression. Even with optimal current therapy, the heart failure pursues a relentless course.

There are many therapeutic interventions for heart failure that show a great deal of promise. These treatments include advanced small molecular therapies; therapy with modified peptides and aptamers; therapies that modify RNA translation, including those that employ the cellular RNA interference machinery; classical gene therapy, and cell therapy. An abbreviated review of some of the most interesting of these interventions follows (**Fig. 8**).

New Small Molecule Therapies

As has been noted, current therapeutic medical options for cardiac failure consist primarily of small molecular weight drugs. Small molecular weight drugs have several advantages that ensure that they will remain part of the therapeutic armamentarium: they typically have oral bioavailability; they can be designed to access intracellular targets; and they can be produced with high purity at relatively low cost.

Identifying small molecular weight compounds that have a positive effect on disease processes and at the same time do not exhibit unwanted

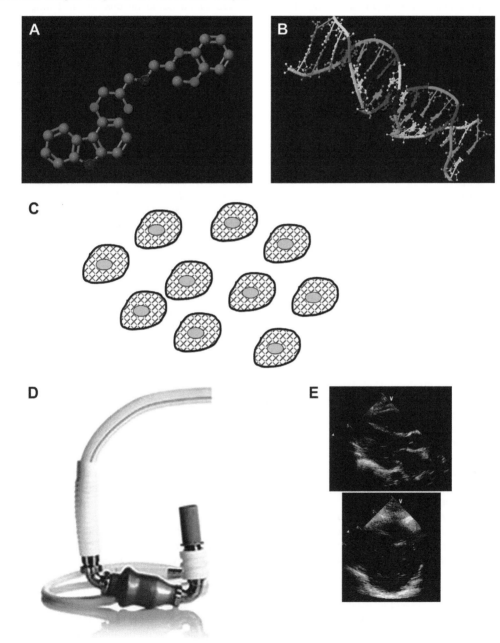

Fig. 8. Multiple therapeutic options are available for patients with heart failure. These options include (*A*) small molecule therapy (eg, Carvedilol) (*B*) gene therapy, (*C*) cell therapy, (*D*) ventricular assist device (VAD; Heart-Matell), and, (*E*) heart transplantation (echocardiogram of heart transplant shown). (VAD photo *courtesy of Throratec Corp; with permission.*)

toxicity has proven difficult. The number of combinatorial possibilities of potential small molecule medications is truly massive. Exhaustive evaluation of these possibilities is not feasible, regardless of the institutional resources available. High-throughput testing methods are required to screen just a small fraction of the conceivable small molecule drug structures. It follows that a critical part of small molecule drug development is reduction of the vast potential matrix of possible drugs to an approachable sparse matrix that can be reasonably evaluated.

One obvious potential approach to restrict the search space for new drug moieties is to limit chemical compound libraries using rule-based algorithms, such as those developed by Lipinski[128,129] and Veber,[130] that exclude chemicals with known toxic tendencies. Another historically highly useful approach is to screen for naturally occurring compounds with biologic activity and to base designs on them.[131] An obvious and related approach is to employ knowledge from the structure of compounds with documented biologic activity to design new compounds with structural similarities.

Chemogenomics is a developing discipline that may speed drug discovery. Chemogenomics has been defined as the study of libraries of chemical compounds against families of functionally related proteins.[132–135] Chemogenomics employs modern genomics, proteomics, transcriptomics, and metabolomics technologies to evaluate the overall effect of agents selected from the compound libraries. Chemogenomics can be performed in the reverse fashion, corresponding to a target-based strategy. With this type of chemogenomic approach, gene sequences of interest are typically cloned, inserted into a host organism, and screened against the library for efficacy of target binding. Chemogenomics can also be performed in the forward manner, corresponding to a system-based strategy for drug discovery, in which organisms are exposed to elements of the library and then assayed for desired phenotypic change in a high-throughput manner. Both reverse and forward chemogenomics approaches can be combined to give additional power to drug development.

When knowledge is available about drug structure or binding site configuration, in silico computer tools can be employed to further restrict the drug search space. A great deal of utility in focusing drug structure selection can certainly be gained from computer databases and in silico methods. However, extensive biochemical and biologic testing is necessary in any effort at drug discovery after the initial project phase.

Fragment-based drug discovery is yet another drug discovery approach that is becoming widely utilized.[136] Fragment-based drug discovery was originated by Rosenberg and Fesik, who noted that high-throughput screening of a compound library at Abbott Laboratories was unsuccessful at identifying substances that bound with high affinity to the multidomain protein BCL-XL.[137] These investigators hypothesized that such a substance could be created in 2 steps. First, they identified 2 fragment molecules of simple structure that bound to adjacent but not overlapping locations on the targeted receptor surface. The 2 fragments were then linked together with synthetic chemistry to produce a composite molecule that bound more strongly than either fragment because of summation of the binding energies of its parts. The investigators performed iterative rounds of optimization with nuclear magnetic resonance and were successful in producing a molecule, ABT-737, with high binding specificity for BCL-XL. Fragment-based drug discovery has the advantage of starting with very small molecular weight compounds. The sequence space of these compounds is relatively much smaller than the typical drug library, and thus it can be more exhaustively searched with actual experiments.

Although positive results have been obtained using small molecule drug therapies in patients with heart failure and although small molecules have some good medicinal features, small molecule drugs have intrinsic limitations as a class. Even when small molecule drugs are designed to bind selectively to known protein binding sites, they may also bind nonspecifically to off-target sites to a greater or lesser extent.[60] The off-target binding is not necessarily bad in the context of pharmacologic therapy. Indeed, drugs that promiscuously bind at multiple sites can be more effective at causing perturbation of typical scale-free biologic networks than drugs that bind in a more selective manner. However, the off-target effects can also be unwanted and toxic.

It is uncertain whether deliberate design of individual small molecular drugs with multiple desirable effects will be possible.[138] The drugs that we currently employ that in fact have such multiple salutary effects have often had the additional effects noted by serendipity after initial development. A good example is the angiotensin receptor inhibitor class of medications, which were originally designed as antihypertensives, but were later noted to have antiproliferative actions that serve to reduce adverse myocardial remodeling. Another good example is, of course, the β-blocker medicine class. These drugs were initially developed as antianginal agents and were originally thought to be contraindicated in patients with heart failure. Later studies showed that the early recommendations were in error and that β-blockers were in fact efficacious in heart failure.

Protein Therapies

Proteins are the only other structural class of therapeutic molecules in common use. Large protein molecules have an advantage in that they can incorporate much greater structural information than typical small molecular weight drugs. Designed proteins could potentially bind to the whole range of the human proteome. Unfortunately, therapeutic proteins are not easily deliverable to intracellular targets in most cases. Thus, therapy with designed proteins is limited to targets that are either secreted or located on the cell surface.

Therapy with Modified Peptides

Small molecule drugs generally act as ligands to protein binding sites. Because small drug molecules usually contain less than 100 atoms, they have only a relatively small surface area. Proteins typically envelop their small molecule ligands in a pocket containing hydrophobic amino acid side chains. This enclosure maximizes the hydrophobic bonding between protein and ligand and stabilizes the ligand-protein complex. If a protein is to be druggable, it must generally have an invagination incorporating hydrophobic amino acids. In addition, this invagination must be located at a position on the protein where it is accessible to solvents. Only about 3000 of the estimated 25,000 proteins encoded by the human genome have such a hydrophobic pocket. Hence, only about 12% of the proteins produced by the human genome can be effectively targeted with standard small molecule drugs.[139–141] Included among the "non-druggable" proteins are a large number of enhancers and other proteins that produce their biologic function via intracellular protein-protein interactions. Many of these proteins are attractive targets for therapy.

One might think that small peptides would be a logical and natural choice for targeting the large portion of the human proteome not druggable by standard small molecule therapy. However, peptides have definite limitations as drugs. Because they do not have the large stabilizing mass of a complete protein, peptides typically do not have a stable 3-dimensional structure. Rather, they rapidly and stochastically change conformation from one of a large variety of isomeric configurations to another on a nanosecond time scale. This property gives them relatively poor receptor binding properties, makes them more susceptible to proteolytic enzymes, and because it exposes their backbone amides to water, reduces their ability to cross the outer cell membrane.

However, it is possible to chemically modify natural peptides so that desirable conformations are locked in place, or "stapled."[142,143] These "stapled peptides" are a new class of drugs that have a great deal of promise. Although they are very new, significant experimental successes have been obtained with them.[144]

Aptamers

DNA or RNA oligonucleotides, and peptides can be created to bind to specific target molecules. Such molecules are termed aptamers.[145] DNA and RNA aptamers have significant potential as therapeutic tools, as ligands to direct therapeutic payloads to specific cellular targets, and as biosensors. Noncoding RNA sequences also have the capability to act as riboswitches, binding to small molecules, subsequently undergoing conformation change and then affecting transcription and translation.

Aptamers are typically produced by a selection and amplification process known as SELEX (Systematic Evolution of Ligands by Exponential Enrichment). This process starts with synthesis of a large oligonucleotide library. Library sequences are exposed to the target ligand. Sequences that do not bind are removed, typically by affinity chromatography. Bound sequences are then eluted and amplified by the polymerase chain reaction. The process then repeats until an aptamer is selected with the desired binding properties. Aptamers have significant advantages over antibodies in several respects. Aptamers can target molecules for which antibodies are difficult to produce. Because they are produced by chemical synthesis, they can be highly purified, eliminating batch-to-batch variation. Aptamers are amenable to chemical modification to enhance stability, and have low immunogenicity. Their diagnostic and therapeutic potential is just beginning to be explored, but multiple uses are being investigated, and one aptamer drug for glaucoma has been approved by the Food and Drug Administration (FDA).

Manipulation of the Genetic Code and its Expression

Targeting the production of proteins by manipulation of the genetic code is an alternative therapeutic option to targeting the proteome itself.[146] The primary code for protein production resides on DNA and is translated into the secondary RNA code before the transcription of RNA into the actual protein. Manipulation of either DNA or RNA, or both, can affect the protein product.

Genetic therapy via manipulation of DNA or RNA or both, and/or their expression is particularly attractive for treatment of inherited genetic cardiomyopathy and viral cardiomyopathy. These cardiomyopathies are important causes of heart failure, and have a relatively well understood etiology with an underlying genetic basis. Thus, for these types of heart failure, it might be possible to design specific treatments addressing causation, rather than simply trying to counter the downstream consequences of an unknown primary cause.

The classic notion of gene therapy involves insertion of DNA into the cell nucleus. The inserted DNA is then transcribed into mRNA and translated therapeutic protein. However, such therapy can often be performed using RNA as a primary effector. Eukaryotic cells contain machinery that greatly facilitates sequence-specific posttranscriptional control of gene expression via shortchain RNA molecules. This process, originally discovered in C elegans by Andrew Fire and Craig Mello, is called RNA interference.[147] Fire and Mello demonstrated that double-stranded RNA (dsRNA) sequences could cause dramatic silencing of homologous gene expression. In mammalian cells, lengthy chains of double-stranded RNA initiate a generalized shutdown of transcription and translation, which is thought to be an antiviral response, and which is toxic to the cells. However, Elbashir and colleagues[148] found that relatively short chains of dsRNA that were 21 to 23 nucleotides long could stop expression of specific mammalian genes without provoking a harmful response. Such short chains of dsRNA are called siRNA. RNA interference has been widely employed investigationally to inactivate gene expression. Recent studies suggest that gene expression can also be activated by short chains of dsRNA under certain circumstances. Therapy based on the RNA interference phenomenon has a great deal of promise if effective delivery mechanisms for such therapy can be developed.

There are multiple intrinsic barriers that can prevent efficacious intravenous genetic therapy. These barriers include: the tendency of some types of therapeutic particles to aggregate in the blood, nuclease activity of serum, uptake by the reticuloendothelial system, uptake by untargeted cells in general, exclusion by tight endothelial cell junctions (eg, blood-brain and blood-heart barriers), exclusion by the membrane of the target cell, the nucleases of the endosomes/lysosomes of the target cell, entrapment by the endosomes/lysosomes of the target cell, undesired exocytosis by the target cell, and humoral and cellular immune reactions. For genetic therapy that requires transcription to implement its effect, there are additional barriers. These barriers include inefficient transport of therapeutic vector to the nucleus, inefficient transcription of therapeutic genes, and inactivation of therapeutic genes by the target cell.[149]

Although cellular uptake of genetic information can occur subsequent to administration of naked DNA or RNA, efficiency of this transfer is usually very low. Therefore, DNA or RNA intended for gene therapy is typically administered in conjunction with a vector to facilitate targeting of the nucleic acids. Either viral or nonviral vectors can be employed. Viruses are composed of an outer protein coat, termed the capsid, and an inner genetic payload. Viral protein capsids contain complex molecular machinery that enhances cellular binding, internalization, and delivery of the viral nucleic acids.

Currently available nonviral vector designs have not been able to match the sophistication of the viral capsid machinery, and consequently the cellular transfection efficacy of nonviral vectors is substantially less than that of viral vectors.[150] Obviously there are safety issues that pertain to viral deployment. Such issues include viral replication, insertional mutagenesis, tissue-specific targeting, and immunogenicity. These issues can be substantively addressed by appropriate nanomolecular engineering of viruses to convert them into gutted hybrid nanoparticle vectors, although a great deal of progress remains to be made before routine clinical use is possible.

However, there is also a great deal of continued interest in nonviral vectors. Nonviral vectors have the potential advantages of being easier to manufacture in a standardized manner, of having relatively low immunogenicity, and of having no possibility of recombination with DNA sequences in the host to produce a replication-competent virus. Cationic liposome-nucleic acid complexes have been employed experimentally with significant successes. More complicated designs of these liposomes that incorporate ligands designed to bind to cellular receptors and thereby target-specific tissues are under evaluation.[151] Polymers and dendrimers have also been utilized as vectors for nonviral gene delivery.

Multiple virus types can be effectively employed for gene delivery.[152] Adenovirus, adeno-associated virus, and retroviruses, including lentiviruses, are the major viruses that have been used. Adenoviruses have the advantage of having relatively large capacity and the ability to efficiently transfect many tissues. The major limitations of adenovirus vectors are immunogenicity and the transient nature of the adenovirus transfection. For some applications, however, a transient transfection is desirable. Retroviruses can also efficiently transfect many tissues. Retroviruses can provide stable expression of administered genes, at the cost of possible insertional mutagenesis. Lentiviruses, a subtype of retrovirus, are particularly good at transducing cells that are not dividing.

Initial human investigations with adenoviral and retroviral vectors demonstrated some successes. However, serious safety concerns became apparent in some of these early trials. Use of first-generation adenoviral vectors was associated with the death of a patient.[153] Leukemia developed in several children treated with retroviral gene therapy for X-linked severe combined immunodeficiency.[154] There is optimism that these safety issues with adenoviral and retroviral vectors can be successfully resolved with technical improvements to the vectors. Nonetheless, continued careful scrutiny of these and all other vectors for gene therapy will be necessary.

Much recent research with viral vectors for gene therapy has centered around adeno-associated virus (AAV) agents.[155] Adeno-associated viruses have multiple potential advantages as vehicles for gene delivery. These viruses have not been demonstrated to cause disease in humans; they can transduce nondividing cells and slowly dividing cells, a property that is necessary for delivery of gene therapy to mature cardiomyocytes. Recent advances in technology have allowed production of recombinant gene therapy vectors manufactured from adeno-associated virus (rAAV) that do not contain viral genes. Such vectors obviously will not provoke cellular immune responses directed against viral genes, although immune responses can still be produced against the protein of the viral capsid or against the transgene itself. In addition, rAAV vectors with strong tissue tropisms have been identified. AAV serotype 9 has been found to have a particularly strong affinity for cardiac tissue.[156] Adaptive techniques have been employed to further accentuate the tropism of rAAV vectors for cardiomyoctyes.[157] Strong affinity of gene therapy vectors for heart cells will reduce the necessary dosage of these vectors and also reduce off-target transduction outside the heart.

There is a plethora of potential targets for gene therapy. In patients with monogenic cardiomyopathic disorders causative for heart failure, an obvious target is the abnormal gene. In some cases, it may be possible to correct these diseases by simple overexpression of normal wild-type protein. It is not yet possible to perform definitive correction of monogenic cardiomyopathies in intact animals by excising the abnormal genes and replacing them with normal wild-type genes via homologous recombination, although techniques that might make such a procedure feasible are under development.[158] In autosomal dominant genetic cardiomyopathy, knockdown of the abnormal gene with RNA interference methods might prove to be effectively curative. In selected cases, it may be possible to interfere with translation of mRNA so that exons containing harmful mutations are skipped. The resultant truncated proteins may be substantially functional. Investigational studies of exon skipping suggest that many variants of Duchenne muscular dystrophy might someday be effectively palliated by this technique.[159–161]

Patients with virally induced cardiomyopathic heart failure also have a known genetic source for their heart failure. There is considerable interest in antiviral therapy that employs RNA interference to block expression of essential viral proteins. It does seem that it will be necessary to simultaneously inhibit expression of multiple such proteins in order to avoid mutational escape of the virus, particularly viruses whose replication is error-prone.[162]

The majority of patients have heart failure without a currently definable genetic cause. However, gene therapy targeting of known final common pathways of myocardial derangement in heart failure may prove to be effective in treating these patients.[163,164] Such therapy has shown promise in investigational animal models, and has sometimes even yielded dramatic results. Cardiac calcium cycling and myocardial β-adrenergic receptor signaling are well known to exhibit malfunction in heart failure.[165] Multiple studies in experimental animals have targeted different facets of these 2 systems.

Sympathetic regulation of the heart is an essential part of its underlying control mechanism. The catecholamines epinephrine and norepinephrine predominantly mediate this regulation via adrenergic receptors located on the cardiomyocytes. The β1 and β2 cardiac adrenergic receptor subtypes are the predominant cardiac adrenergic receptors, with the subtype β1 representing approximately 75% to 80% of the expressed myocyte receptors, with the remainder being mostly β2.[166] β-adrenergic receptors (βARs) are a subgroup of the large family of heterotrimeric guanine nucleotide (G) protein-coupled receptors (GPCR). The receptors are activated by agonist binding, which causes the GPCR to undergo a conformational change from inactive to active form. This change results in stimulation of adenylyl cyclase, cyclic adenosine monophosphate production, and enhancement of cardiac chronotrophy and inotropy.

The activation of βARs is regulated to prevent overstimulation. One mechanism of this regulation is mediated by serine/threonine kinases termed G-protein coupled receptor kinases (GRKs). A type of GRK, GRK2, phosphorylates both β1AR and β2ARs, causing receptor desensitization.[167] In failing human hearts, β1ARs are selectively lost and both β1ARs and β2ARs are desensitized. Furthermore, experimental data suggest that GRK2 protein levels are elevated in incipient heart failure.

A peptide derived from the carboxy terminal region of GRK2 called βARKct has been demonstrated to effectively inhibit GRK2.[168] Multiple studies in mice and larger animals have demonstrated that transgenic expression of βARKct has a favorable effect on heart failure, and can even abolish it in some experimental preparations. For example, Rengo and colleagues[169] delivered adeno-associated virus type 6 (AAV6) vectors by direct intramyocardial injection to a rat model of chronic heart failure. The AAV6 vectors had been engineered to express βARKct. The rats sustained substantial global improvement in cardiac function, which was more than that produced by β-blocker treatment alone. Not all studies with βARKct have shown benefit, suggesting that significant unappreciated system complexity is present. However, the generally favorable studies have greatly encouraged further investigation. There are many additional potential targets in the β-adrenergic receptor signaling pathways, and a number are being actively investigated as sites for gene therapy.

Calcium is the fundamental regulator of excitation-contraction coupling, which is the process responsible for the cyclical muscular contraction of the heart.[170] Calcium is stored in the sarcoplasmic reticulum (SR) and is released when extracellular calcium moves into the cell via the voltage-dependent L-type calcium channel. The calcium release from the SR occurs via the ryanodine receptor through a calcium-dependent change in its configuration. The calcium that is released from the SR binds to the myofilament protein troponin C, initiating the sarcomere contraction. Cardiac relaxation requires calcium removal from the cytosol, so that calcium can be dissociated from troponin C and so that the myofilaments can be deactivated. Calcium is primarily transported out of the cytosol and back into the SR by action of sarco/endoplasmic reticulum calcium adenosine triphosphatase (ATPase) (SERCA2a Ca^{2+}-ATPase), although the sarcolemmal Na-Ca exchange (NCX) transporter plays a significant role.

Calcium cycling during excitation contraction coupling becomes deranged during cardiac failure.[53,54] One particular feature of this derangement is loss of activity of SERCA2a Ca^{2+}-ATPase and NCX upregulation. This loss of activity causes a decrease in SR Ca^{2+} levels.

One obvious potential for gene therapy in heart failure is to produce upregulation of SERCA2a Ca^{2+}-ATPase production. Several investigators have demonstrated beneficial results with transfer of viral vectors expressing SERCA2a Ca^{2+}-ATPase to animal models of heart failure.[146] Although the results have not been uniformly positive, augmentation of cardiac SERCA2a Ca^{2+}-ATPase in heart failure continues to be a widely investigated gene therapy approach, and human trials have been initiated.

The calcium regulatory protein S100A1 has been a recent target of cardiac gene therapy. S100A1 augments Ca^{2+} release during systole and stabilizes the ryanodine receptor during diastole.[171] Increasing cardiac cellular S100A1 is another obvious strategy for gene therapy for heart failure. It has been successfully tested in small and large animal models. For example, Pleger and colleagues[172] employed retroinfusion of AAV9 vector expressing S100A1 in a pig model of chronic left ventricular failure. Fourteen weeks after treatment, the treated pigs demonstrated an average left ventricular ejection fraction of 61% ± 3.7% versus 39% ± 2.1% for untreated pigs. Left ventricular end diastolic diameter was 3.43 ± 0.1 cm for treated pigs versus 4.45 ± 0.1 cm for controls. Dp/dt$_{max}$ was 1526 ± 83 mm Hg/s for treated pigs versus 983 ± 81 mm Hg/s for controls. This therapy is also being readied for human trials.

Despite substantial successes in demonstrating proof of concept,[173] we should not underestimate the inherent difficulties in moving gene therapy into the clinic. There are considerable targeting difficulties and very real concerns regarding insertional mutagenesis. In addition, the very robust human humoral and cellular immune response system provides a substantial challenge to gene therapy,[174] just as it continues to do for transplant therapy.

Stem Cells and Dilated Cardiomyopathies

Dilated cardiomyopathies are a major cause of heart failure syndromes.[2,175] Dilated cardiomyopathy is often a familial genetic disorder caused by mutations in the genes encoding cytoskeletal proteins. However, other genetic origins are possible. Dilated cardiomyopathy may result from multiple myocardial infarctions and subsequent fibrosis and remodeling. Viral myocarditis or cardiotoxic chemotherapeutic agents can produce dilated cardiomyopathy. The end result of these processes is a paucity of functioning myocytes. Thus, in its essence, dilated cardiomyopathy is a myocyte deficiency disorder.[176,177] It follows that the symptoms of dilated cardiomyopathy could be alleviated by myocyte replacement or regeneration therapy. Such therapy might prove to be a very advantageous alternative to cardiac transplant or mechanical assist devices for many patients.

Conventional approaches to the treatment of dilated cardiomyopathy have not included an effort to increase the number of functioning myocytes, despite the widespread recognition that myocyte deficiency is a core problem in dilated cardiomyopathy. For this reason we do not yet have robust techniques to produce such increases, and the traditionally accepted theory that the adult heart is a terminally differentiated organ has tended to discourage research in this area.

However, it is evident that large amounts of normally functioning heart muscle can be produced from a few progenitor cells under the proper circumstances, because this phenomenon occurs routinely as a part of every normal child's development. It follows that one potential avenue, and possibly the best, to radically improve treatment for patients with dilated cardiomyopathy is to discover how we can help them regenerate their heart.

The heart was thought to be a terminally differentiated organ for many years.[178,179] This dogma was founded on the belief that adult cardiac myocytes could not enter the cell cycle. It was supported by experimental observations that myocardial cell mitosis was difficult to demonstrate in mature hearts, even those exhibiting enlargement and hypertrophy. Further support was lent by the finding that cardiomyocyte cell lines with well-differentiated features could not be established in continuous culture. Finally, it was clear that even after substantial myocardial insults, such as myocardial infarction, hearts underwent little spontaneous repair in humans and experimental mammals. Thus, mammalian postnatal hearts were not thought to have regenerative capacity.

It now seems clear that myocyte death and regeneration are continually taking place, albeit at a slow pace in normal individuals.[178,179] This paradigm change in thinking is based first on observations of histologic morphometric examination demonstrating an increase in cardiac myocyte number from birth to adulthood in humans and rodents. Calculation of the rate of required new myocyte production from the morphometric data demonstrated that a very low rate of myocardial cell proliferation, unlikely to be detected by routine microscopic assessment for mitotic figures, would account for the observed increase in cell number from birth to adulthood. Second, biochemical and cytological marker studies of cell cycling and DNA synthesis, including studies using bromodeoxyuridine (BrdU) labeling and the nucleolus Ki67 cell proliferation marker, suggested strongly that new myocardial cells were being formed, even in normal adult animals. In addition, data from carbon[14] incorporation into human cardiac DNA during historical atmospheric nuclear weapons testing suggested that cardiomyocyte turnover is taking place, at a rate that gradually decreases with age, from 1% annually at age 25 to 0.45% annually at age 75 years.[180]

However, the previously accepted dogma does not appear to be completely incorrect. The evidence suggests that large, fully differentiated cardiac myocytes undergo cell division only rarely. These larger cells appear to preferentially undergo hypertrophy rather than mitosis. Myocardial proliferative activity appears to originate almost solely from a population of relatively small myocardial progenitor cells that do not exhibit the usual phenotypic characteristics of cardiac myocytes, but are capable of developing into mature myoctyes.[181,182]

Multiple endocrine, paracrine, and juxtacrine cell-cell interaction factors are known to promote and alter myocardial development.[183–185] Many of these factors can be expected to influence myocardial regeneration. Experience with investigations in molecular cardiac embryology unequivocally indicates that appropriate development of cardiac stem cells will not occur without a sustaining niche or cellular milieu.[186,187]

Factors responsible for the propensity of the heart to remodel in dilated cardiomyopathy will also undoubtedly influence the development of cardiac stem cells inserted into cardiomyopathic hearts. The mechanisms regulating cardiac remodeling in dilated cardiomyopathy have not been completely elucidated. However, the extracellular matrix is increasingly thought to play a crucial role, and there is a realization that the extracellular matrix itself is a dynamic tissue that changes in response to local environmental stimuli.

Changes in the extracellular cardiac matrix are primarily mediated by the balance of between the activity of the degradative matrix metalloproteinase (MMP) enzymes and their multifunctional inhibitors, the tissue inhibitors of metalloproteinases (TIMPs).[188–190] Cardiac cellular structure itself changes with the remodeling process. In eccentric hypertrophy both cardiomyocyte diameter and length increase proportionately, so that ventricular wall thickness and volume increase in tandem. As cardiac failure becomes decompensated, myocytes elongate without a concomitant increase in diameter. These cellular changes indicate a process of active internal reorganization of myofibrils and sarcomeres within the cardiomyocytes. The renin-angiotensin-aldosterone system, the sympathetic nervous system, and the inflammatory response are all known to play roles in the remodeling process.

There are many tissues from which stem cells can be isolated, including bone marrow, skeletal muscle, fat, and even the myocardium.[191–193] Stem cells from these differentiated tissues are termed "adult stem cells." Undifferentiated stem cells, termed pluripotent, can be isolated from embryonic tissues and indefinitely propagated in culture. A significant amount of experimental data does suggest that undifferentiated stem cells have an inherently greater capacity to expand and regenerate tissues than differentiated stem cells. However, undifferentiated stem cells may also form tumors or other unwanted tissue types. Furthermore, there are major ethical and logistic impediments associated with the use of human pluripotent stem cells derived from embryos. Finally, immunologic barriers prevent the ready use of pluripotent stem cells derived from a donor that is genetically different than the recipient.

Recent major technical advances have made it possible to induce differentiated somatic cells to become pluripotent.[194–198] Such induced pluripotent stem cells, termed iPS cells, have great potential advantages. Because they can be derived from readily available somatic tissues such as skin, fat, or blood, there are minimal impediments to their acquisition. Furthermore, as with adult stem cells, they are not immunologically rejected by their donor.

At the present time it is unclear what stem cell type will prove to be the most advantageous for achieving myocardial regeneration or even whether the best stem cell based therapeutic strategy might be stimulation of endogenous myocardial stem cells. However, it is very clear that an enhanced ability to characterize the mechanisms of stem cell development in the myocardial milieu is a prerequisite to therapeutic advances.[199,200] Reporter gene technology is a promising means to this end.

Effective heart muscle regeneration in patients with dilated cardiomyopathy will have 3 principal requirements. First, it will be necessary to positively affect the dynamic equilibrium between production of the new cardiac cells and the loss of the old cells by senescence, apoptosis, phagocytosis, or necrosis. The set point for this dynamic equilibrium appears to progressively shift towards cell loss in dilated cardiomyopathy at a much more rapid rate than it does with normal aging. Second, improvement in cardiac cellular functioning will need to be achieved. Finally, effective regeneration strategies will necessitate modifications of the gross and microscopic architecture of the myocardium, to reverse deleterious remodeling patterns.

If introduction of stem cells into the myocardium is to be effective in regenerating myocardium, it will be important to determine how they should be isolated, expanded, and, if necessary, genetically modified. Another important concern will be to determine how they should be introduced. Introducing cells in an optimal manner is a very important consideration, because a high proportion of stem cells introduced with current techniques die shortly after introduction. Furthermore, if the injected cells do not properly integrate into the myocardial syncytium, the results are not necessarily beneficial, even if the cells live.[201–203]

As with gene therapy, cell therapy has demonstrated substantial success in several animal models. Multiple early human trials have now been performed, primarily with autologous bone marrow cells, and primarily in the setting of acute myocardial infarction.[204–206] These trials have demonstrated the feasibility and safety of myocardial administration of stem cell therapy in humans. The majority of these trials have been successful in demonstrating a positive functional effect. However, the enhancement of cardiac function obtained has been relatively small on average, although some cases of dramatic improvement have occurred. Furthermore, the therapeutic benefits have often found to be secondary to incompletely defined paracrine effects rather than the hoped-for regeneration of new myocardium. It is clear that this field is in its infancy, and much investigational work will be needed to delineate the role of stem cell therapy in patients with heart failure.

THOUGHTS REGARDING DEVELOPMENT OF NEW MEDICAL THERAPIES

Because of the demographic importance of heart failure, there have been multiple efforts to add to the repertoire of medical therapy for this illness. Unfortunately, these attempts have had only limited success to date, at least in the sense of producing new therapies that restore patients to a normal or near-normal physiologic state and prognosis. Why has it been so difficult to produce effective medical treatments for heart failure?

There are undoubtedly other reasons for the paucity of efficacious new heart failure therapies,[207] but one important problem has been neglect of the systemwide effects of proposed therapeutic modalities. Early physicians dosed their patients with naturally available substances and recorded the results. As medicine became more scientific, animal models of disease were introduced and employed as primary screens. In both cases, initial testing was system based, that is, it was performed in complex living systems.

The development of biochemistry and molecular biology made possible the design of chemical compounds and macromolecules to specifically interact with known biologic targets. The possibility of such design made pharmacologic research in general a much more intellectually satisfying endeavor and facilitated a rational approach to treatment development, as opposed to strict empiricism. Thus, target-based strategies for pharmaceutical investigation became the norm.

However, because of the highly networked, nonlinear and very dynamic nature of biology, the consequences of interventions at the molecular and cellular level inherently have limited predictability at the level of the organism.[208–211] Even if a carefully fashioned drug or macromolecule performs the anticipated action on a designated biologic target, the intended effect on the experimental animal or patient may be thwarted by an unanticipated adaptational change in an alternate networked pathway or pathways or by a rare variant genetic polymorphism.

Moreover, no drug has perfect specificity. There are always off-target effects that must be reckoned with. Occasionally these off-target effects can be beneficial, but in many instances they are deleterious. In addition, the diverse nature of the genome, inherited epigenome, acquired epigenome, and environmental exposure history of human patients causes further unpredictability when a drug advances into routine clinical usage. The same types of considerations apply to gene therapy and to stem cell therapy.

Any conceivable therapeutic regimen will encounter both nonresponders and some individuals that will be worsened by the treatment. Although pharmacogenomic screening prior to treatment shows much promise, epigenetic and environmental differences will always cause variable response rates, as twin studies strongly suggest. It will be important to identify patients who are not being helped at the earliest opportunity, so that they can be transitioned to alternative therapy.

How can therapeutic research best proceed? The authors are not by any means advocating rejection of molecular targeting per se. Molecular actions are the underlying basis of biologic function, and one cannot have true understanding without understanding molecular mechanisms. As an analogy, one cannot truly understand radios without some appreciation of how transistors work. However, a basic knowledge of circuit diagrams is an even more fundamental requirement.[212]

Rather, the authors suggest that in additional to targeting specific molecules, the targeting should extend to the targeting of important interaction networks and final common pathways, and the flux though these networks and pathways. In most cases, the authors hypothesize that multiple perturbations with drugs and in selected cases RNA interference, gene therapy, and cell therapy will be required to achieve desirable modifications at these higher levels of biologic organization. Many of our most successful medications, initially thought to have single mechanisms of action, have lately been found to in fact affect multiple targets simultaneously. As an analogy, early attempts to target the human immune deficiency virus via single mechanisms were largely ineffective.[213] When physicians began to deliberately give therapy that simultaneously interfered with multiple aspects of the virus life cycle, dramatic successes were obtained.[214]

Furthermore, there is a great need to develop realistic integrative and quantitative computer models of pathophysiology as it relates to heart failure. Animal models, cell culture systems, and in vitro mechanistic experiments are vital for progress in the therapy for heart failure, as are the gold standards of patient experience and clinical trials. However, as predictive computer models have become essential to the success of engineering projects, so they must become an essential part of clinical and basic research in heart failure. Biologic diagrams, though important and useful in assisting with scientific understanding, are typically naïve from the engineering standpoint, in that they are generally not quantitative and that they generally do not incorporate critical feedback loops.

Just as making major modifications to an airliner design is a complex engineering project, heart failure therapy is also in many respects a complex engineering project. The ability to model gives engineers the capability to test multiple hypotheses and to quantitatively assess many scenarios without the expense and time of empirical experimental appraisal. Modeling does not replace empirical evaluations such as wind tunnel assessments and test flights. Indeed, engineers are very cognizant of the fact that models often contain substantial conceptual fallacies and often require revision because of unanticipated problems. However, modeling allows expensive and time consuming empirical testing to be reserved for critical questions and final confirmation. Modern aeronautic engineers would not consider giving up their numerical computer models and basing their initial designs on trial and error. Modern physicians should not be limited to trial and error either.[24,25,215,216]

A variety of advanced network analysis techniques can successfully be applied for modeling of human disease.[217–219] These methods include Bayesian classification, nonlinear differential equations coupled with multiple linear regression, cellular automata, and reverse engineering. These approaches provide straightforward quantitative ways to deal with the large number of interactive relationships between the components of biologic organisms.

One impediment that does constrain modeling, at least with respect to humans, is the wide individual variation in the general population.[220,221] This limitation can in principle be addressed by frequent and detailed individualized feedback with advanced biomarker panels and molecular imaging, so that the models are constantly validated with data and well correlated with biologic reality.

CARDIAC RESYNCHRONIZATION THERAPY

There have been multiple studies in adults that have demonstrated beneficial effects of biventricular cardiac pacing to resynchronize contraction in heart failure patients with a wide QRS complex and consequent electrical dyssynchrony.[222–225] Typically a transvenous approach is utilized, and the left ventricle is paced by a lead placed in a branch of the coronary sinus. In a substantial number of patients improvement has been demonstrable, with relief of symptoms, improvement in ejection fraction, and evidence of reverse cardiac remodeling. These responding patients can often be continued on medical therapy and at least temporarily avoid transplantation. Unfortunately there are also a substantial number of nonresponders to cardiac resynchronization therapy (CRT).[224,226] At present, there is no generally accepted technique to predict which patients will respond and which will not,[227] although a recent study suggests that sophisticated MRI methods might be helpful in this regard.[228] Furthermore, the positive cardiac functional improvement from CRT, when it occurs, is typically modest, and much less than the functional improvement that occurs subsequent to ventricular mechanical support or cardiac transplant.[229]

There are many anatomic variants that can occur in patients with pediatric and congenital heart disease. Some of these patients have systemic right ventricles or even single ventricles. As a result, it is difficult to make direct correlations with the adult resynchronization experience. The feasibility of CRT has been demonstrated in patients with pediatric and congenital cardiac disease, although highly variable coronary sinus anatomy can preclude transvenous resynchronization. An international, multicenter, retrospective evaluation of 103 patients demonstrated an increase in ejection fraction of the systemic ventricle of 12.8 ± 12.7 percentage ejection fraction units subsequent to CRT. There were several complications from the resynchronization procedures, however, with 2 deaths. Of 18 patients who underwent CRT while listed for transplant list, only 3 improved sufficiently to allow delisting.[230]

Some investigators have raised concerns about the use of right ventricular pacing in patients with bradycardia, whether or not they have normal systolic function of the systemic ventricle.[231] These concerns are controversial, however. Left ventricular dysfunction in pediatric patients with congenital atrioventricular block who have been paced is an unusual occurrence, even when these patients have been paced for over 10 years.[232]

At present there are no clear guidelines for CRT in patients with pediatric and congenital heart disease.[233] The procedure is relatively costly, requires considerable operator time and expertise, and is not without risk. However, some patients do seem to benefit. More clinical research is needed to find the appropriate patient population for CRT.

END-STAGE HEART FAILURE

Heart failure is a progressive disease.[1,234] Treatment to block the effects of neurohormonal activation and reduce tendencies toward ventricular remodeling have reduced the rate of progression of the disease and have probably reduced the tendency toward arrhythmic death. However, typical patients still deteriorate and eventually present with severe hemodynamic compromise. Intravenous inotropic infusions in such patients may ameliorate symptoms but are associated with higher rates of mortality in comparison with placebo.[3,235] Oral inotropic agents have also been found to increase mortality in these patients.[236] Multiple studies demonstrate that there is a very high near-term mortality for heart failure patients dependent on inotropic infusion for symptomatic relief, with 1-year survival rates of 25% or less.[4,237] The alternative therapeutic options for such patients are mechanical support and transplantation with a cardiac allograft. Some patients have successfully undergone ventricular assist device replacement as a "bridge to recovery."[238,239] In this scenario the heart is rested and allowed to recover. The device is then explanted. Aggressive pharmacologic therapy to produce maximal remodeling and the β-2 receptor agonist clenbuterol are sometimes administered. Temporary ventricular assist device replacement has been quite successful in allowing cardiac recovery from acute heart failure secondary to viral myocarditis or postcardiopulmonary bypass myocardial stunning. However, the success rate following chronic heart failure has been limited.

Cardiac transplant has been successful in providing additional years of life for a substantial number of patients with pediatric and congenital heart disease and end-stage heart failure, although the very real successes of this therapy are tempered with the need for immunosuppression and the problem of chronic graft rejection.

Of course, there will always be only a limited number of human heart donors. However, the population of patients with end stage heart failure is steadily increasing. Two potential future options for patients who are unable to obtain cardiac allografts are xenotransplantation and destination therapy with a cardiac assist device.

XENOTRANSPLANTATION

One potential solution to the limited number of cardiac allografts is to transplant organs from animals. Pigs have been suggested as the most suitable animal for xenotransplant production. Initial experiments with xenotransplantation demonstrated that the immunologic barriers to acceptance of these transplants greatly exceeded those to allotransplantation. Hyperacute rejection mediated by natural anti-αGal xenoreactive antibodies was determined to be a major factor in primate rejection of pig xenotransplants. A major technical advance was achieved by development of genetically engineered pigs, which do not express the αGal xenoepitope.[240] However, multiple other impediments to successful xenotransplantation remain; these include additional immune mechanisms, both humoral and cellular, as well as nonimmune mechanisms such as incompatibilities between pig and human coagulation systems. Further research and development is required before cardiac xenotransplants will be ready for human trials.[241]

CARDIAC ASSIST DEVICES FOR DESTINATION THERAPY

The first generation of cardiac assist devices was intended to serve as a bridge to cardiac transplant. These pulsatile devices were pneumatically driven from external consoles via transcutaneous lines. The devices facilitated patient survival for many months while awaiting transplant, although typical implantation time was 50 to 60 days. In 2001 a randomized trial in 129 end-stage heart failure patients not eligible for cardiac transplantation was performed comparing medical therapy to left ventricular assist device (LVAD) therapy.[237] The device employed was the HeartMate, produced by Thoratec. This multicenter trial, the REMATCH trial, demonstrated a dramatic reduction of mortality in the patient group treated with the LVAD. Symptoms of heart failure were substantially reduced in the group treated with device therapy in comparison with the medically treated group. Survival was 52% in the LVAD group versus 25% in the medically treated group at 1 year. On the strength of this study, the Heart-Mate was approved for destination therapy by the FDA.

During the ensuing 8 years, substantial improvements have occurred in LVAD technology. Experimental data has been obtained suggesting that substantial benefit can be derived from LVADs without the necessity for pulsatile flow. Miniaturized second-generation continuous-flow LVAD devices have been designed with a simplified mechanism that uses only one moving part. The new LVADs are much more mechanically reliable than the older pulsatile devices. Power to the device is now electrical. Very recently a comparative trial of the older HeartMate device to the second-generation HeartMate II device has been completed.[242,243] This study demonstrated a substantial advantage of the HeartMate II device over the older HeartMate device, largely because of the much greater mechanical reliability of the newer device and the consequently lower reoperation rate. As a matter of fact, there were no primary pump or bearing failures in the HeartMate II devices over the 2-year course of the study. Associated strokes did occur in patients receiving both types of devices, but the incidence (0.13 strokes per patient year) in the second-generation device is comparable to medically treated patients with heart failure who have atrial fibrillation. Infections did continue to occur, although in reduced number in the HeartMate II. Rehospitalizations were much less common with the continuous flow pump. Functional capacity was substantially increased by the LVAD treatment, with a nearly doubled 6-minute walk distance.

In another publication, results of a trial with a separate type of second-generation LVAD, the Jarvik 2000, were described.[244] A new power delivery technology has been developed for this device that is resistant to infection and relies on a skull pedestal implant. One of the LVAD recipients described in this publication has had an event-free survival of 7.5 years.

The results with the new LVADs are clearly exciting. The technology still has considerable room for improvement. The studies described were performed in adults. There is a need for such devices to be optimized for small pediatric patients. There is expectation that the devices can eventually be completely internalized and receive power wirelessly. Such internalization could further reduce the incidence of infection and enhance the quality of life of patients. There is a need to determine appropriate calibration of anticoagulant therapy in individual patients so that stroke incidence can be further reduced. There is a need to find improved techniques to deal with concomitant right ventricular failure, when this problem is present. There are certainly cost considerations, although some estimates suggest that the yearly cost of LVAD destination therapy compares favorably with the yearly cost of renal dialysis. But even the current systems clearly offer substantial benefits over medical therapy for end-stage heart failure. For selected patients, LVADs may even be a superior alternative to cardiac allograft transplantation.

REFERENCES

1. Mann DL, Bristow MR. Mechanisms and models in heart failure: the biomechanical model and beyond. Circulation 2005;111(21):2837–49.
2. Towbin J, Bowles N. The failing heart. Nature 2002; 415(6868):227–33.
3. Hunt SA, Abraham WT, Chin MH, et al. 2009 Focused update incorporated into the ACC/AHA 2005 guidelines for the diagnosis and management of heart failure in adults. J Am Coll Cardiol 2009;53(15):e1–90.
4. Nohria A, Lewis E, Stevenson LW. Medical management of advanced heart failure. JAMA 2002;287(5):628–40.
5. Mudd JO, Kass DA. Tackling heart failure in the twenty-first century. Nature 2008;451(7181): 919–28.
6. Morales DLS, Dreyer WJ, Denfield SW, et al. Over two decades of pediatric heart transplantation: how has survival changed? J Thorac Cardiovasc Surg 2007;133(3):632–9.
7. Hsu DT, Pearson GD. Heart failure in children: part I: history, etiology, and pathophysiology. Cir Heart Fail 2009;2(1):63–70.
8. Hsu DT, Pearson GD. Heart failure in children: part II: diagnosis, treatment, and future directions. Cir Heart Fail 2009;2(5):490–8.
9. Bolger AP, Coats AJS, Gatzoulis MA. Congenital heart disease: the original heart failure syndrome. Eur Heart J 2003;24(10):970–6.
10. Brooks PA, Penny DJ. Management of the sick neonate with suspected heart disease. Early Hum Dev 2008;84(3):155–9.
11. d'Udekem Y, Cheung MMH, Setyapranata S, et al. How good is a good Fontan? Quality of life and exercise capacity of Fontans without arrhythmias. Ann Thorac Surg 2009;88(6):1961–9.
12. Schadt EE, Sachs A, Friend S. Embracing complexity, inching closer to reality. Sci STKE 2005;2005(295):pe40.
13. Baltimore D. 50,000 Genes, and we know them all (almost). New York Times paper. June 25, 2000 edition.
14. Noble D. Claude Bernard, the first systems biologist, and the future of physiology. Exp Physiol 2008;93(1):16–26.
15. Noble D. Genes and causation. Philos Transact A Math Phys Eng Sci 2008;366(1878):3001–15.
16. Hatchwell E, Greally JM. The potential role of epigenomic dysregulation in complex human disease. Trends Genet 2007;23(11):588–95.
17. Peaston AE, Whitelaw E. Epigenetics and phenotypic variation in mammals. Mamm Genome 2006;17(5):365–74.
18. Fraga MF, Ballestar E, Paz MF, et al. Epigenetic differences arise during the lifetime of monozygotic twins. Proc Natl Acad Sci U S A 2005;102(30):10604–9.
19. Adams K. Systems biology and heart failure: concepts, methods, and potential research applications. Heart Fail Rev 2010;15(4):371–98.
20. Kitano H. Systems biology: a brief overview. Science 2002;295(5560):1662–4.
21. Ideker T, Galitski T, Hood L. A new approach to decoding life: systems biology. Annu Rev Genomics Hum Genet 2001;2:343–72.

22. Ouzounis C, Mazière P. Maps, books and other metaphors for systems biology. Biosystems 2006; 85(1):6–10.

23. Robson B. The dragon on the gold: myths and realities for data mining in biomedicine and biotechnology using digital and molecular libraries. J Proteome Res 2004;3(6):1113–9.

24. Noble D. Systems biology and the heart. Biosystems 2006;83(2–3):75–80.

25. Bassingthwaighte J, Hunter P, Noble D. The Cardiac Physiome: perspectives for the future. Exp Physiol 2009;94(5):597–605.

26. Han J-DJ, Bertin N, Hao T, et al. Evidence for dynamically organized modularity in the yeast protein-protein interaction network. Nature 2004; 430(6995):88–93.

27. Roguev A, Bandyopadhyay S, Zofall M, et al. Conservation and rewiring of functional modules revealed by an epistasis map in fission yeast. Science 2008;322(5900):405–10.

28. Towbin J. The role of cytoskeletal proteins in cardiomyopathies. Curr Opin Cell Biol 1998;10(1): 131–9.

29. Bowles N, Bowles K, Towbin J. The "final common pathway" hypothesis and inherited cardiovascular disease. The role of cytoskeletal proteins in dilated cardiomyopathy. Herz 2000;25(3):168–75.

30. Zanzoni A, Soler-López M, Aloy P. A network medicine approach to human disease. FEBS Lett 2009; 583(11):1759–65.

31. Barabási A-L, Oltvai ZN. Network biology: understanding the cell's functional organization. Nat Rev Genet 2004;5(2):101–13.

32. Jeong H, Tombor B, Albert R, et al. The large-scale organization of metabolic networks. Nature 2000; 407(6804):651–4.

33. Watts DJ, Strogatz SH. Collective dynamics of 'small-world' networks. Nature 1998;393(6684): 440–2.

34. Barabasi A, Albert R. Emergence of scaling in random networks. Science 1999;286(5439): 509–12.

35. Albert R. Scale-free networks in cell biology. J Cell Sci 2005;118(Pt 21):4947–57.

36. Alon U. An introduction to systems biology. Boca Raton (FL): Chapman & Hall/CRC; 2007.

37. Buchman TG. The community of the self. Nature 2002;420(6912):246–51.

38. Towbin JA, Bowles NE. Dilated cardiomyopathy: a tale of cytoskeletal proteins and beyond. J Cardiovasc Electrophysiol 2006;17(8):919–26.

39. Toyo-Oka T, Kawada T, Nakata J, et al. Translocation and cleavage of myocardial dystrophin as a common pathway to advanced heart failure: a scheme for the progression of cardiac dysfunction. Proc Natl Acad Sci U S A 2004;101(19): 7381–5.

40. Badorff C, Lee GH, Lamphear BJ, et al. Enteroviral protease 2A cleaves dystrophin: evidence of cytoskeletal disruption in an acquired cardiomyopathy. Nat Med 1999;5(3):320–6.

41. Vatta M, Stetson SJ, Perez-Verdia A, et al. Molecular remodelling of dystrophin in patients with end-stage cardiomyopathies and reversal in patients on assistance-device therapy. Lancet 2002;359(9310):936–41.

42. Vatta M, Stetson SJ, Jimenez S, et al. Molecular normalization of dystrophin in the failing left and right ventricle of patients treated with either pulsatile or continuous flow-type ventricular assist devices. J Am Coll Cardiol 2004;43(5):811–7.

43. Mohapatra B, Vick GW, Fraser CD, et al. Short-term mechanical unloading and reverse remodeling of failing hearts in children. J Heart Lung Transplant 2010;29(1):98–104.

44. Phillips R, Kondev J, Theriot J. Network organization in space and time. Physical biology of the cell. New York: Garland Science; 2009. p. 721–74.

45. Kurakin A. Scale-free flow of life: on the biology, economics, and physics of the cell. Theor Biol Med Model 2009;6:6.

46. Goldberger AL. Non-linear dynamics for clinicians: chaos theory, fractals, and complexity at the bedside. Lancet 1996;347(9011):1312–4.

47. Goldberger AL. Giles F. Filley lecture. Complex systems. Proc Am Thorac Soc 2006;3(6):467–71.

48. Alligood KT, Sauer TD, Yorke JA. Chaos: an introduction to dynamical systems. New York: Springer-Verlag; 2000.

49. Poon CS, Merrill CK. Decrease of cardiac chaos in congestive heart failure. Nature 1997;389(6650): 492–5.

50. Arzeno NM, Kearney MT, Eckberg DL, et al. Heart rate chaos as a mortality predictor in mild to moderate heart failure. Conference proceedings: Annual International Conference of the IEEE Engineering in Medicine and Biology Society 2007; 2007:5051–4.

51. Del Monte F, Hajjar RJ. Intracellular devastation in heart failure. Heart failure reviews 2008;13(2): 151–62.

52. Liew C-C, Dzau VJ. Molecular genetics and genomics of heart failure. Nat Rev Genet 2004;5(11): 811–25.

53. Kranias EG, Bers DM. Calcium and cardiomyopathies. Subcell Biochem 2007;45:523–37.

54. Bers DM. Altered cardiac myocyte Ca regulation in heart failure. Physiology 2006;21:380–7 (Bethesda, MD).

55. Schadt EE, Lum PY. Thematic review series: systems biology approaches to metabolic and cardiovascular disorders. Reverse engineering gene networks to identify key drivers of complex

disease phenotypes. J Lipid Res 2006;47(12): 2601–13.

56. Pearl J. Causality: models, reasoning, and inference. New York: Cambridge University Press; 2000.

57. Roth BL, Sheffler DJ, Kroeze WK. Magic shotguns versus magic bullets: selectively non-selective drugs for mood disorders and schizophrenia. Nat Rev Drug Discov 2004;3(4):353–9.

58. Bianchi MT, Pathmanathan J, Cash SS. From ion channels to complex networks: magic bullet versus magic shotgun approaches to anticonvulsant pharmacotherapy. Med Hypotheses 2009; 72(3):297–305.

59. Goh K-I, Cusick ME, Valle D, et al. The human disease network. Proc Natl Acad Sci U S A 2007; 104(21):8685–90.

60. Yildirim MA, Goh K-I, Cusick ME, et al. Drug-target network. Nat Biotechnol 2007;25(10):1119–26.

61. Stevenson LW, Perloff JK. The limited reliability of physical signs for estimating hemodynamics in chronic heart failure. JAMA 1989;261(6):884–8.

62. Solomon SD, Stevenson LW. Recalibrating the barometer: is it time to take a critical look at noninvasive approaches to measuring filling pressures? Circulation 2009;119(1):13–5.

63. Setoguchi S, Stevenson LW. Hospitalizations in patients with heart failure: who and why. J Am Coll Cardiol 2009;54(18):1703–5.

64. Chow EY, Beier BL, Francino A, et al. Toward an implantable wireless cardiac monitoring platform integrated with an FDA-approved cardiovascular stent. J Interv Cardiol 2009;22(5): 479–87.

65. Najafi N, Ludomirsky A. Initial animal studies of a wireless, batteryless, MEMS implant for cardiovascular applications. Biomed Microdevices 2004;6(1):61–5.

66. Goettsche T, Graefe M, Osypka P. New diagnostics with wireless pressure monitoring. Med Device Technol 2008;19(5):23–5.

67. Reichelt S, Fiala J, Werber A, et al. Development of an implantable pulse oximeter. IEEE Trans Biomed Eng 2008;55(2 Pt 1):581–8.

68. Zile MR, Bennett TD, St John Sutton M, et al. Transition from chronic compensated to acute decompensated heart failure: pathophysiological insights obtained from continuous monitoring of intracardiac pressures. Circulation 2008;118(14): 1433–41.

69. Adamson PB, Magalski A, Braunschweig F, et al. Ongoing right ventricular hemodynamics in heart failure: clinical value of measurements derived from an implantable monitoring system. J Am Coll Cardiol 2003;41(4):565–71.

70. Gerszten RE, Wang TJ. The search for new cardiovascular biomarkers. Nature 2008;451(7181):949–52.

71. Braunwald E. Biomarkers in heart failure. N Engl J Med 2008;358(20):2148–59.

72. Rocchiccioli JP, McMurray JJV, Dominiczak AF. Biomarkers in heart failure: a clinical review. Heart Fail Rev 2010;15(4):251–73.

73. Dries DL. Relevance of molecular forms of brain natriuretic peptide for natriuretic peptide research. Hypertension 2007;49(5):971–3.

74. Horwich TB, Patel J, MacLellan WR, et al. Cardiac troponin I is associated with impaired hemodynamics, progressive left ventricular dysfunction, and increased mortality rates in advanced heart failure. Circulation 2003;108(7):833–8.

75. Jessup M, Brozena S. Heart failure. N Engl J Med 2003;348(20):2007–18.

76. Cicoira M, Rossi A, Bonapace S, et al. Independent and additional prognostic value of aminoterminal propeptide of type III procollagen circulating levels in patients with chronic heart failure. J Card Fail 2004;10(5):403–11.

77. Seddon M, Looi YH, Shah AM. Oxidative stress and redox signalling in cardiac hypertrophy and heart failure. Heart 2007;93(8):903–7.

78. Shantsila E, Watson T, Lip GYH. Endothelial progenitor cells in cardiovascular disorders. J Am Coll Cardiol 2007;49(7):741–52.

79. Werner N, Kosiol S, Schiegl T, et al. Circulating endothelial progenitor cells and cardiovascular outcomes. N Engl J Med 2005;353(10):999–1007.

80. Balconi G, Lehmann R, Fiordaliso F, et al. Levels of circulating pro-angiogenic cells predict cardiovascular outcomes in patients with chronic heart failure. J Card Fail 2009;15(9):747–55.

81. Valgimigli M, Rigolin GM, Fucili A, et al. CD34+ and endothelial progenitor cells in patients with various degrees of congestive heart failure. Circulation 2004;110(10):1209–12.

82. Schmidt-Lucke C, Rössig L, Fichtlscherer S, et al. Reduced number of circulating endothelial progenitor cells predicts future cardiovascular events: proof of concept for the clinical importance of endogenous vascular repair. Circulation 2005; 111(22):2981–7.

83. Povsic TJ, Zavodni KL, Kelly FL, et al. Circulating progenitor cells can be reliably identified on the basis of aldehyde dehydrogenase activity. J Am Coll Cardiol 2007;50(23):2243–8.

84. Greenberg B. Molecular imaging of the remodeling heart: the next step forward. JACC Cardiovasc Imaging 2008;1(3):363–5.

85. Mann DL. Molecular imaging and the failing heart: through the looking glass. JACC Cardiovasc Imaging 2009;2(2):199–201.

86. van den Borne SWM, Isobe S, Zandbergen HR, et al. Molecular imaging for efficacy of pharmacologic intervention in myocardial remodeling. JACC Cardiovasc Imaging 2009;2(2):187–98.

87. Jaffer FA, Libby P, Weissleder R. Molecular imaging of cardiovascular disease. Circulation 2007;116(9):1052–61.

88. Cheong B, Muthupillai R, Wilson J, et al. Prognostic significance of delayed-enhancement magnetic resonance imaging. Survival of 857 patients with and without left ventricular dysfunction. Circulation 2009;120(21):2069–76.

89. Vick GW. The gold standard for noninvasive imaging in coronary heart disease: magnetic resonance imaging. Curr Opin Cardiol 2009;24(6):567–79.

90. Korngold EC, Jaffer FA, Weissleder R, et al. Noninvasive imaging of apoptosis in cardiovascular disease. Heart Fail Rev 2008;13(2):163–73.

91. Sosnovik DE, Schellenberger EA, Nahrendorf M, et al. Magnetic resonance imaging of cardiomyocyte apoptosis with a novel magneto-optical nanoparticle. Magn Reson med 2005; 54(3):718–24.

92. Shaw SY. Molecular imaging in cardiovascular disease: targets and opportunities. Nat Rev Cardiol 2009;6(9):569–79.

93. Mulder WJM, Cormode DP, Hak S, et al. Multimodality nanotracers for cardiovascular applications. Nat Clin Pract Cardiovasc Med 2008;5(Suppl 2): S103–11.

94. Ly HQ, Frangioni JV, Hajjar RJ. Imaging in cardiac cell-based therapy: in vivo tracking of the biological fate of therapeutic cells. Nat Clin Pract Cardiovasc Med 2008;5(Suppl 2):S96–102.

95. Beer M, Seyfarth T, Sandstede J, et al. Absolute concentrations of high-energy phosphate metabolites in normal, hypertrophied, and failing human myocardium measured noninvasively with (31) P-SLOOP magnetic resonance spectroscopy. J Am Coll Cardiol 2002;40(7):1267–74.

96. Neubauer S. The failing heart—an engine out of fuel. N Engl J Med 2007;356(11):1140–51.

97. Golman K, Petersson JS, Magnusson P, et al. Cardiac metabolism measured noninvasively by hyperpolarized ^{13}C MRI. Magn Reson Med 2008; 59(5):1005–13.

98. Jaffer F, Weissleder R. Seeing within: molecular imaging of the cardiovascular system. Circ Res 2004;94(4):433–45.

99. Capecchi MR. Gene targeting in mice: functional analysis of the mammalian genome for the twenty-first century. Nat Rev Genet 2005;6(6):507–12.

100. Tsien R. Imagining imaging's future. Nat Rev Mol Cell Biol 2003;(Suppl):SS16–21.

101. Zernicka-Goetz M, Pines J, McLean Hunter S, et al. Following cell fate in the living mouse embryo. Development 1997;124(6):1133–7.

102. Chun HJ, Wilson KO, Huang M, et al. Integration of genomics, proteomics, and imaging for cardiac stem cell therapy. Eur J Nucl Med Mol Imaging 2007;34(S1):20–6.

103. Gibbons GH, Liew CC, Goodarzi MO, et al. Genetic markers: progress and potential for cardiovascular disease. Circulation 2004;109(25 Suppl 1):IV47–58.

104. Geisterfer-Lowrance AA, Kass S, Tanigawa G, et al. A molecular basis for familial hypertrophic cardiomyopathy: a beta cardiac myosin heavy chain gene missense mutation. Cell 1990;62(5):999–1006.

105. Towbin JA, Lowe AM, Colan SD, et al. Incidence, causes, and outcomes of dilated cardiomyopathy in children. JAMA 2006;296(15):1867–76.

106. Towbin JA, Hejtmancik JF, Brink P, et al. X-linked dilated cardiomyopathy. Molecular genetic evidence of linkage to the Duchenne muscular dystrophy (dystrophin) gene at the Xp21 locus. Circulation 1993;87(6):1854–65.

107. Hershberger RE, Lindenfeld J, Mestroni L, et al. Genetic evaluation of cardiomyopathy—a Heart Failure Society of America practice guideline. J Card Fail 2009;15(2):83–97.

108. Pereira NL, Weinshilboum RM. Cardiovascular pharmacogenomics and individualized drug therapy. Nat Rev Cardiol 2009;6(10):632–8.

109. McNamara DM. Emerging role of pharmacogenomics in heart failure. Curr Opin Cardiol 2008; 23(3):261–8.

110. Feldman DS, Carnes CA, Abraham WT, et al. Mechanisms of disease: beta-adrenergic receptors—alterations in signal transduction and pharmacogenomics in heart failure. Nat Clin Pract Cardiovasc Med 2005;2(9):475–83.

111. Investigators B-BEoST. A trial of the beta-blocker bucindolol in patients with advanced chronic heart failure. N Engl J Med 2001;344(22):1659–67.

112. Liggett SB, Mialet-Perez J, Thaneemit-Chen S, et al. A polymorphism within a conserved beta(1)-adrenergic receptor motif alters cardiac function and beta-blocker response in human heart failure. Proc Natl Acad Sci U S A 2006; 103(30):11288–93.

113. Liggett SB, Cresci S, Kelly RJ, et al. A GRK5 polymorphism that inhibits beta-adrenergic receptor signaling is protective in heart failure. Nat Med 2008;14(5):510–7.

114. Dorn GW, Liggett SB. Mechanisms of pharmacogenomic effects of genetic variation within the cardiac adrenergic network in heart failure. Mol Pharmacol 2009;76(3):466–80.

115. Cresci S, Kelly RJ, Cappola TP, et al. Clinical and genetic modifiers of long-term survival in heart failure. J Am Coll Cardiol 2009;54(5):432–44.

116. Gibbs R. Deeper into the genome. Nature 2005; 437(7063):1233–4.

117. Schuster SC. Next-generation sequencing transforms today's biology. Nat Methods 2008;5(1):16–8.

118. Schadt EE. Molecular networks as sensors and drivers of common human diseases. Nature 2009; 461(7261):218–23.

119. Gabriel SB, Schaffner SF, Nguyen H, et al. The structure of haplotype blocks in the human genome. Science 2002;296(5576):2225–9.

120. Consortium IH, Frazer KA, Ballinger DG, et al. A second generation human haplotype map of over 3.1 million SNPs. Nature 2007;449(7164):851–61.

121. Manolio TA, Brooks LD, Collins FS. A HapMap harvest of insights into the genetics of common disease. J Clin Invest 2008;118(5):1590–605.

122. Hirschhorn JN. Genomewide association studies—illuminating biologic pathways. N Engl J Med 2009;360(17):1699–701.

123. Goldstein DB. Common genetic variation and human traits. N Engl J Med 2009;360(17):1696–8.

124. Bodmer W, Bonilla C. Common and rare variants in multifactorial susceptibility to common diseases. Nat Genet 2008;40(6):695–701.

125. Schork NJ, Murray SS, Frazer KA, et al. Common vs. rare allele hypotheses for complex diseases. Curr Opin Genet Dev 2009;19(3):212–9.

126. Loscalzo J. Association studies in an era of too much information: clinical analysis of new biomarker and genetic data. Circulation 2007;116(17):1866–70.

127. Shaddy RE, Penny DJ. Chronic heart failure: physiology and treatment. In: Anderson RH, Baker E, Redington A, et al, editors. Paediatric cardiology. Churchill Livingstone. 3rd Edition; 2009. p. 257–68.

128. Lipinski CA, Lombardo F, Dominy BW, et al. Experimental and computational approaches to estimate solubility and permeability in drug discovery and development settings. Adv Drug Deliv Rev 2001;46(1-3):3–26.

129. Lipinski C, Hopkins A. Navigating chemical space for biology and medicine. Nature 2004;432(7019):855–61.

130. Veber DF, Johnson SR, Cheng HY, et al. Molecular properties that influence the oral bioavailability of drug candidates. J Med Chem 2002;45(12):2615–23.

131. Li JW-H, Vederas JC. Drug discovery and natural products: end of an era or an endless frontier? Science 2009;325(5937):161–5.

132. Wuster A, Madan Babu M. Chemogenomics and biotechnology. Trends Biotechnol 2008;26(5):252–8.

133. Cases M, Mestres J. A chemogenomic approach to drug discovery: focus on cardiovascular diseases. Drug Discov Today 2009;14(9–10):479–85.

134. Jacoby E. Chemogenomics: drug discovery's panacea? Mol BioSyst 2006;2(5):218–20.

135. Maréchal E. Chemogenomics: a discipline at the crossroad of high throughput technologies, biomarker research, combinatorial chemistry, genomics, chemoinformatics, bioinformatics and artificial intelligence. Comb Chem High Throughput Screen 2008;11(8):583–6.

136. Hajduk PJ, Greer J. A decade of fragment-based drug design: strategic advances and lessons learned. Nat Rev Drug Discov 2007;6(3):211–9.

137. Bruncko M, Oost TK, Belli BA, et al. Studies leading to potent, dual inhibitors of Bcl-2 and Bcl-xL. J Med Chem 2007;50(4):641–62.

138. Hopkins AL, Mason JS, Overington JP. Can we rationally design promiscuous drugs? Curr Opin Struct Biol 2006;16(1):127–36.

139. Hopkins AL, Groom CR. The druggable genome. Nat Rev Drug Discov 2002;1(9):727–30.

140. Russ AP, Lampel S. The druggable genome: an update. Drug Discov Today 2005;10(23-24):1607–10.

141. Sakharkar MK, Sakharkar KR, Pervaiz S. Druggability of human disease genes. Int J Biochem Cell Biol 2007;39(6):1156–64.

142. Verdine GL, Walensky LD. The challenge of drugging undruggable targets in cancer: lessons learned from targeting BCL-2 family members. Clin Cancer Res 2007;13(24):7264–70.

143. Kutchukian PS, Yang JS, Verdine GL, et al. All-atom model for stabilization of alpha-helical structure in peptides by hydrocarbon staples. J Am Chem Soc 2009;131(13):4622–7.

144. Moellering RE, Cornejo M, Davis TN, et al. Direct inhibition of the NOTCH transcription factor complex. Nature 2009;462(7270):182–8.

145. Dausse E, Da Rocha Gomes S, Toulmé J-J. Aptamers: a new class of oligonucleotides in the drug discovery pipeline? Curr Opin Pharmacol 2009;9(5):602–7.

146. Vinge LE, Raake PW, Koch WJ. Gene therapy in heart failure. Circ Res 2008;102(12):1458–70.

147. Fire A, Xu S, Montgomery MK, et al. Potent and specific genetic interference by double-stranded RNA in *Caenorhabditis elegans*. Nature 1998;391(6669):806–11.

148. Elbashir SM, Harborth J, Weber K, et al. Analysis of gene function in somatic mammalian cells using small interfering RNAs. Methods 2002;26(2):199–213.

149. Vaughan EE, DeGiulio JV, Dean DA. Intracellular trafficking of plasmids for gene therapy: mechanisms of cytoplasmic movement and nuclear import. Current Gene Therapy 2006;6(6):671–81.

150. Lyon AR, Sato M, Hajjar RJ, et al. Gene therapy: targeting the myocardium. Heart 2008;94(1):89–99.

151. Templeton NS. Nonviral delivery for genomic therapy of cancer. World J Surg 2009;33(4):685–97.

152. Gray SJ, Samulski RJ. Optimizing gene delivery vectors for the treatment of heart disease. Expert Opin Biol Ther 2008;8(7):911–22.

153. Cotrim AP, Baum BJ. Gene therapy: some history, applications, problems, and prospects. Toxicol Pathol 2008;36(1):97–103.

154. Davé UP, Jenkins NA, Copeland NG. Gene therapy insertional mutagenesis insights. Science 2004; 303(5656):333.

155. Mccarty DM, Young SM, Samulski RJ. Integration of adeno-associated virus (AAV) and recombinant AAV vectors. Annu Rev Genet 2004;38:819–45.

156. Inagaki K, Fuess S, Storm TA, et al. Robust systemic transduction with AAV9 vectors in mice: efficient global cardiac gene transfer superior to that of AAV8. Mol Ther 2006;14(1):45–53.

157. Kwon I, Schaffer DV. Designer gene delivery vectors: molecular engineering and evolution of adeno-associated viral vectors for enhanced gene transfer. Pharm Res 2008;25(3):489–99.

158. Pruett-Miller SM, Connelly JP, Maeder ML, et al. Comparison of zinc finger nucleases for use in gene targeting in mammalian cells. Mol Ther 2008;16(4):707–17.

159. Lu QL, Mann CJ, Lou F, et al. Functional amounts of dystrophin produced by skipping the mutated exon in the mdx dystrophic mouse. Nat Med 2003;9(8):1009–14.

160. Goyenvalle A, Vulin A, Fougerousse F, et al. Rescue of dystrophic muscle through U7 snRNA-mediated exon skipping. Science 2004; 306(5702):1796–9.

161. McClorey G, Moulton HM, Iversen PL, et al. Antisense oligonucleotide-induced exon skipping restores dystrophin expression in vitro in a canine model of DMD. Gene Ther 2006;13(19):1373–81.

162. Brake OT, Hooft KT, Liu YP, et al. Lentiviral vector design for multiple shRNA expression and durable HIV-1 inhibition. Mol Ther 2008;16(3):557–64.

163. Ly H, Kawase Y, Yoneyama R, et al. Gene therapy in the treatment of heart failure. Physiology 2007; 22:81–96 (Bethesda, MD).

164. Davis J, Westfall MV, Townsend D, et al. Designing heart performance by gene transfer. Physiol Rev 2008;88(4):1567–651.

165. Pleger ST, Boucher M, Most P, et al. Targeting myocardial beta-adrenergic receptor signaling and calcium cycling for heart failure gene therapy. J Card Fail 2007;13(5):401–14.

166. Brodde OE, Michel MC. Adrenergic and muscarinic receptors in the human heart. Pharmacol Rev 1999;51(4):651–90.

167. Hausdorff WP, Caron MG, Lefkowitz RJ. Turning off the signal: desensitization of beta-adrenergic receptor function. FASEB J 1990;4(11):2881–9.

168. Akhter SA, Eckhart AD, Rockman HA, et al. In vivo inhibition of elevated myocardial beta-adrenergic receptor kinase activity in hybrid transgenic mice restores normal beta-adrenergic signaling and function. Circulation 1999;100(6):648–53.

169. Rengo G, Lymperopoulos A, Zincarelli C, et al. Myocardial adeno-associated virus serotype 6-betaARKct gene therapy improves cardiac function and normalizes the neurohormonal axis in chronic heart failure. Circulation 2009;119(1):89–98.

170. Bers DM. Cardiac excitation-contraction coupling. Nature 2002;415(6868):198–205.

171. Kraus C, Rohde D, Weidenhammer C, et al. S100A1 in cardiovascular health and disease: closing the gap between basic science and clinical therapy. J Mol Cell Cardiol 2009;47(4): 445–55.

172. Pleger ST, Shan C, Kziencek J, et al. Retroinfusion-facilitated inotropic aav9-s100a1 gene therapy restores global cardiac function in a clinically relevant pig heart failure model. Circulation 2008;118: S792.

173. Suckau L, Fechner H, Chemaly E, et al. Long-term cardiac-targeted RNA interference for the treatment of heart failure restores cardiac function and reduces pathological hypertrophy. Circulation 2009;119(9):1241–52.

174. Hasbrouck NC, High KA. AAV-mediated gene transfer for the treatment of hemophilia B: problems and prospects. Gene Ther 2008;15(11):870–5.

175. Dec G, Fuster V. Idiopathic dilated cardiomyopathy. N Engl J Med 1994;331(23):1564–75.

176. Nakamura T, Schneider MD. The way to a human's heart is through the stomach: visceral endoderm-like cells drive human embryonic stem cells to a cardiac fate. Circulation 2003;107(21):2638–9.

177. Oh H, Wang SC, Prahash A, et al. Telomere attrition and Chk2 activation in human heart failure. Proc Natl Acad Sci U S A 2003;100(9):5378–83.

178. Nadal-Ginard B, Kajstura J, Leri A, et al. Myocyte death, growth, and regeneration in cardiac hypertrophy and failure. Circ Res 2003;92(2):139–50.

179. Anversa P, Leri A, Rota M, et al. Concise review: stem cells, myocardial regeneration, and methodological artifacts. Stem Cells 2007;25(3):589–601.

180. Bergmann O, Bhardwaj RD, Bernard S, et al. Evidence for cardiomyocyte renewal in humans. Science 2009;324(5923):98–102.

181. Urbanek K, Cesselli D, Rota M, et al. Stem cell niches in the adult mouse heart. Proc Natl Acad Sci U S A 2006;103(24):9226–31.

182. Bearzi C, Rota M, Hosoda T, et al. Human cardiac stem cells. Proc Natl Acad Sci U S A 2007;104(35): 14068–73.

183. Schneider MD, Gaussin V, Lyons KM. Tempting fate: BMP signals for cardiac morphogenesis. Cytokine Growth Factor Rev 2003;14(1):1–4.

184. Nakamura T, Sano M, Songyang Z, et al. Wnt- and beta-catenin-dependent pathway for mammalian cardiac myogenesis. Proc Natl Acad Sci U S A 2003;100(10):5834–9.

185. Gnecchi M, He H, Liang OD, et al. Paracrine action accounts for marked protection of ischemic heart by Akt-modified mesenchymal stem cells. Nat Med 2005;11(4):367–8.

186. Parmacek MS, Epstein JA. Pursuing cardiac progenitors: regeneration redux. Cell 2005;120(3): 295–8.

187. Olson EN, Schneider MD. Sizing up the heart: development redux in disease. Genes Dev 2003; 17(16):1937–56.

188. Fedak PWM, Verma S, Weisel RD, et al. Cardiac remodeling and failure: from molecules to man (Part I). Cardiovasc Pathol 2005;14(1):1–11.

189. Fedak PWM, Verma S, Weisel RD, et al. Cardiac remodeling and failure From molecules to man (Part II). Cardiovasc Pathol 2005;14(2):49–60.

190. Fedak PWM, Verma S, Weisel RD, et al. Cardiac remodeling and failure: from molecules to man (Part III). Cardiovasc Pathol 2005;14(3):109–19.

191. Dimmeler S, Zeiher A, Schneider M. Unchain my heart: the scientific foundations of cardiac repair. J Clin Invest 2005;115(3):572–83.

192. Gersh BJ, Simari RD, Behfar A, et al. Cardiac cell repair therapy: a clinical perspective. Mayo Clin Proc 2009;84(10):876–92.

193. Segers VFM, Lee RT. Stem-cell therapy for cardiac disease. Nature 2008;451(7181):937–42.

194. Okita K, Ichisaka T, Yamanaka S. Generation of germline-competent induced pluripotent stem cells. Nature 2007;448(7151):313–7.

195. Kaji K, Norrby K, Paca A, et al. Virus-free induction of pluripotency and subsequent excision of reprogramming factors. Nature 2009;458(7239): 771–5.

196. Boland MJ, Hazen JL, Nazor KL, et al. Adult mice generated from induced pluripotent stem cells. Nature 2009;461(7260):91–4.

197. Martinez-Fernandez A, Nelson TJ, Yamada S, et al. iPS programmed without c-MYC yield proficient cardiogenesis for functional heart chimerism. Circ Res 2009;105(7):648–56.

198. Zhao X-y, Li W, Lv Z, et al. iPS cells produce viable mice through tetraploid complementation. Nature 2009;461(7260):86–90.

199. Frangioni JV, Hajjar RJ. In vivo tracking of stem cells for clinical trials in cardiovascular disease. Circulation 2004;110(21):3378–83.

200. Schroeder T. Imaging stem-cell-driven regeneration in mammals. Nature 2008;453(7193):345–51.

201. Ly HQ, Nattel S. Stem cells are not proarrhythmic: letting the genie out of the bottle. Circulation 2009;119(13):1824–31.

202. Macia E, Boyden PA. Stem cell therapy is proarrhythmic. Circulation 2009;119(13):1814–23.

203. Schenke-Layland K, MacLellan WR. Induced pluripotent stem cells: it's like déjà vu all over again. Circulation 2009;120(15):1462–4.

204. Yousef M, Schannwell CM, Köstering M, et al. The BALANCE Study: clinical benefit and long-term outcome after intracoronary autologous bone marrow cell transplantation in patients with acute myocardial infarction. J Am Coll Cardiol 2009; 53(24):2262–9.

205. Forrester JS, Makkar RR, Marbán E. Long-term outcome of stem cell therapy for acute myocardial infarction: right results, wrong reasons. J Am Coll Cardiol 2009;53(24):2270–2.

206. Martin-Rendon E, Brunskill SJ, Hyde CJ, et al. Autologous bone marrow stem cells to treat acute myocardial infarction: a systematic review. Eur Heart J 2008;29(15):1807–18.

207. Krum H, Tonkin A. Why do phase III trials of promising heart failure drugs often fail? The contribution of "regression to the truth". J Card Fail 2003;9(5): 364–7.

208. Sams-Dodd F. Target-based drug discovery: is something wrong? Drug Discov Today 2005;10(2): 139–47.

209. Sams-Dodd F. Drug discovery: selecting the optimal approach. Drug Discov Today 2006; 11(9–10):465–72.

210. van der Greef J, McBurney RN. Innovation: rescuing drug discovery: in vivo systems pathology and systems pharmacology. Nat Rev Drug Discov 2005;4(12):961–7.

211. Kubinyi H. Drug research: myths, hype and reality. Nat Rev Drug Discov 2003;2(8):665–8.

212. Lazebnik Y. Can a biologist fix a radio?—Or, what I learned while studying apoptosis. Cancer Cell 2002;2(3):179–82.

213. Concorde: MRC/ANRS randomised double-blind controlled trial of immediate and deferred zidovudine in symptom-free HIV infection. Concorde Coordinating Committee. Lancet 1994;343(8902):871–81.

214. Palella FJ, Delaney KM, Moorman AC, et al. Declining morbidity and mortality among patients with advanced human immunodeficiency virus infection. HIV Outpatient Study Investigators. N Engl J Med 1998;338(13):853–60.

215. Noble D. The rise of computational biology. Nat Rev Mol Cell Biol 2002;3(6):459–63.

216. Noble D. Modeling the heart. Physiology 2004;19: 191–7 (Bethesda, MD).

217. Morel NM, Holland JM, van der Greef J, et al. Primer on medical genomics. Part XIV: Introduction to systems biology—a new approach to understanding disease and treatment. Mayo Clin Proc 2004;79(5):651–8.

218. Loscalzo J, Kohane I, Barabasi A-L. Human disease classification in the postgenomic era: a complex systems approach to human pathobiology. Mol Syst Biol 2007;3:124.

219. Alon U. Network motifs: theory and experimental approaches. Nat Rev Genet 2007;8(6):450–61.

220. Cohn JN. The fallacy of the mean. J Card Fail 2001; 7(2):103–4.

221. Jackson DB. Clinical and economic impact of the nonresponder phenomenon—implications for

systems based discovery. Drug Discov Today 2009;14(7–8):380–5.

222. Bristow MR, Saxon LA, Boehmer J, et al. Comparison of Medical Therapy P, and Defibrillation in Heart Failure (COMPANION) investigators. Cardiac-resynchronization therapy with or without an implantable defibrillator in advanced chronic heart failure. N Engl J Med 2004;350(21):2140–50.

223. Anand IS, Carson P, Galle E, et al. Cardiac resynchronization therapy reduces the risk of hospitalizations in patients with advanced heart failure: Results From the Comparison of Medical Therapy, Pacing and Defibrillation in Heart Failure (COMPANION) Trial. Circulation 2009; 119(7):969–77.

224. Bax JJ, Abraham T, Barold SS, et al. Cardiac resynchronization therapy: part 1—issues before device implantation. J Am Coll Cardiol 2005; 46(12):2153–67.

225. Bax JJ, Abraham T, Barold SS, et al. Cardiac resynchronization therapy: part 2—issues during and after device implantation and unresolved questions. J Am Coll Cardiol 2005; 46(12):2168–82.

226. Díaz-Infante E, Mont L, Leal J, et al. Predictors of lack of response to resynchronization therapy. Am J Cardiol 2005;95(12):1436–40.

227. Beshai JF, Khunnawat C, Lin AC. Mechanical dyssynchrony from the perspective of a cardiac electrophysiologist. Curr Opin Cardiol 2008;23(5):447–51.

228. Bilchick KC, Dimaano V, Wu KC, et al. Cardiac magnetic resonance assessment of dyssynchrony and myocardial scar predicts function class improvement following cardiac resynchronization therapy. JACC Cardiovasc Imaging 2008;1(5): 561–8.

229. Wilson SR, Givertz MM, Stewart GC, et al. Ventricular assist devices the challenges of outpatient management. J Am Coll Cardiol 2009;54(18): 1647–59.

230. Dubin AM, Janousek J, Rhee E, et al. Resynchronization therapy in pediatric and congenital heart disease patients: an international multicenter study. J Am Coll Cardiol 2005;46(12):2277–83.

231. Yu C-M, Chan JY-S, Zhang Q, et al. Biventricular pacing in patients with bradycardia and normal ejection fraction. N Engl J Med 2009;361(22): 2123–34.

232. Kim JJ, Friedman RA, Eidem BW, et al. Ventricular function and long-term pacing in children with congenital complete atrioventricular block. J Cardiovasc Electrophysiol 2007;18(4):373–7.

233. Dubin AM. Resynchronization in pediatrics who needs it? J Am Coll Cardiol 2005;46(12):2290–1.

234. Ammar KA, Jacobsen SJ, Mahoney DW, et al. Prevalence and prognostic significance of heart failure stages: application of the American College of Cardiology/American Heart Association heart failure staging criteria in the community. Circulation 2007;115(12):1563–70.

235. Elis A, Bental T, Kimchi O, et al. Intermittent dobutamine treatment in patients with chronic refractory congestive heart failure: a randomized, double-blind, placebo-controlled study. Clin Pharmacol Ther 1998;63(6):682–5.

236. Reddy S, Benatar D, Gheorghiade M. Update on digoxin and other oral positive inotropic agents for chronic heart failure. Curr Opin Cardiol 1997; 12(3):233–41.

237. Rose EA, Gelijns AC, Moskowitz AJ, et al. Group REoMAftToCHFRS. Long-term mechanical left ventricular assistance for end-stage heart failure. N Engl J Med 2001;345(20):1435–43.

238. Lahpor J. State of the art: implantable ventricular assist devices. Current opinion in organ transplantation 2009;14(5):554–9.

239. Hon JKF, Yacoub MH. Bridge to recovery with the use of left ventricular assist device and clenbuterol. Ann Thorac Surg 2003;75(6 Suppl):S36–41.

240. Ekser B, Cooper DK. Update: cardiac xenotransplantation. Curr Opin Organ Transplant 2008; 13(5):531–5.

241. Pierson RN. Current status of xenotransplantation. JAMA 2009;301(9):967–9.

242. Slaughter M, Rogers J, Milano C, et al. Investigators HeartMate II. Advanced heart failure treated with continuous-flow left ventricular assist device. N Engl J Med 2009.

243. Fang J. Rise of the machines—left ventricular assist devices as permanent therapy for advanced heart failure. N Engl J Med 2009; 361(23):2241–51.

244. Westaby S, Siegenthaler M, Beyersdorf F, et al. Destination therapy with a rotary blood pump and novel power delivery. Eur J Cardiothorac Surg 2010;37(2):350–6.

Index

Note: Page numbers of article titles are in **boldface** type.

doi:10.1016/S1551-7136(10)00091-7
1551-7136/10/$ – see front matter

United States Postal Service

Statement of Ownership, Management, and Circulation
(All Periodicals Publications Except Requestor Publications)

1. Publication Title	2. Publication Number	3. Filing Date
Heart Failure Clinics of North America	0 2 5 - 0 5 5	9/15/10

4. Issue Frequency	5. Number of Issues Published Annually	6. Annual Subscription Price
Jan, Apr, July, Oct	4	$193.00

7. Complete Mailing Address of Known Office of Publication (Not printer) (Street, city, county, state, and ZIP+4®)

Elsevier Inc.
360 Park Avenue South
New York, NY 10010-1710

Contact Person
Stephen Bushing
Telephone (Include area code)
215-239-3688

8. Complete Mailing Address of Headquarters or General Business Office of Publisher (Not printer)

Elsevier Inc., 360 Park Avenue South, New York, NY 10010-1710

9. Full Names and Complete Mailing Addresses of Publisher, Editor, and Managing Editor (Do not leave blank)

Publisher (Name and complete mailing address)

Kim Murphy, Elsevier, Inc., 1600 John F. Kennedy Blvd. Suite 1800, Philadelphia, PA 19103-2899

Editor (Name and complete mailing address)

Barbara Cohen-Kligerman, Elsevier, Inc., 1600 John F. Kennedy Blvd. Suite 1800, Philadelphia, PA 19103-2899

Managing Editor (Name and complete mailing address)

Catherine Bewick, Elsevier, Inc., 1600 John F. Kennedy Blvd. Suite 1800, Philadelphia, PA 19103-2899

10. Owner (Do not leave blank. If the publication is owned by a corporation, give the name and address of the corporation immediately followed by the names and addresses of all stockholders owning or holding 1 percent or more of the total amount of stock. If not owned by a corporation, give the names and addresses of the individual owners. If owned by a partnership or other unincorporated firm, give its name and address as well as those of each individual owner. If the publication is published by a nonprofit organization, give its name and address.)

Full Name	Complete Mailing Address
Wholly owned subsidiary of	4520 East-West Highway
Reed/Elsevier, US holdings	Bethesda, MD 20814

11. Known Bondholders, Mortgagees, and Other Security Holders Owning or Holding 1 Percent or More of Total Amount of Bonds, Mortgages, or Other Securities. If none, check box ☐ None

Full Name	Complete Mailing Address
N/A	

12. Tax Status (For completion by nonprofit organizations authorized to mail at nonprofit rates) (Check one)
The purpose, function, and nonprofit status of this organization and the exempt status for federal income tax purposes:
☐ Has Not Changed During Preceding 12 Months
☐ Has Changed During Preceding 12 Months (Publisher must submit explanation of change with this statement)

PS Form 3526, September 2007 (Page 1 of 3 (Instructions Page 3)) PSN 7530-01-000-9931 PRIVACY NOTICE: See our Privacy policy in www.usps.com

---

13. Publication Title	14. Issue Date for Circulation Data Below
Heart Failure Clinics of North America	July 2010

15. Extent and Nature of Circulation		Average No. Copies Each Issue During Preceding 12 Months	No. Copies of Single Issue Published Nearest to Filing Date
a. Total Number of Copies (Net press run)		550	500
b. Paid Circulation (By Mail and Outside the Mail)	(1) Mailed Outside-County Paid Subscriptions Stated on PS Form 3541. (Include paid distribution above nominal rate, advertiser's proof copies, and exchange copies)	89	95
	(2) Mailed In-County Paid Subscriptions Stated on PS Form 3541 (Include paid distribution above nominal rate, advertiser's proof copies, and exchange copies)		
	(3) Paid Distribution Outside the Mails Including Sales Through Dealers and Carriers, Street Vendors, Counter Sales, and Other Paid Distribution Outside USPS®	32	25
	(4) Paid Distribution by Other Classes Mailed Through the USPS (e.g. First-Class Mail®)		
c. Total Paid Distribution (Sum of 15b (1), (2), (3), and (4))	►	121	120
d. Free or Nominal Rate Distribution (By Mail and Outside the Mail)	(1) Free or Nominal Rate Outside-County Copies Included on PS Form 3541	73	68
	(2) Free or Nominal Rate In-County Copies Included on PS Form 3541		
	(3) Free or Nominal Rate Copies Mailed at Other Classes Through the USPS (e.g. First-Class Mail)		
	(4) Free or Nominal Rate Distribution Outside the Mail (Carriers or other means)		
e. Total Free or Nominal Rate Distribution (Sum of 15d (1), (2), (3) and (4))	►	73	68
f. Total Distribution (Sum of 15c and 15e)	►	194	188
g. Copies not Distributed (See instructions to publishers #4 (page #3))	►	356	312
h. Total (Sum of 15f and g)	►	550	500
i. Percent Paid (15c divided by 15f times 100)	►	62.37%	63.83%

16. Publication of Statement of Ownership
☐ If the publication is a general publication, publication of this statement is required. Will be printed in the October 2010 issue of this publication. ☐ Publication not required

17. Signature and Title of Editor, Publisher, Business Manager, or Owner

Stephen R. Bushing
Stephen R. Bushing – Fulfillment Inventory Specialist

Date
September 15, 2010

I certify that all information furnished on this form is true and complete. I understand that anyone who furnishes false or misleading information on this form or who omits material or information requested on the form may be subject to criminal sanctions (including fines and imprisonment) and/or civil sanctions (including civil penalties).

PS Form 3526, September 2007 (Page 2 of 3)

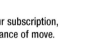